Communication, Relationships and Care

This book will be invaluable to practitioners and managers across all health and social care settings, – it illuminates communication against the backdrop of personal and professional relationships, intensely emotional situations and in our organisational lives. It will challenge, inform and empower . . .

Professor Hilary Brown, Canterbury Christ Church, University College

I can't think of anyone who works in social care who wouldn't benefit from this book. This book develops understanding of communication and skills in using it to best effect.

Linda Farthing, former Programme Director for Surestart in Milton Keynes and a critical reader for the course

Communication and relationships have become an increasing focus of attention in debates about the future of health and social care. People working in care services are being encouraged to improve communication processes, to develop more participatory relationships with service users, and to work more closely in partnership with other professionals.

This Reader provides a comprehensive collection of literature that aims to enable those involved in care services, as workers, carers or service users, to reflect on their everyday interactions and to situate them in wider contexts. Including new material from the frontline of research and practice, as well as some classic readings, this wide-ranging volume emphasises the need to see interpersonal communication as embedded in relationships, and to take account of issues of power and diversity, as well as the emotional dimension of care work. Covering both health and social care, the Reader is divided into four sections, focusing on:

- concepts and contexts;
- analysing aspects of communication;

- the person in the process;
- communication and relationships in organisations.

Communication, Relationships and Care will be an essential resource for students of social work, nursing, health and social policy, and for all involved in health and social care services, whether as professionals, carers or service users. It is a set book for The Open University's second level undergraduate course Communication and Relationships in Health and Social Care (K205).

Martin Robb, Sheila Barrett, Carol Komaromy and **Anita Rogers** are all lecturers in the School of Health and Social Welfare at The Open University.

Communication, Relationships and Care

A Reader

Edited by Martin Robb, Sheila Barrett,
Carol Komaromy and Anita Rogers

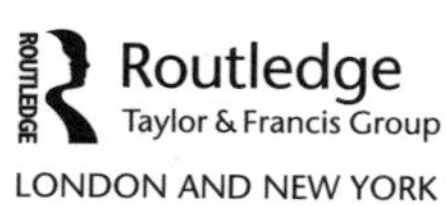

LONDON AND NEW YORK

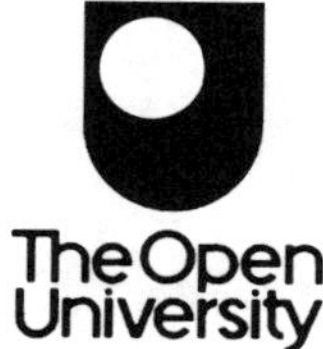

First published 2004
by Routledge
11 New Fetter Lane, London EC4P 4EE

Simultaneously published in the USA and Canada
by Routledge
29 West 35th Street, New York, NY 10001

Routledge is an imprint of the Taylor & Francis Group

Typeset in 10/12 Sabon by Wearset Ltd, Boldon, Tyne and Wear
Printed and bound in Great Britain by TJ International Ltd, Padstow, Cornwall

British Library Cataloguing in Publication Data
A catalogue record for this book is available from the British Library

Library of Congress Cataloging in Publication Data
A catalog record for this book has been requested

ISBN 0-415-32659-1 (hbk)
ISBN 0-415-32660-5 (pbk)

Open University Course: Communication and Relationships in Health and Social Care (K205)

This Reader forms part of The Open University course Communication and Relationships in Health and Social Care, a 60 points second level undergraduate course.

Opinions expressed in the Reader are not necessarily those of the Course Team or of The Open University.

If you are interested in studying this course or working towards a related degree or diploma please write to the Information Officer, School of Health and Social Welfare, The Open University, Walton Hall, Milton Keynes, MK7 6AA, UK. Details can also be reviewed on our web page http://www.open.ac.uk.

CONTENTS

INTRODUCTION

Martin Robb

Communication and relationships have become an increasing focus of attention in debates about the future of health and social care services. Enquiries into a number of high-profile tragedies and scandals have highlighted apparent failures in communication, and have led to calls for changes in the nature of relationships, both between care professionals and between service providers and service users (for example: Department of Health 1991; Newham Area Child Protection Committee 2002). At the same time, pressure from service users themselves, together with the consumerism encouraged by the partial marketisation of care services, has brought a new emphasis on participation and partnership in relationships within services (Clarke and Newman 1997).

Plans for reform of the health service and of social care have included strategies both for improving communication processes between providers and the public, and for breaking down barriers between different groups of care professionals (e.g., Department of Health 2000; General Social Care Council 2002). People working at all levels in care services are being encouraged to improve their interpersonal communication skills, while developing better communication processes is now seen as fundamental to improving the quality of services (Cameron 2000). Workers across the care sector increasingly find themselves working in multi-professional teams and in partnerships between different agencies.

There is a need for resources to support those on the frontline of care services, as they come under increasing pressure to improve communication and transform relationships within services. But there is also a need to place these demands for improvement in a wider context and subject them to critical scrutiny. Resources that enable workers, carers and service users to reflect on the complexity and diversity of their everyday interactions, rather than simply providing a 'quick fix' solution, have been thin on the ground until recently. Many existing publications on communication in the health and social care field tend to be straightforward skills manuals which risk decontextualising interpersonal communication. On the other hand, much academic writing on communication and relationships in the context of care has failed to connect with the practical needs of staff and service users. This volume aims to supply the need for a wide-ranging resource that links theory to practice, encouraging those involved in health and social care to see their interactions in wider contexts. The Reader is comprehensive in its concern with both caring relationships and with professional and inter-professional relationships. It covers both health and social care, respecting the differences between care sectors and the variety of relationships that exist within them, while at the same time exploring commonalities and shared issues. Aimed primarily at those with a frontline role in health and social care, the Reader also includes material that will be found useful by managers, educators and policy-makers, as well as by service users and those with a general interest in the quality of health and social care services.

This Reader is unusual in not promoting a particular theoretical approach to interpersonal communication, but instead presenting material from a range of perspectives, including behaviourist, psychodynamic and humanistic, as well as more recent social constructionist and postmodern approaches to its subject. However, the organisation and selection of material reflects an underlying emphasis on communication as situated in, and shaped by, different kinds of contexts. At the most fundamental level, the title of the Reader argues for viewing interpersonal communication in the context of continuing relationships, whether caring or professional, and emphasises the interaction between the two. In different ways, the readings in the Reader all draw attention to the importance of different kinds of context, whether personal, institutional, or more widely social and cultural. As part of this focus, key issues of power, diversity and difference recur throughout the Reader. At the same time, however, there is also an emphasis on the personal and emotional dimensions of communication and relationships in the context of care.

USING THE READER

The Reader has been designed to be used by a variety of readers. Students on a wide range of courses in health and social care, particularly at undergraduate level, should find the readings included here an invaluable aid to their studies. The Reader is also a set text for the Open University course Communication and Relationships in Health and Social Care (K205), which aims to encourage those involved in health care, social work and social care to reflect critically on their everyday interactions and relationships and to develop their practice.

The Reader is divided into four parts, each of which includes a selection of readings on a particular topic. The introduction to each part provides an overview of its contents, draws attention to links between chapters, and briefly describes each of the readings. The chapters included in *Part I* introduce some of the key concepts that will be developed throughout the Reader, while at the same time situating communication and relationships in a range of contexts. *Part II* analyses some key aspects of interpersonal communication in care settings, focusing on key issues of power, diversity and difference and examining the importance of language and the body in communication. In *Part III* there is a shift to the more personal and affective dimension of caring relationships, as different readings consider the attitudes, attributes and skills that individuals bring to the process of communication, as well as the emotional impact of relationships on those involved. Finally, *Part IV* broadens the focus to explore communication and relationships in health and social care organisations, with chapters discussing the impact of the organisational context at the individual, group and institutional levels, and considering issues of organisational culture and leadership.

This Reader has grown out of debates and discussions in the K205 course team at the Open University. Members of the team have suggested items for inclusion and have helped with editing, while the editors have made a final selection and written introductory material. Besides the four editors, other course team members involved in this process have been Ann Brechin, Jenny Douglas, Linda Finlay, Liz Forbat, Anne Fletcher and Janet Seden. Caroline Malone, the course manager, has played a key role in co-ordinating the preparation of the Reader, while Val O'Connor has provided secretarial support. Finally, thanks are due to the authors of the chapters reproduced here for allowing their work to be used.

REFERENCES

Cameron, D. (2000) *Good to Talk? Living and Working in a Communication Culture*, London: Sage.

Clarke, J. and Newman, J. (1997) *The Managerial State: Power, Politics and Ideology in the Remaking of Social Welfare*, London: Sage.

Department of Health (1991) *Child Abuse; a Study of Inquiry Reports 1980–1989*, London: The Stationery Office.

Department of Health (2000) *The NHS Plan: A Plan for Investment, a Plan for Reform*, London: The Stationery Office.

General Social Care Council (2002) *Code of Practice for Social Care Workers and Code of Practice for Employers of Social Care Workers*, London: Crown Copyright.

Newham Area Child Protection Committee (2002) *Ainlee: Born: 24.06.1999: Died: 07.01.2002*, Chapter 8 Review.

PART I

CONCEPTS AND CONTEXTS

INTRODUCTION

Martin Robb

The chapters included in Part I introduce some of the key concepts, or ways of thinking about communication and relationships, that are developed in different ways throughout the Reader. They also place interpersonal communication in care settings in the personal, institutional and social contexts that help to shape them.

The first two chapters engage with the question of what is meant by 'communication' and 'relationships' in the context of health and social care. Although Chapter 1, 'Communicating humans . . . but what does that mean?' by social anthropologist Ruth Finnegan, does not make specific reference to care, its approach has important implications for thinking about interactions in care settings. Finnegan argues that communication is a basic human process, rather than a separate or specialist activity, and one that embraces a wide range of activities and uses a multitude of resources. In this view, communication is also an interactive process, in which those involved jointly construct the meaning of their interactions. In Chapter 2, 'Relationship-based social policy: personal and policy constructions of "care"', researchers Jeanette Henderson and Liz Forbat use examples from their own and others' research in the area of informal care to present a view of care as fundamentally relational. Like Finnegan, they emphasise the active involvement of all participants in the process, at the same time challenging fixed views of the roles played by 'carers' and 'cared for'. Instead, they pursue the idea that the roles played by people in caring relationships are many-sided and complex, with an important emotional dimension.

The second pair of readings builds on these introductory chapters by focusing on communication in two different contexts, while also exploring the ways in which contexts shape communication. In Chapter 3, 'Giving voice to the lifeworld', by Barry *et al.*, the authors, who are all involved in different ways in medical education, discuss communication between doctors and patients in general practice. The research reported on here uses the work of the medical sociologist Mischler, who called the voice of the doctor the 'voice of medicine' and that of the patient the 'voice of the life-world'. The study reveals the complex use of these two voices and discusses different communication strategies used by doctors and patients. Chapter 4, 'Life choices: making antenatal screening decisions' by writers and researchers Carol Komaromy and Angela Russell, is based on a study of the way that pregnant women and their supporters make decisions about screening. It explores the ways in which different elements of context, both personal and institutional, frame the decision-making process.

The next three readings engage with some of the ways in which the context of interpersonal relations in care services is changing. One of the main developments in health and social care in recent years has been a move away from relationships based on paternalism and towards a degree of service user participation. In Chapter 5, 'Experience and meaning of user involvement: some explorations from a community mental health project', researchers Carole Truman and Pamela Raine make use of their own study of a community mental health project to explore the meanings of user involvement for those taking part, as well as some of the barriers to meaningful participation. A key element of changing practice in interpersonal communication in care services, and in society more generally, has been the growing influence of counselling as a model. In Chapter 6, 'Cultural and historical origins of counselling' John McLeod, an established writer and teacher in this field, situates the growth of counselling in its cultural and historical context. Viewing counselling as bound up with developments in western societies in the last century, McLeod argues for regarding it as one approach among many, rather than as a universal panacea. Following on from this discussion, Chapter 7, 'Communication culture: issues for health and social care' by Deborah Cameron, an academic and writer on language and social issues, takes a critical look at the increasing emphasis on 'communication skills' in care services.

Another important area of change is in ideas about communication and relationships. Elsewhere in this Reader, a range of theoretical perspectives on interpersonal relations is represented, including humanist approaches (see Chapter 19, by Carl Rogers) and psychodynamic perspectives (see Chapters 30, by William Halton and 32, by Jon Stokes). In Chapter 8, 'Postmodernism and the teaching and practice of interpersonal skills', Helen Jessup and Steve Rogerson draw on their experience of teaching interpersonal skills to social work students as they challenge these largely psychological approaches. Basing their critique on the theoretical work of Michel Foucault and the radical educational practice of Paolo Freire, Jessup and Rogerson advocate what they describe as a postmodern approach to teaching interpersonal skills – one that is oriented to radical social change. The final reading in this part of the book explores the implications for practice of adopting this kind of critical theoretical approach. In Chapter 9, 'Practising reflexivity', Carolyn Taylor and Susan White, who are also involved in social work education, argue that a truly reflective approach to practice involves being critically aware of the values and assumptions that we bring to our interactions and relationships.

CHAPTER 1

COMMUNICATING HUMANS . . . BUT WHAT DOES THAT MEAN?

Ruth Finnegan

Like other living creatures human beings interconnect with each other. When you come to think about it, this is actually something remarkable – that individual organisms are not isolated but have active and organised ways of connecting with others outside themselves; that we can reach out to others beyond the covering envelopes of our own skins.

How do we do it? And what resources do humans have at their disposal for achieving this? The answer is in a way simple: we work through the resources of our bodies and of our environment. Unpacking that short statement is less easy, however. It leads into a vast and wonderful field of the complex resources that human beings draw on to interconnect with each other...

Rather than plunging at once into definitional issues let us start with four short examples. [...]

COMMUNICATION AND HUMAN INTERCONNECTEDNESS

Three people are standing around discussing a recent event they all feel strongly about. They are interchanging spoken comments, partly taking turns, partly interrupting, capping and overlapping each other, and formulating their annoyance and surprise through gesture and body positions as

Source: *Communicating*, London: Routledge, 2002.

well as words. One shows round a memo, pointing to specific bits of it, additionally inflaming their anger. They gasp, tut-tut or 'hm' from time to time in acknowledgement or agreement (partial at least) with each other's comments and actions, or as a way of expressing ironic or mock-incredulous reactions. One is more lukewarm, but all three show their active involvement through mutually recognised actions like eye contact, direction of their gaze, body movements, facial expressions, postures, and occasional touches. They move in to stand closer, and increasingly formulate and build up a shared sense of indignation about what had happened.

Face-to-face interaction among a small number of people is one obvious instance but not of course the only context for communicating. Take another example. Among the highlights of the year among the Limba rice farmers of northern Sierra Leone in the 1960s were the rites surrounding boys' initiation into manhood. The night before the boys were taken off to be secluded in the bush there was a grand and public ritual thronged with hundreds of people from throughout the chiefdom. The boys wore the special garb traditional for these rituals, an obligatory mark of the occasion. All through the night they displayed their prowess in special dances, incredibly vigorous and demanding with powerful gymnastic gyrations and hand-springs. Expert drummers sounded out the emotive patterned beats appropriate for the occasion, engaging both dancers and spectators over the long hours with their body-stirring rhythms. Whistles were blown, songs sung, and the crowds, above all the principals in the rite, contributed their shouts and movements. Every now and then friends or relatives rushed up to touch one of the dancers or give a gift in token of their support and admiration. Speeches of welcome and admonition were made by local dignitaries. Fires and lamps lightened the gloom, itself part of the atmosphere. So too was the olfactory ambience from the aromas of food, palm wine, closely touching crowds and perspiring dancers. Through these colourful performances people marked the public validation of the boys' approaching status-change, a major occasion for the community, enacted through these highly specific and recognised multisensory processes. Individuals signalled their personal allegiances and involvement, the boys demonstrated their fitness for elevation to manhood, and through their speeches the elders conveyed both their own leading positions and what they presented as the age-old values of *malimba ma*, 'the Limba way'. All these multiple communicative processes were mediated not through publication in writing but through publicly shared and multifaceted enactment.

Humans also interconnect at greater distances – not so easy perhaps but made possible through our ingenious uses of material objects and technologies. So as a third example consider a personal letter and photograph sent through the post. Simple at first sight, this again has multiple dimensions, though in different ways from the other two cases. The visual marks on the material page – written words, format, punctuation, handwriting – are one obvious dimension. But others matter too. Even before the letter is opened up, the envelope and its handwritten address visibly declare its specific character not only to the named addressee but also to others in the household where it is delivered. The appearance and feel of the paper and the layout on the page are relevant too, accepted conventions which in this case clearly indicate personal intimacy not officialese. So are the handwriting, the non-verbal visual signs (a squiggle of a diagram, x's at the end (for kisses), exclamation marks), the crackle of paper and envelope, and, not least, the enclosed photograph, a human-made artefact which also plays its part. The communicating is experienced in the context of (more, or less) shared understandings and associations between the various participants – participants who include not only letter writer and addressee but in this case a number of other people involved in different ways and at various removes, including others in the recipient's household among whom the letter is mentioned or read aloud, the photograph circulated, or the interpretations formulated – some more interested or more directly involved than others. And if time passes and the letter and photograph are looked at again, other forms of interconnecting may come into play for those later users. The specific ways in which people engage in 'mediated' communicating of this kind vary with different individuals, contexts and conventions. But the communicative process is always likely to be more complex than just a chunk of information transmitted once-and-for-all by fixed marks on a sheet of paper.

The final short example is one where the enactors were involved in yet further temporal and spatial dimensions beyond the momentary occasion: the memorial service for the British Poet Laureate Ted Hughes in May 1999, a large-scale ritual in Westminster Abbey drawing on the multiple resources conventionally deployed on such occasions. There were jointly sung hymns; choir anthems; a visually colourful procession; organ, piano and guitar playing; the olfactory and spatial ambience of the building; the closely-pressed throng; spoken and read words; and a ringingly declaimed oration. And then came the dead poet's unseen voice reciting 'Fear no more the heat of the sun', with all its resonating associations for an English-speaking gathering.

> *One by one, line by line, the looking stopped and the listening went on: 'The sceptre, learning, physic must, all follow this and come to dust' … And now for a few moments, he was back with us. It was as though he was moving from the pews of the living into the poets' corner of the dead … The crowd that flowed away out of the Abbey was both different from and the same as the one which arrived.*
>
> (Stothard 1999: 24)

The occasion drew not only on written and remembered words, first formulated centuries ago and long handed-down through people's creative chains of experience, but also on recent auditory technology for storing and transmitting recorded sounds, all set within a multidimensional process with its plurality of participants.

These four short cases … assume a view of 'communicating' that is not confined to linguistic or cognitive messages but also includes experience, emotion and the *un*spoken. Communicating is envisaged as creative human process rather than transport of data or meeting of 'minds', and goes beyond the preoccupation with 'information' and 'the information revolution' typical of much current discussion. It encompasses the many modes of human interacting and living, both near and distant – through smells, sounds, touches, sights, movements, embodied engagements and material objects.

These interconnecting processes are necessary ones for collective human life. We humans are notably social animals. We live in interacting groups, larger or smaller depending on the context and purpose. Through these we bring up our children, order our affairs, make decisions (the disputed and disastrous as well as the happy ones), express ourselves, share out our complementary tasks, our space and our material resources, avoid (more or less) treading on each other's toes, conduct our lives, and collaborate in the joint enterprises of collective living. Humans are dependent on webs of interconnectedness for their basic modes of growth and livelihood as well as the rich arts and practices of human cultures. In a whole series of organised ways we formulate and share information, ideas, activities, experiences, resources and emotions, and in so doing – for good or ill – engage interactively with each other.

Human creatures call on a vast array of resources for this interconnecting: the examples above represent only the minutest sample of the amazingly diverse ways in which they do so. We use gestures, sounds, writing, images, material objects, bodily contacts, supported by the more or less agreed conventions through which we variously recognise such usages as purposive forms of interaction and mutual influence. Through activating our voices, touches and movements we can share wishes or emotions with others; make visible movements of our bodies to encounter or avoid each other in public places; utilise pictorial displays, visually codified graphics, and three-dimensional artefacts to interconnect over space or time. Deploying these communicative resources is fundamental to our human existence. […]

This is to take a broad view of communication which includes all the channels open to human interaction, whether auditory, visual, kinesic, proxemic, tactile or olfactory. Humans are not solely intellectual or rational creatures, and their communication through human-made artefacts and through their facial expressions, dress or bodily positionings form as relevant a part of their dynamic interacting as verbally-articulated sentences. Human beings, in short, draw on a multitude of resources to interconnect with each other and in so doing interactively create their human world. […]

COMMUNICATING – A MULTIPLE, RELATIVE AND EMERGENT PROCESS

[...] The position in this chapter could be summarised by saying that communication is here taken to be a dynamic interactive process made up of the organised, purposive, mutually-influential and mutually-recognisable actions and experiences that are created in a variety of modes by and between active participants as they interconnect with each other.

This formulation naturally carries the ambiguities and opacities of any attempt to encapsulate a complex and controversial notion in a relatively short form of words. It is certainly not intended as a forever definitive account. But it does take a stand on the interpretation and relevance of certain issues that recurrently feature in contrasting approaches to communication. Three aspects could do with further comment.

First, it lacks the sharp focus of some definitions and, fuzzy at the edges, cannot provide an unambiguous distinction between communicating and other forms of human behaviour. Its breadth and apparent impreciseness are in fact positive properties. This is a 'bundle definition'. In other words, 'communicating' is not one single once-and-for-all thing which you either have or don't have, but a bundle of features, themselves graduated rather than absolute. A process that can be described as communicating may be more, or less, purposive, organised and conscious; more or less mutually influential or recognisable; work simultaneously or sequentially on multiple levels; develop and change during its temporal process; draw on relatively standardised systems or on less widely agreed or only partially shared conventions; and involve more, or less, explicit interacting among the enactors who (to different degrees and in different ways) participate more (or less) creatively in the process and at greater or lesser temporal or spatial distance from each other.

Communication in this view is a relative process with multiple features each of which may in any given case be present to a greater or lesser extent – a multidimensional spectrum of acting and experiencing, not a bounded entity. And just because the spectrum *is* multifaceted the boundaries between communicative and non-communicative action are not absolute. Perhaps all human action involves some degree of communicating, but in some cases only minimally. Other cases are clearer, with a strong input from all the elements mentioned. In other cases yet again, some may be clearly in play, others weak or absent. It is a multifaceted matter of degree.

This relative quality is also relevant for what has proved a difficulty in many theories of communication – a consistent framework for both personal small-scale interaction and communicating across space and time. The perspective here might appear better for close embodied interaction than for more distant situations. But human communication *does* also take place over distance (this too being a matter of degree) in organised, purposive and (more, or less) mutually recognisable ways. It may be mediated through material artefacts rather than in tangible bodily co-presence but still involves human interconnecting through, for example, pictures, books, buildings or, more recently, auditory records. [...]

There are indeed multiply diverse resources through which people interconnect across generations and between different cultures and geographical areas as well as nearby, doing so with a greater or lesser degree of active and creative involvement. It is not an all or nothing matter.

A second point may seem too obvious to need stating: humans use a *variety* of modes to connect with each other. This is another way of emphasising the point, repeatedly made above, that human communicating is not confined just to one mode. Humans draw on manifold resources. There are not only the direct actions of people's bodies – a versatile and marvellous resource indeed, from frowns or bows to sign languages and dance – but also the multifarious sum of human-made media like clothing, books, calligraphic systems, sculptures, textiles, paintings (of 'doom', 'human varieties' and much else), musical instruments, recording devices, set-piece performances, fragrances, broadcasting systems, computer screens and an infinitude of others. Humans have used all these forms to interconnect both face-to-face and at a distance...

Finally, the phrase '*as they interconnect with each other*' is crucial. Communication is a dynamic and emergent process: a dimension of human activity not a separate entity. This emphasis on 'mutuality' and 'interconnectedness' may give an unduly harmonious and optimistic impression (a reasonable criticism of some pragmatist approaches). But looking to the modes through which humans actively interconnect need not carry assumptions about whether this is done in a friendly, hostile, self-interested or self-sacrificial manner (to mention just some possibilities), any more than we can assume that human interconnections always end up to the benefit or mutual understanding of the many rather than few. The focus here is on the process of human interconnectedness not its 'good' or its 'bad' effects in any given case. To quote Birdwhistell's phrase, communication can indeed be understood as the 'dynamic aspect of human interconnection' (1968: 27). It is found in the actions and experiences created by and through people as they interact, affective no less than cognitive. It includes interacting at a distance as well as bodily co-presence at a given temporal moment, and not just messages transmitted from one party to another but all the multidimensional contacts going on within and among groups of people, all the emergent processes through which people mutually – and to multiply varying degrees – interconnect with each other. This is a wide perspective on communication, and, in consequence, on humanity. It enlarges the scope beyond information-transfer and linguistic articulation to encompass all the modes exploited in our active human sociality.

REFERENCES

Birdwhistell, R.L. (1968) 'Communication', in Sills 3: 24–29.

Sills, D.L. (ed.) (1968) *International Encyclopedia of the Social Sciences*, 17 vols, New York: Macmillan and Free Press.

Stothard, P. (1999) 'The moment that changed a memorial', London: *The Times* 14 May: 24.

CHAPTER 2

RELATIONSHIP-BASED SOCIAL POLICY: PERSONAL AND POLICY CONSTRUCTIONS OF 'CARE'

Jeanette Henderson and Liz Forbat

INTRODUCTION

'Care' has received a lot of attention in recent years in legislation, policy and practice. In the UK, the Carers (Recognition and Services) Act 1995 (DoH 1995) and the strategy document *Caring about Carers: A National Strategy for Carers* (DoH 1999a) have been introduced. In England and Wales, Standard 6 of the *National Service Framework for Mental Health* (DoH 1999b) focuses on the needs of 'carers' who 'play a vital role in helping look after service users' (1999b: 69). It goes on to note that 'caring can be rewarding [but] the strains and responsibilities of caring can also have an impact on carers' own mental and physical health' (1999b: 69). Care has been placed at centre stage and policy has sought to outline who carers are, what they do and what support they might need. The 1995 Carers Act has furthered each of these goals, while also seeking to satisfy the influential carer lobby. [...]

This Chapter seeks to problematise some of the assumptions made about care, and part of this lies in the terms and labels applied to people involved in informal care relationships. Traditionally, terms that have been used to refer to the recipients of care are 'dependent', 'service user' or 'cared-for'. To us, each of these terms is unsatisfactory, implying a passivity and lack of agency in the care relationship. The use of the terms care, carer, cared-for, caree and so on remain contested as long as they imply a

Source: *Critical Social Policy*, November 2002, 73 22 (4).

simplistic association with a loss in agency. For lack of better labels, we use these terms, but suggest that each should be read as though it is in quotation marks. To maintain this troubling of labels, we alternate terms and hope that this is received as problematising the use of language and adding to the debate rather than as a distraction from our argument.

CONSTRUCTING CARE

The social construction of 'carers' and 'community care' has been traced back to the 1601 Poor Law by Bytheway and Johnson (1998) who suggest that this was a distinct point where care first became the concern of the state. Carers became a discrete social category with distinctive needs. More recently, the growth of carer-focused support organisations has helped establish the idea that the provision of informal care warrants attention because of the relationship between burden and carers. Care is constructed as being both normal within families and as warranting additional support from government.

This latter point is clearly reflected in the most recent, carer legislation, *Caring about Carers* (DoH 1999a). The increasing professionalisation of informal care has perpetuated a narrow focus on the carer. The recognition of the *relationship* between carer and cared-for ... is largely absent. Additionally, policy does not recognise the shifting balance of care relationships. Care is often reciprocal; the fixed identities constructed in policy do not reflect the complexity and mutuality of many relationships.

Research and support organisations that prioritise 'the carer' have been compounded by constructions of care provision as unidirectional (see, e.g., Bytheway and Johnson 1998). The carer is seen to provide whatever is needed, often at great personal sacrifice and cost, and bears a heavy burden. The National Strategy constructs carers as experiencing stress and as having their independence curtailed. Opie (1993) suggests that talk of stress in care relationships requires more explanation than has traditionally been offered, since the term has become debased through overuse. The constructions of loss of independence for the carer and inevitable dependency for the cared-for have facilitated the way carers' needs have been prioritised.

Feminist theorists have long argued the influence of dependency on assumptions about compromised citizenship, indicating a need to look critically at this label (Graham 1983; Morris 1991). Dependency and care can no longer be viewed as two sides of the same coin, and the dialectic of dependence/independence needs to be examined critically. To be dependent is not necessarily associated with impairment, but can be seen as a more commonplace feature of social life and interpersonal relations. As Brechin (1998: 6) notes, 'everyone is dependent upon some care from others throughout life for both physical and emotional health development'. The importance of this relational component of care is missing consistently from legislation, policy and research.

The National Strategy constructs carers in a number of distinct ways, and it is worth pausing on this document to identify how this is achieved. The opening three pages construct carers in the following ways: as family members; as aware of their own identities as carers; as co-workers; and as commodities. The following passage of the Strategy presents carers as being clients in their own right, with their own care needs:

> *Carers play a vital role – looking after those who are sick, disabled, vulnerable or frail. The Government believes that care should be something which people do with pride. We value the work that carers do. So we are giving new support to carers. Carers care for those in need of care. We now need to care about carers.*
>
> (DoH 1999a: 11)

The opening paragraphs develop a sense of shared responsibility for carers and a feeling that caring touches all our lives. This is accomplished alongside a notion of the shared financial burden that comes with statutory care. Elsewhere, the document upholds the sanctity of family care while asserting that caring can be troubled and that stress can be a potential outcome. [...]

LOCATING THE RELATIONSHIP IN INFORMAL CARE

For many people, the central component of their relationship is not care, but interpersonal dynamics. That is, while care is an element of the relationship, it is not an overriding or defining characteristic. This rings true on an intuitive level and is supported in the following quotations. To reiterate, however, the importance of the interpersonal or relational component of care exchanges is not an understanding that is woven through policy. Policy either circumvents people's own 'meanings' in informal care provision or focuses largely on care as the defining feature of a relationship (if the relationship is considered at all). Participants in our studies constructed the relationship as central:

> *For us during the period I was either high or low, there wasn't really an opportunity to put things behind us. It was a different relationship, and at no time was it our normal relationship until I actually became well at the end of the period. Then once I became well after a time we*

could actually start to put to bed some of the nasty things we said to each other or did to each other. The bits that destroyed parts of our relationship and we could start to build them back up again. I think if you're either manic or depressed there's no opportunity then to really get the relationship back together again. All you're doing is breaking it down all the time.

(Teresa: JH)[5]

I was being pushed in that direction even before the term [carer] was invented. It was something you were supposed to do, turn into some sort of policeman/nurse in the situation. Obviously there is always going to be a bit of that and you have to make sure that disasters don't occur when she's ill. But it was her who explained to me just how damaging that was. How I would turn from being her husband into her carer and that would be the end of it. Neither of us wanted that to happen at all. So she said to me if you want to carry on being my husband you mustn't do that. I resisted that furiously, I thought bloody cheek. This mad woman telling me what and what not to do, but of course she was right, absolutely right. I gradually learned to relate to her even when she's really ill, or to try to. And not to take up this semi-professional mask of the carer at all. It seems to work.

(Richard: JH)

The following quotation comes from a man who has a diagnosis of bipolar disorder and creates immediately a case for prioritising the meaning of the pre-existing relationship over any need for care:

Although Val's endurance has been called upon in a more profound way than I would have hoped at various times, I see it to be an extension of our basic relationship. I don't think that she suddenly when I'm ill steps into a different status or because I have a long-term illness. I don't think of her as having a different status to the normal day-to-day normal man and wife.

(Peter: JH)

Care is constructed as part of a continuum of their marital relationship. The provision of care is constructed as something that would have to be 'stepped into' in order to ring true of his experiences. The repetition of the word 'normal' when referring to the support he receives bolsters the proposition that care is not something to be demarcated from the interpersonal relationship in which it occurs.

The next quotation comes from Peter's wife:

> *I've lived with it for so long. We've been married for 31 years this year and Peter's been diagnosed for the past 28 years, to me it's actually part of our everyday life ... Giving Peter the best support and giving the children the best support that they can have.*
>
> (Val: JH)

The meaning of care provision is thus subsumed by the interpersonal. Orienting to a gendered interpretation of care here, another level of analysis becomes possible, most clearly marked out by her reference to their children. The normality of care being part of the relationship may reflect the assertion that men are looked after all their lives while women assume the responsibility of caring (for both men and children). Men caring for women may not have the same degree of normativity, and may thus be more likely to be conceived as something additional to the relationship. Fisher (1994) presents a critique of the General Household Survey, expressing similar concerns. The survey, he suggests, underestimated the number of male carers because of a lack of clarity over a prompt question. The survey asked about 'extra family responsibilities' which, Fisher suggests, was clearly open to interpretation since men may experience caring as 'women's work' and hence respond positively to the question, whereas women may not.

The process of self-identification as 'carer' or 'caree' is complicated when the more predominant expression of the process is given over to family members such as daughter, son, wife, father, daughter-in-law, brother or sister. The provision of care within a family setting has implications for the gendered take-up of identities of carer and caree. This is, therefore, another feature of the complexity of informal care which is not apparent in policy.

The centrality of the relationship is apparent in the following passage. This account is extremely powerful, not least because of the passion with which it is articulated and the inequity of the impact of illness on relationships throughout the whole family:

> *I feel that it's grossly unfair. It's grossly unfair. I often wonder what I must have done in my last life. I must have been a commandant of a death camp if not something a bit worse, it's really unfair. I think the whole thing leaves the other person out in the cold. You have the person that's affected getting all the attention and this, that and the other and here we have the rest of the family that's affected not getting any attention or help. I've spoken to people like the support workers.*

> *I think that is one of the worst arrangements I've ever come across, is 'we can only speak to you if we have permission'. I think it's a load of crap. I don't think it helps anybody but I think the whole thing is really unfair.*
>
> (Martin: JH)

The tension between the meaning of the illness for this participant and the difficulties in accessing services is brought out with the swipe at carer's assessment (under the 1995 Act). This extract illustrates forcefully the implications of the prerequisite conditions of assessment, the effect on the carer and the subsequent impact that is then felt *within the relationship*. Where the need for care is understood by support services to take precedence over the situation (relationship) in which it is provided, the result is a reaction against this blinkered vision – deeming it to be wholly inappropriate.

The tension is echoed in the talk of Martin's partner. She expresses the importance of the relationship by rejecting the labels of carer and care:

JH: What about with you and Martin?

SALLY: I don't accept at all that he's responsible for my care. I won't have it.

JH: Why do you say that?

SALLY: Because I'm my carer. I don't want a carer. I don't want it or expect it. I get right annoyed when everybody refers to him as my carer because he's not my carer. I'm my own carer and I don't want anybody else to take responsibility because I can take it for myself.

JH: So what is he?

SALLY: My husband. Not a carer at all. I don't think you can be both, not and have a proper relationship.

Subsuming the importance of the interpersonal in the relationship, the focus of the interaction is shifted onto the meaning and impact of care itself. This seems not to reflect the reality of people's experiences. Certainly the two extracts above indicate a mismatch between a straightforward conceptualisation of relationships being totally explicable in terms of care.

One impact of understanding care dyads purely in terms of the provision/receipt of care is in bolstering a professionalised carer role. This locates the two people as associated primarily as a consequence of one's need for care and the other's role in its provision. Carers become conduits of home care knowledge to professionals employed by health and social services. This monitoring and observational role adds weight to Heaton's proposition that there has been an increased visibility of informal care through the extension of the medical gaze. People may become solely defined as carers, reducing any recognition of the interpersonal relationship and fostering a more professional role.

Professionalising carers reduces the need for trained professionals and, hence, there are fiscal reprieves for the government. However, as illustrated above, there is a resistance to increasing the specialism and role of informal carers and a continued expression of the importance of relationship over role.

One central differential feature between relationship (that of partner, child or parent) and role (as carer or caree) lies in the emotional versus professional components. Relationships create space for emotions to be expressed and managed. [...]

CONCLUSION

In this chapter, we have presented a critique of some current social policy pertaining to informal care. Quotations taken from our research illustrate the importance of eliciting accounts from both carer and caree. This approach enhances a reflection on policy. In particular, the quotations illustrate how people in informal care relationships talk about the importance of interpersonal issues, the process of care and the emotional labour involved.

The quotations have been drawn from interviews with members of care dyads and presented in such a way that the reader is able to draw their own conclusions as to the symmetry or overlap between different participants' constructions. We propose that research methods that include both the voices of carer and caree are able to explore areas that other methods cannot reach. There is a value in being able to look at accounts of care exchanges from both perspectives in order to get to grips with the complexities and challenges in informal care.

Interviews from both studies pointed to several themes that are not represented in government thinking on informal care. Initially this was focused at the level of resisted or unwanted identities – characterised in variations of the oft-quoted 'I'm not a carer – she's my wife'. The resistance to the label carer (and indeed caree) is about the meaning for those speakers, that is, the meanings of the labels that are used to describe people involved in a care relationship. The terms care, carer and caree prevent the construction of assistance being expressed as a normal component of the relationship. The terms suggest 'otherness', which places meaning outside of the interpersonal arena. This highlights a tension between meanings conveyed in policy and those constructed by care participants in their lives.

Social policy supports the assumption that care giving or care receipt is a normative component of family life, while paradoxically indicating that it is something that requires special consideration, resources and legislation. Policy chooses not to reflect the voices of both sides of the care relationship and, indeed, often fails to incorporate any recognition of the importance of the relationship itself in how people construct meanings of their situation.

There is the potential to address this lack of recognition by developing multifaceted care policies that recognise care as a contested concept. In addition to including views from the Carers' National Association in policy consultations, views from user organisations could also be sought. This would go some way to enabling the development of integrated policies and a diversity of approach that would meet needs as outlined in the personal constructions of care presented here.

Emotional labour has been identified in the care literature, as well as our own interviews, to be a key component to the care giving and care receiving experience. Social policy at present demonstrates no insight into this, which compounds the lack of awareness of the complexities and differing layers of relationships.

It is, of course, nonsense to expect social policy to reference directly each and every possible and potential influence and outcome of a care relationship. What we suggest, however, is that there are some pervasive and important aspects to care relationships that are systematically overlooked. There is room for policy to incorporate fluidity in care provision, with both people taking on the roles of carer and caree. There is also room to present an understanding of the process and emotional aspects of informal care, and to acknowledge the overriding importance of the relationship over the care, allowing for relationship-based social policy.

NOTE

1 References in parentheses refer to the participant's pseudonym and the research from which it was taken. The following descriptions are intended to give readers some context to the quotes used in this article:

Teresa is a white, middle-class heterosexual woman who was given a diagnosis of bipolar disorder. Teresa considers that her partner Daniel was her carer for a period of time, but that she has also been his carer.

Richard is a middle-class, white heterosexual man who does not identify himself as a carer of his partner Elaine.

Martin is a white working-class man who is unsure of the identity of carer accorded to him by professionals. Sally is Martin's partner. She is a white working-class woman who has been given a diagnosis of bipolar disorder. Sally does not consider Martin to be her carer.

Val and Peter are both white, middle-class and heterosexual. Peter was given a diagnosis of bipolar disorder many years ago. Peter and Val see the role of carer as shifting, depending on the circumstances at the time.

REFERENCES

Brechin, A. (1998) 'What makes for good care?', in Brechin, A., Walmsley, J., Karz, J. and Peace, S. (eds) *Care Matters*, London: Sage, 170–185.

Bytheway, B. and Johnson, J. (1998) 'The social construction of carers', in Symonds, A. and Kelly, A. (eds) *The Social Construction of Community Care*, London: Macmillan, 241–253.

DoH (Department of Health) (1995) *Carers (Recognition and Services) Act*, London: Stationery Office.

DoH (Department of Health) (1999a) *Caring about Carers: A National Strategy for Carers*, London: Stationery Office.

DoH (Department of Health) (1999b) *National Service Framework for Mental Health*, London: Stationery Office.

Fisher, M. (1994) 'Man-made Care: Community care and other male carers', *Bristol Journal of Social Work* 24(6): 658–80.

Graham, H. (1983) 'Caring: a labour of love', in Lewis, J. and Meredith, B. *Daughters Who Care: Daughters Caring for Mothers at Home*, London: Routledge.

Morris, J. (1991) *Pride against Prejudice*, London: The Women's Press.

Opie, A. (1993) 'The discursive shaping of social work records: organisational change, professionalism, and client "empowerment"', *International Review of Sociology* 3: 167–189.

CHAPTER 3

GIVING VOICE TO THE LIFEWORLD. MORE HUMANE, MORE EFFECTIVE MEDICAL CARE? A QUALITATIVE STUDY OF DOCTOR–PATIENT COMMUNICATION IN GENERAL PRACTICE

Christine A. Barry, Fiona A. Stevenson, Nicky Britten, Nick Barber and Colin P. Bradley

INTRODUCTION

The voice of the lifeworld refers to the patient's contextually-grounded experiences of events and problems in her life. These are reports and descriptions of the world of everyday life expressed from the perspective of a 'natural attitude'. The timing of events and their significance are dependent on the patient's biographical situation and position in the social world. In contrast, the voice of medicine reflects a technical interest and expresses a 'scientific attitude'. The meaning of events is provided through abstract rules that serve to decontextualise events, to remove them from particular personal and social contexts.

(Mishler 1984: 104)

Source: *Social Science & Medicine* 53 (2001): 487–505.

In 'The Discourse of Medicine: Dialectics of Medical Interviews' Elliot Mishler employs concepts from Jurgens Habermas' Theory of Communicative Action, to make sense of the patterns of communication between doctors and their patients, in hospitals and private practice in America in the mid-1970s. In this chapter we revisit the concepts with reference to a sample of British consultations recorded in general practice in the late 1990s. We have found the concepts to be very useful in teasing out the dynamics at play in medical communication and we have found support for Mishler's typologies of consultation. We have also uncovered evidence of different patterns of communication. We find support for Mishler's notion of a better model of medical care where space is given to the lifeworld, although we take issue with his terminology, in particular his use of the word inhumane.

Before presenting our data we will summarise the theoretical concepts of Habermas and show how these have been applied by Mishler, and others using his work.

THE THEORY OF COMMUNICATIVE ACTION

Habermas' theory of Communicative Action[1] posits a dialectical struggle between two types of rationality, which in turn produces two different types of world (Habermas 1984). On the one hand, is communicative or value rationality, which inhabits the lifeworld, and on the other is purposive rationality, which inhabits the system. Habermas's project is a moral one and he sees the dangers of the growth of the system as threatening to engulf the lifeworld. The lifeworld is situated within value rationality and involves the contextually grounded experiences of everyday events, expressed in what Schutz has labelled the natural attitude (Schutz 1962). Within this world action is oriented to understanding and is defined by moral considerations. [. . .]

MISHLER'S VOICE OF MEDICINE AND VOICE OF THE LIFEWORLD

Mishler (1984) has drawn on Habermas's concepts and applied them specifically to the world of medicine (one aspect of the technocratic system in late 20th century western society). [. . .]

Where the voice of medicine is used in a purely scientific context, and has no hidden agendas it can be seen as undistorted. However, in dealing with patients, science-based medicine operates on a number of hidden assumptions which could be seen as distortions of the lifeworld [. . .]

These distorted patterns of the voice of medicine are incompatible with the more natural, undistorted communication patterns of the voice of the lifeworld. The voice of medicine has doctors maintaining control within a power imbalance. As a result the coherent and meaningful accounts of patients are suppressed. The result is a struggle in the consultation between the very different modes of the two voices and resulting disruption and fragmentation of communication. This struggle is sometimes invisible.

Mishler does not highlight one of the strengths of Habermas's theory. The struggle need not signify any lack of moral intent on the part of the doctor. His theory allows for doctors to act in good faith, and satisfy patients' expectations, and yet still to be capable of systematically distorted communication without either party being aware of any problem, as is often the case in studies of patient satisfaction.

Mishler (1984) proposes that if doctors were able to use more ideal speech interactions the resultant care would become both more humane and more effective. The examples he gives are listening, asking open-ended questions, translating technical language into the voice of the lifeworld and negotiating a sharing of power. Mishler (1984) develops these ideas through the analysis of 25 interactions between doctors and patients. These represent a subset of a collection of American consultations, in hospitals and private practice, recorded by Howard Waitzkin and his colleagues in the mid-1970s (Waitzkin 1991).

Mishler found there to be a typical pattern of communication, which he labelled the Unremarkable Interview. Conducted wholly in the voice of medicine, a basic structural unit of discourse is repeated throughout the interview. This comprises

- a request from the doctor;
- a response from the patient;
- a post-response assessment (sometimes implicit) followed by a new request; and
- optionally a request for clarification or elaboration of the patient's response [. . .]

In saying that any medical encounter without the voice of the lifeworld was inhumane and ineffective, Mishler could be seen to be making very judgmental statements about medicine. Inhumane is a very powerful word that could imply unfeeling, uncivilised behaviour, and possibly even violations of human rights. It is highly unlikely, however, that these were the connotations Mishler wanted to convey [. . .]

METHODS

The data reported here were collected as part of a Department of Health funded project, 'Improving doctor–patient communication about drugs'. The aim was to conduct an in-depth exploration of the expectations and perceptions of patients prior to consulting a general practitioner, to relate these to the behaviour of GPs and patients in the consultation and to describe the consequences with regard to any medicines prescribed.

SAMPLE

We conducted a total of 62 case studies, comprising 62 patients visiting 20 doctors in the midlands and south-east England. [. . .]

Each case study consisted of patient interviews before and after a consultation, doctor interviews about these consultations and transcribed recordings of the consultations ... From this total, it was only feasible given the considerable depth of analysis to analyse 35 case studies in full. [. . .]

The 35 case studies consisted of 17 male and 18 females ranging from three months (accompanied by mother) to 80 years of age and including a range of socio-economic groups. Thirty-four classified themselves of white ethnic origin. Eleven were attending surgeries without appointments and 24 had made prior appointments to see their doctor. Eleven of the patients had psychological presenting problems (although eight of these also had physical presenting problems), 24 had solely physical presenting problems. [. . .]

FINDINGS: THE VOICES OF MEDICINE AND OF THE LIFEWORLD

In our 35 case studies we found four broadly different patterns of communication according to whether the voice of medicine or the voice of the lifeworld was used and by whom, doctor or patient. We have labelled these groups Strictly Medicine, Lifeworld Blocked, Lifeworld Ignored, and Mutual Lifeworld. The first two groups seem similar to those noted by Mishler (1984) so for reasons of space we will give more detailed examples of the Lifeworld Ignored group, which is qualitatively different to the patterns noted by Mishler. [. . .]

LIFEWORLD BLOCKED

The Lifeworld Blocked occurred in eight consultations with seven doctors. These appear similar to those consultations where Mishler reports seeing glimpses of the lifeworld. These glimpses were immediately suppressed as a result of the doctor using the structural sequence of question control illustrated above. These consultations had less successful outcomes. We rated three as outcome category 4 with significant problems. Most of these patients were consulting for chronic physical problems.

Figure 3.1 shows an example of two points early on in a consultation where a patient talks in the voice of the lifeworld but is silenced by the voice of medicine. Krystof Blyntz[2] a 77-year-old retired scientist was suffering with chronic renal failure and heart problems, most recently angina. For the previous two weeks he had swollen legs with red patches. Dr Williams was unsure about the cause and asked Krystof to return after a week. Krystof, as well as attending at the doctor's request, had an agenda of his own. He had doubts about the angina diagnosis, wanting to know why it had started and what the prognosis was. He had questions about the dosage of medication and the reasons for a blood test. In general, he was very worried about his condition and worried about dying (he did in fact die six months after fieldwork). The two excerpts in Figure 3.1 hint at these worries. [...]

After the consultation, Krystof was still not sure if it was angina, still did not know why it started and was worried it might be something more serious. He was left feeling very vulnerable about his health, and his life expectancy. There were also more bio-medical problematic outcomes such

---

Krystof is very ill and worried about dying as he alludes to twice in his opening lines. He is also struggling to make sense of the angina, how he got it, and how will it progress as shown in the second excerpt (GP20, P51)

002	M	D	Now sit down. <looks at notes> How are you?
003	L	P	**Er still surviving**
004	M	D	Has it [got any better
005	LM	P	**[Surviving. That's right**. Well this thing I had on my- on my leg you remember
134	L	P	**As er er as I say angina is is something that is m- I picked up somewhere**
1- er			**last year I think**.
135	M	D	Yes <uses computer>
136	L	P	**I have never had it before in my life**
137	M	D	<uses computer>
138		P	**((sigh))**
139	M	D	And when you wake up and go off to the loo are you feeling breathless then?

Figure 3.1 The Lifeworld Blocked.

as Krystof's misunderstanding that he should double his dose of isosorbide when the higher quantity had been prescribed to lengthen the time between prescriptions. In our view if Krystof's lifeworld concerns had been taken up some of these problem outcomes may have been reduced. [...]

LIFEWORLD IGNORED

The Lifeworld Ignored is a group of seven consultations with six doctors. Here the patients talked either exclusively or for a large amount of the consultation in the voice of the lifeworld. However, the doctors completely ignored this and conducted the whole of their communication in the voice of medicine. Most of these patients had chronic physical problems and this group had the worst outcomes of any group. We rated five of the seven in the poorest outcome category 4. Patients and doctors seemed to be operating at odds to each other. Patients often seemed relaxed and happy to chat away in the voice of the lifeworld about their concerns while doctors stayed rigidly inside the biomedical format. Six of the patients in this group knew their doctor well and had been on their list for between two and ten years. Perhaps this was a factor in allowing patients to feel able to introduce the concerns of the lifeworld.

Steve (P31), a 24-year-old accountant had been a patient for five years on the list of Dr. Caroline Edwards (GP10) a 38-year-old doctor in an urban fundholding practice with four partners. He was presenting with an ongoing nine-month-old problem of repeated pilonodal cysts between his buttocks. His main concerns, apart from the pain, were needing to drive long distances with his job and as a result having to take time off work, and interference with his sports activities. As well as frustration with his situation, Steve was fairly angry as he had visited another doctor at the practice the day before and got no action on his situation. He was desperate to get something done.

The excerpts from this consultation, shown in Figure 3.2, show points at which the doctor's replies in the voice of medicine seem very disjointed against the patient's voicing of his lifeworld concerns. This pattern reoccurs at six points during the consultation, mostly in the first half. It is as though the patient tries valiantly to be listened to on his terms but slowly gives up and retreats into the voice of medicine. The doctor uses general interjections such as 'right' 'sure' and 'absolutely'. These might be taken as representing a habitual style of communication that is meant to indicate listening and encouraging the patient to talk, and perhaps indicative of good communication skills to the doctor. However, the way in which these interjections seem to be used here is more as a way of vetting information in order to dismiss the lifeworld and seek voice of medicine information with which to continue the consultation, or to interrupt if only lifeworld is forthcoming. So the listening may be there, but is selective. Steve manages

022	**L**	**P**	**Er but during the night er er, I don't know how- what you say, it burst or something**
023			Right. [Right
024	**L**	**P**	**[I've got a hole in my back and it was pouring out with blood and =**
025		D	[Right. Right. Right.
026	**L**	**P**	**[(unintelligible on tape) and I'm in quite a lot of pain**
027	M	D	Right. Just getting the timescale [sorted out,
028		P	[yeah
029	M	D	so it's been over 9 months?
030–047	M	*Consultation continued in voice of medicine by patient and doctor, text omitted*	
048	**L**	**P**	**I can't do any sports, I do a lot of travelling with work**
049		D	Sure. Yeah.
050	**L**	**P**	**and I just don't know where I am from [one day to the next.**
051	M	D	[Did you go you up to the out-patient clinic following on from that at all. Were you actually referred?
052–073	M	*Consultation continued in voice of medicine by patient and doctor, text omitted*	
074	**L**	**P**	**but with the [travelling I d- I do eight-over eighteen miles a day**
075		D	[Yeah. Sure. Sure.
076	**L**	**P**	**And that's just going to work and then if I have to travel from work**
077	M	D	.hh Can I just take a look?
078–094	M	*Consultation continued in voice of medicine by patient and doctor, text omitted*	
095	**L**	**P**	**It was just last night when it went and I thought well it's Sod's Law isn't it, the day after [you've been to the doctor.**
096		D	[Oh absolutely. Absolutely.
097	M		You hadn't had any antibiotics or anything had you?
098–187	M	*Consultation continued in voice of medicine by patient and doctor, text omitted*	
188	**L**	**P**	**I'm er having time off work with it and it's not-**
189	M	D	Do you have trouble with antibiotics at all?
190–359	M	*Consultation continued in voice of medicine by patient and doctor, to end, text omitted*	

Figure 3.2 The Lifeworld Ignored.

to voice some of his lifeworld problems but these are never truly acknowledged, accepted, discussed or empathised with.

Compared to those consultations where once the lifeworld is blocked it does not re-emerge, patients like Steve are notable in their repetition of their lifeworld concerns. Steve's worries are being voiced but not dealt with and he keeps trying again and again to get his frustration acknowledged. There seems little attentiveness or responsiveness on the part of the doctor towards the patient's needs to be heard and understood.

Patients in this group were motivated to press on with the voice of the lifeworld because they had strong feelings about their situations. Six of them were struggling with chronic problems with no easy solutions. These included gout, arthritis, asthma and gynaecological problems. The feelings here were so strong that they were breaking through the barriers of the technocratic medicine in spite of the question structure and control tactics of the doctors concerned. Steve, while not entirely happy, did achieve his wanted referral to hospital so his outcomes on the surface seem good. Psychologically, however, Steve was left feeling angry and unheard. Other patients in this group fared even worse with outcomes.

As well as failing to recognise the patient as unique, the ensuing structure of the interview appears less than effective. Steve's repeated return to his unacknowledged problems continually interrupted the flow of the doctor's biomedical agenda. It appears like a battle field. Had the doctor entered the lifeworld early on in the consultation and really acknowledged Steve's position, perhaps the later necessary medical questions could have been conducted more efficiently. [...]

DISCUSSION

In 1984 Elliot Mishler suggested that there was an 'Unremarkable Interview' format for consultations between doctors and patients. He showed how doctors use strategic and manipulative methods in the consultation to maintain control of the dialogue. As a result medical communication was conducted almost entirely in the voice of medicine and the voice of the lifeworld was suppressed and fragmented. This pattern of communication fits very well with Habermas' ideas about the system rationalisation and colonisation of the lifeworld. It could be said that doctors are using distorted communication in a success oriented, purposive rational action (albeit unconsciously in all probability). Mishler concludes that for more effective and more humane medical care to be present that doctors would need to employ more balanced forms of communication oriented to achieving greater levels of understanding.

In the late 1990s within this sample of 35 British general practice consultations, we have found support for Mishler's Unremarkable Interview format. The voice of the lifeworld is totally absent or fleeting in those consultations we have labelled Strictly Medicine and Lifeworld Blocked. The control structures imposed by the doctors in these encounters are strong.

However, we have also found that about half the consultations studied did not fit this format, with far more use of the voice of the lifeworld. Where this was purely on the side of the patients, Lifeworld Ignored, this appears to produce dysfunctional consultations. Where it was used by both doctors and patients, Mutual Lifeworld, we begin to see a glimpse of Habermas' ideal speech interaction which is contextually grounded in everyday events and where there is an emphasis on working together to reach understanding through negotiation. [...]

In our sample, the voice of the lifeworld was used by doctors and encouraged in patients primarily in psychological consultations. (The consultations studied by Mishler were mainly for physical presenting conditions.) However, most of the patients with Mutual Lifeworld consultations had physical as well as psychological presenting problems and it may have been that in a different type of consultation only their physical symptoms would have emerged as the business of the consultation. [...]

Being generalists, general practitioners have less structured routines to rely on, than psychiatric medical staff. The tools of the flow-chart, decision-tree format of diagnostic questions and physical examination aimed at diagnosis of physical conditions, are not as available for psychological problems, for GPs whose interest does not specifically lie in psychiatric illness. Therefore, the voice of the lifeworld is seen as legitimate discourse by general practitioners for the psychological consultation. [...]

The Lifeworld Ignored consultations showed most evidence of an active dialectical struggle between the two voices. Here patients repeatedly returned to the concerns of the lifeworld and doctors repeatedly ignored them. This produced the most problematic consultations of all. The fact that a patient is willing to resist the strength of the doctor's control and keep repeating a lifeworld issue might suggest that this issue is one about which they feel very strongly. If patients continue to mention lifeworld concerns, it suggests their needs have not been heard and they feel compelled to try again in the hope of being heard. These consultations had very poor outcomes and may provide a message for doctors hoping to improve on this situation.

This pattern of consultation is similar to one identified by Byrne and Long (1976) as dysfunctional consultations. They identified the problem arising when the doctor was trying to move the patient towards closure while the patient was trying to bring the doctor back to the stage of identifying and defining the problem. Our findings suggest that the reason the patient might have felt their problem had not been sufficiently defined was because of the exclusion of the lifeworld. [...]

The problem seems to lie with the patients with chronic, ostensibly physical conditions whose lifeworld concerns, including psychological responses to their condition, are seen as invalid and irrelevant to the consultation. This seems to be the area that might benefit the most from allowing the voice of the lifeworld more space. If doctors want to pay more attention to the lifeworld they might need more training to be attentive to the glimpses or flashes of the lifeworld that they seem to be quashing (Balint and Norell 1973). They might also need new skills for dealing with the lifeworld once the space has been opened up.

CONCLUSION

Mishler's theoretical ideas about the dialectical struggle between the voice of medicine and the voice of the lifeworld, provide a useful way of looking at doctor – patient communication. Through a more complex data collection strategy we have been able to elaborate on this idea to show more complex relations than he was able to illustrate from the use of consultation data alone.

Our analysis has shown that the doctors here seemed to switch their communication strategy depending on whether they perceived the patient to be presenting with physical or psychological problems. Where they employed the Strictly Medicine discourse for acute physical problems this appeared to be a successful strategy. As long as there were not hidden concerns, patients did not suffer from exclusion of the lifeworld, and outcomes of the consultation were good.

Where the doctors adopted the voice of the lifeworld in the Mutual Lifeworld consultations, for patients with psychological problems, this also appeared to be a successful strategy, even when patients were also suffering from physical conditions.

The real problems seem to lie in the consultations where patients were consulting about chronic physical problems. To patients these conditions were a lifeworld issue. However, the doctors seemed to see them as a physical issue requiring the voice of medicine, and the blocking or ignoring of the voice of the lifeworld as a nuisance or an inconvenience.

Some of the doctors in this study demonstrated the capacity to operate in both voices but did not always apply the voice of the lifeworld. This would suggest that if doctors could be sensitised to the importance of dealing with the concerns of the lifeworld with patients with chronic physical conditions as well as psychological conditions, it may be possible to obtain better care for patients.

As the role of the GP changes with the rise of chronic illness in an ageing population GPs may have to change their notions of success from purely technical considerations to include their patients feeling understood, listened to and treated like whole and unique human beings. However, there will be a need for structural reforms to provide a suitable framework within which GPs can be supported to offer this type of care.

ACKNOWLEDGEMENTS

The study was funded by the Department of Health as part of the Prescribing Research Initiative. Any views expressed in this paper are those of the authors, not the Department of Health. Christine Barry is supported by an NHS Health Services Research Fellowship. Dr Stevenson is supported by Sir Siegmund Warburg's Voluntary Settlement.

We would like to thank all the participating receptionists, doctors and patients. We are grateful to delegates at the 1999 BSA Medical Sociology Conference and Eliot Mishler for comments on an earlier version of the paper, and for the comments of the anonymous referees.

NOTES

1 Useful introductions to the theory of communicative action as applied to medicine can be found in Porter (1998) and Scambler (1987).
2 All names and identifying information have been changed to preserve anonymity.

REFERENCES

Balint, E. and Norell, J.S. (eds) (1973) *Six Minutes for the Patient. Interactions in General Practice Consultation*, London: Tavistock Publications.

Byrne, P.S. and Long, B.E.L. (1976) *Doctors Talking to Patients. A Study of the Verbal Behaviour of General Practitioners Consulting in their Surgeries*, London: HMSO.

Habermas, J. (1984) *The Theory of Communicative Action, Reason and the Rationalization of society* 1, London: Heinemann.

Mishler, E.G. (1981) 'Viewpoint: Critical perspectives on the biomedical model', in Mishler, E.G., AmaraSingham, L.R., Hauser, S.T., Liem, S.D., Osherson, R. and Waxler, N.E. (eds), *Social Contexts of Health, Illness and Patient Care*, Cambridge: Cambridge University Press.

Mishler, E.G. (1984) *The Discourse of Medicine. The Dialectics of Medical Interviews*, Norwood, NJ: Ablex.

Porter, S. (1998) *Social Theory and Nursing Practice*, London: Macmillan.

Scambler, G. (1987) 'Habermas and the power of medical expertise', in Scambler, G. (ed.) *Sociological Theory and Medical Sociology*, London: Tavistock, 165–193.

Schutz, A. (1962) *Collected Papers, I. The Problem of Social Reality*, The Hague: Martinus Nijhoff.

Waitzkin, H. (1991) *The Politics of Medical Encounters. How Patients Deal With Social Problems*, New Haven, CT: Yale University Press.

CHAPTER 4

LIFE CHOICES: MAKING ANTENATAL SCREENING DECISIONS

Carol Komaromy and Angela Russell

This chapter is based on some of the findings from an Open University study that explored the way that women make antenatal screening decisions. The idea for this study grew out of reflections from my practice as a midwife in the 1990s on the way those women and their supporters make these decisions. Angela was employed as the full-time researcher on the project.

Pregnant women who attend antenatal 'booking interviews' for midwifery and obstetric care are presented with a series of choices. The main decision that a woman will make with her midwife or GP at this early meeting, usually around the twelfth week of pregnancy, is about place of birth. But women also have to make a series of choices throughout the antenatal period, which involves them in a complex process of decision-making that is both practical and ethical (Davis 1999; Ewart 2000; Holt 1996). The study findings were rich and diverse and there were many more factors involved in the decision making process than we had anticipated. Here we focus on just a few of these that form part of the context of decisions. We have restricted our discussion to just one screening test – that for Down's syndrome.

First we set the scene by exploring the complexity of Down's syndrome screening (Cuckle 1998; Quaglierini 1997). We then draw upon observational data to continue setting the scene with what happens at the booking interview. This is followed by an exploration of some of the factors that influence screening decisions.

BACKGROUND TO THE STUDY

In my experience as a midwife, many women are familiar with the existence of Down's syndrome or Trisomy 21, and that it is possible to screen for this condition, where a person has an additional chromosome. A test is routinely offered to pregnant women and is one of a series of different screening choices that they have to make. The nature of test results, however, involves women in the need to understand quite abstract notions of risk probability and this is something that most women seem to be unprepared for.

Pregnant women in the UK are routinely offered an AFP[1] screening test for Down's syndrome between 16 and 20 weeks into their pregnancy. This test measures the amount of alpha feta protein in the blood and this level, at this stage in the pregnancy, combined with an estimate of risk based on the woman's age, provides a prediction of the probable risk of her baby having Down's syndrome. Those women whose results indicate a 'high' probability of the risk of Down's syndrome, are offered a further diagnostic test called an amniocentesis. This is an invasive procedure in which a specimen of amniotic fluid from the uterus is taken and genetically screened for the presence of Down's syndrome cells. Although the test is deemed to be 99 per cent accurate it carries between a one and two per cent risk of miscarriage. Women then have to make a difficult choice about whether or not to endanger the life of the foetus. But, if the result is positive, then women will be offered a 'therapeutic' termination of the pregnancy.

There are several difficulties for a woman who is offered these screening choices. If a woman undergoes an AFP blood test she will not be given a definite diagnosis, only an estimate of the probability that her baby has Down's syndrome. If the risk is greater than 1:250 she will be offered an amniocentesis. If the risk is lower than this she will not be offered a further test, but she could still have an affected child. However, even when a baby has Down's syndrome (or spina bifida) it is not possible to know the extent of the disability in advance, although scans might reveal potential disability. To be asked to decide whether to have a termination with such uncertainty and complex information is, at the least, very difficult. Added to this is the amount of time that a woman has to wait for the results, the possibility of false positives and false negatives and all the other aspects of the pregnancy as well as her own circumstances and experiences. The lack of certainty associated with any test results and the risk of *false* positive results can take an emotional toll and increase the levels of anxiety for potential parents and supporters. It seems to be entirely appropriate that Heyman (2001) has likened this 'decision-making process' to that of stepping onto a risk escalator. Women are invited to have an initial risk assessment and might then be offered more invasive investigations and even ultimately a therapeutic abortion. This complexity and the ethical dilemmas that can result from stepping onto the risk escalator also challenge midwives. On a practical level, midwives need to be able to provide information that is clear and comprehensible. But as already stated, there is a lot of uncertainty and ambiguity in screening test results.

There are wider outcomes of screening for abnormality. One *implication* of screening for Down's syndrome is that the rate of therapeutic abortion has reduced the rise in the incidence of Down's syndrome. This is based on two factors. First, the estimation that 45 per cent of babies with Downs are diagnosed with the condition before birth (Huang 1998). Second, although the incidence of Down's syndrome increases with maternal age and the current (1990–1997) UK trend is for mothers to be older, the prevalence of Downs has not increased at the expected, associated rate. Indeed, between 1990 and 1995, the rate of increase dropped by 14 per cent. It would seem to be likely that many women who are offered a therapeutic abortion agree to this option.

METHODS

The study data was based on observations of antenatal bookings and post-booking research interviews with women and midwives. In all, six midwives and twenty women in three locations participated in the study. Twenty antenatal booking interviews were observed and during the following two-week period, the same pregnant women were interviewed about their experience of the booking interview. Participating midwives were also interviewed after the antenatal booking interviews. Three of the antenatal bookings took place at a hospital antenatal clinic and the remainder was almost equally divided between GP surgeries and women's private homes.

STUDY FINDINGS

An average antenatal booking interview usually lasts for one hour and takes place in either the hospital antenatal clinic, the home of the pregnant woman, or the GPs surgery. A midwife most often conducts it – although she or he is not necessarily the person who will provide care and support to this woman and her family throughout the antenatal period. It is at this interview, most often in the first trimester of pregnancy, that a woman's medical, obstetric and social history is taken. At this time midwives or GPs provide general advice on the pregnancy and such things as diet and lifestyle as it affects the health and wellbeing of the mother and foetus. It is also at this meeting that midwives are expected to make an assessment of risk for mother and foetus – as they evaluate the extent to which the pregnancy and birth can be constructed as a 'normal' event. Screening for abnormality, involves performing a routine physical examination and taking blood and urine tests. If the antenatal interview takes place in a hospital setting, it might also be the time when an ultra sound scan is performed to confirm the viability of the pregnancy and to establish the foetal size and thus estimate the expected date of delivery. Clearly this is a packed hour with much information being exchanged and various basic observations being made.

From the observational data we noted that screening test choices and information about them were offered towards the end of the booking interview, after all the other information had been exchanged. The time taken for this discussion about all of the screening tests on offer took, on average, four minutes. Midwives talked very briefly about screening tests and gave women a leaflet to read to help them to make their decision. If pregnant women knew that they wanted to have the test they then made an appointment with the practice nurse at their GP surgery to take the blood when they would be 16–18 weeks pregnant. So the time in which women were able to make a decision was often very short.

The following is based on interview and observation data recorded at one of the booking interviews. It provides an example of what was discussed in this period of time and how it took place. This example relates to Down's and is therefore only part of the discussion on screening tests.

MAUREEN: Have you thought about screening? About Down's?
ANDREA: It's not one of those that can cause miscarriage?
MAUREEN: I'll give you the date.

She continued to write on the antenatal record.

ANDREA: 'Spose I might as well have it. Is it recommended you have it?
MAUREEN: Think about if you have it done and it came up as high risk. You may have to decide about termination.

She then explained about how risks were calculated depending on the stage of the pregnancy and hormone levels found in the blood test known as the Double Test.

ANDREA: I suppose it's more relevant for older mums.
MAUREEN: You really want to think if you want to do anything about it.

She offered Andrea the leaflet about the test.
Andrea took the leaflet and said to her husband.

ANDREA: We'll have to think about it. I'll talk about it with the doctor.

MAUREEN: Quite often if there is any problem with spina bifida you see it on the scan. I'll see you in 6–7 weeks time in the community. Do blood tests then.

(This conversation about screening took five minutes).

This is just one aspect of a large amount of diverse and complex information that is exchanged at the booking interview. Pregnant women and their supporters are provided with information that relates to different aspects and times in their pregnancy. This can be difficult to assimilate in the short time that this takes place. The way that an interview is managed makes it clear that the midwife follows a routine that is structured by the antenatal record form where obstetric notes are recorded. She asks specific questions and invites pregnant women to provide answers. Our observations revealed that the amount of time that was allocated to women to raise their own issues and concerns was short. Midwives usually rigidly structured the meeting following the booking form and this set the agenda. In none of the interviews was there any attempt made to renegotiate the agenda for the meeting.

Some of the midwives in the study considered that this was reasonable and appropriate. They needed to get to know the woman before discussing this difficult area and therefore this was best done near the end of the meeting. Midwives' views varied about the importance they attached to ensuring that women understood the information that they offered about screening tests. The following quotes from three midwives illustrate this difference:

MIDWIFE A: And I wouldn't leave until I know they understand what I'm telling them.

MIDWIFE C: I'm very aware that on a lot of occasions the women don't erm, rarely understand.

MIDWIFE B: It would help if we knew what the GP had already told the woman about the tests.

One midwife thought women should be informed about choices earlier in the pregnancy and before the 12 week booking interview.

MIDWIFE A: And then us going back and talking to them in more depth about it later, so they've had time to think about it.

However the midwives were in general agreement that there was not enough time to conduct the booking in the fifty minutes allowed since such a large amount of information had to be exchanged. Two midwives expressed this concern thus:

MIDWIFE D: Myself I'd like to see me looking after a small caseload of women giving them time, giving them information that they need, knowing that they can contact me if necessary.

MIDWIFE E: You know there may be huge social problems, there might be financial problems. There might be medical or physical problems. There might be psychological problems and you're expected to deal with all of that emotion, and you know all that problem in a very short time. It's – it's nearly impossible to do it.

Professionals seemed to exert a strong influence in terms of legitimating the need for screening tests for many pregnant women in the study. One woman seemed to be content for the midwife to guide her:

SHARIA: She took some test. I don't know what tests they were. I thought she's the midwife – she knows what she's doing.

It was common for women to express the view that because the tests were routine they were in their best interests. Midwives and 'professional' views were of significant importance in influencing the way those women made screening decisions. But there are other factors that played a role. For example, past experiences and the experiences of friends and family also contributed to women's understanding of screening tests. Jenny told Angela about her friend's experience:

JENNY: I've got a friend at work who has just found out today that she's pregnant. She had the test a couple of weeks ago and it came back as a high risk and they did it again 'cos they were surprised and it came back OK. So, I don't know how accurate they are. So, well, if you think – well – if it comes back with a high result – then you'll ask for it to be done again. But if it comes back with a low result you just trust it don't you?

Some women had experienced the difficulties of caring for a severely disabled child and did not think they would be able to cope.

KIM: [...] but I'd rather make that decision (to terminate) early on before it's fully developed and everything, than to have it born and having to cope with all that afterwards.

Apart from the timing and quality of information given to pregnant women and any supporters at this time, one of the questions that we asked repeatedly during the research period was the extent to which other factors might impact upon the decision-making process. For example, we anticipated that the setting in which the meeting took place would impact upon the quality of the encounter. We speculated that women might be more relaxed in their own home and therefore able to exchange and take in information more easily. However, the greatest cause of interruptions in *all* settings was the presence of demanding toddlers needing frequent attention. In one home although Mary's partner was there to look after their toddler, there was never enough time for there to be an uninterrupted discussion as the toddler was constantly taken in and out of the room in which they were meeting.

The physical symptoms that are associated with pregnancy can also impact upon women's ability to concentrate at this time. Eighteen out of the 20 women in the study complained of feeling very tired and/or nauseous at the time of the booking interview. They told us that they felt unable to concentrate fully on information given to them by their midwives.

There were also psychological factors that impacted upon the context of decision making. For example, for many of the women at such an early stage in the pregnancy, around 12 weeks, the pregnancy did not seem quite 'real'. Half of the women told us that did not want to think too much about what could go wrong when they were just beginning to form an attachment to their baby.

All the study midwives reported that most women did not expect problems and wanted reassurance that the pregnancy was normal. They considered that pregnant women were very vulnerable emotionally. The following quotes illustrate these views.

MIDWIFE C: They, they're – I some sometimes think that they're going to have the test because they feel positive that everything is okay, but they just want to be reassured.

MIDWIFE A: And even some women that are as solid as a rock usually are a bit wobbly when they're pregnant. Especially in the beginning but also, as the pregnancy progresses.

Midwives held strong views about the extent to which women were emotionally capable of making such difficult decisions at this time. At interview all midwives thought that women did not make 'rational' choices about whether to have screening tests.

MIDWIFE E: I believe it is an irrational decision that they will or they won't have the test done.

Values and religious beliefs also influenced decision-making. Some women thought termination was morally wrong.

CARMEN: I could not have a test because I am a committed Christian. I – we – could *never* terminate.

However, there would seem to be dangers inherent in ascribing views associated with culture and beliefs to groups of women in the way that one of the midwives does here:

MIDWIFE B: Asian women have a – are in a culture that they believe that all the tests that we do and all the screening that we do has to be the right thing if the doctor said so.

While another midwife considered that this type of generalisation was clearly unsafe:

MIDWIFE A: And our assumption is because they're Muslim and because they're Asian, they will not have an amniocentesis and they will not go on and have the pregnancy terminated. But we are onto second and third generation Asian women and therefore, sometimes that assumption of how they behave is entirely wrong.

CONCLUSION

There has only been time to provide a snapshot of the views of women and their midwives about antenatal screening for Down's syndrome. Antenatal screening has changed significantly over time and needs to be considered against a background of rapidly changing technology. The routinisation of antenatal decisions makes it more compelling for pregnant women to step onto the 'risk escalator'. At the time of interview only five women declined the test and five were still undecided. Certainly there is a tension between reproductive choice and autonomy when information about screening and its results is complex and ambiguous. Screening choices also present dilemmas at a time which is largely constructed as a positive one of anticipated birth. This study has shown that the quality of information and the way that it is conveyed is just one small part of the context in which women make decisions. The wider reality is that this is just one part of a dynamic experience for pregnant women who will be faced with increasing numbers of complex choices.

NOTE

1 There is a screening test for Down's syndrome that is less invasive and possibly more accurate (Snijders 1998) and this is a nuchal ultrasound scan which measures the thickness of the nuchal fold in the neck of the foetus. However this test was not offered to any of the women in the study. This is because, at the time of the study (2001) the availability of this test varied between regions and Trusts. However, the more that the central political agenda of the NHS National Screening Committee exerts control, the more this is likely to change and for the test to be routinely available on the NHS.

REFERENCES

Cuckle, H. (June 1998) 'Antenatal screening today and in the future', *RCM Midwives Journal* 1: 6.

Davis, A. (March 1999) 'A disabled person's perspective on prenatal screening', *MIDIRS Midwifery Digest* 9: 1.

Ewart, R.M. (2000) 'Primum non nocere and the quality of evidence: rethinking the ethics of screening', *Journal of the American Board of Family Practice* 13, 3: 188–196.

Heyman, B. and Henrikson, M. (2001) *Risk, Age and Pregnancy: A Case Study of Genetic Screening and Pregnancy*, London: Arnold.

Holt, J. (1996) *Screening and the Perfect Baby, Ethics and Midwifery*, Lucy Frith (ed.), Oxford: Reed Educational and Professional Publishing Ltd.

Huang, T. *et al.* (1998) 'Birth prevalence of Down's syndrome'. Letters to the editor, *Journal of Medical Screening* 5: 213–214.

Quaglierini, D. *et al.* (1997) 'Coping with serum screening for Down's syndrome when the result is given as a numeric value', *Prenatal Diagnosis* 18: 816–821.

Snijders R.J.M. *et al.* (1998) 'UK multicentre project on assessment of risk of trisomy 21 by maternal age and fetal nuchal translucency thickness at 10–14 weeks of gestation', *Lancet*, 352; 9125, 343–346.

CHAPTER 5

EXPERIENCE AND MEANING OF USER INVOLVEMENT: SOME EXPLORATIONS FROM A COMMUNITY MENTAL HEALTH PROJECT

Carole Truman and Pamela Raine

INTRODUCTION

User involvement in health service provision is nothing new. There has been a long tradition within the voluntary sector of centring the planning and delivery of services around the needs of users, exemplified by self-help and user-led alternatives to 'mainstream' statutory health and social care services. The philosophy of normalisation, on which many such initiatives were based, sees user involvement in decision-making concerning the services they receive as an individual right, one previously denied to the 'disabled' (Wolfensberger 1972), and offers a fundamental challenge to their exclusion from structures of power (Bowl 1996). However, the incorporation of such ideas into mainstream social care and health provision is relatively recent (and some would argue, partial) (Campbell 1996). In the wake of the government white paper *Caring for People: Community Care in the Next Decade and Beyond* (Department of Health 1989), and the 1990 NHS and Community Care Act, for example, involving service users in the planning and evaluation of their own health and social care has become a central tenet of government policy regarding community care (Biehal 1993; Mort *et al.* 1996; Myers and MacDonald 1996;

Source: *Health and Social Care in the Community* (2002) 10 (3): 136–143.

Harrison *et al.* 1997). This may be seen as the 'official sanctioning of the user voice' (Mort *et al.* 1996: 1133), but one which is perhaps more influenced by consumerism and the ethos of markets than ideas concerning the rights of citizens to participation (Rogers and Pilgrim 1991; Pilgrim and Waldron 1998).

There is a growing acknowledgement among mental health service providers of the need to involve service users in decisions concerning service planning and organisation. The Department of Health, in *The Health of the Nation Key Area Handbook on Mental Illness* (Department of Health 1994), and more recently, the *National Service Framework for Mental Health* (Department of Health 1999), for example, stressed the responsibility of National Health Service (NHS) purchasers and providers, and local authorities to consult with users and their carers about community care plans for this client group. An earlier shift from segregated service provision for the mentally ill in large psychiatric hospitals to more community-based models of treatment encouraged this inclusive approach (Pilgrim and Waldron 1998). However, such advances can be seen to be hard won, following as they do in the wake of vociferous campaigning by the mental health user/survivor movement, seen by some commentators as inspired by the liberation movements of the 1960s and 1970s (Lindow 1994), and fuelled by the influence of the self-help lobby in North America and the Netherlands (Campbell 1996). Campaigning organisations such as Survivors Speak Out, Campaign Against Psychiatric Oppression and Mind have been instrumental in bringing about changes in attitudes towards those suffering from mental illness, and have highlighted both the injustice of their former exclusion from structures of power and their competence as self-advocates (Plumb 1993; Forbes and Sashidharan 1997; Perkins and Repper 1998). The proliferation of user groups within health and social care services in the UK (although there are local variations) is testament to the increasing acceptance of the idea that services should be responsive to their demands (Barnes and Wistow 1994a).

If service users needs and interests are to be central to services, then logically their perspectives should be a central focus within the evaluation of service provision. However, the extent to which this is carried out in practice, and the methods typically used, are both open to question. For example, how can evaluation research embrace the concept of user involvement in a meaningful and valid way? What can evaluative processes tell us about the nature and extent of any involvement taking place? In this chapter, the present authors seek to address such questions by drawing on a piece of evaluative research aimed at exploring the process and outcomes of a community-based exercise facility for people with mental health problems in the North of England. The nature of user involvement is identified in this study which set out to explore:

- the organisational context in which involvement takes place;
- factors which encourage meaningful participation on the part of service users;

- barriers to user involvement; and
- issues of sustainability and continuity relating to user involvement.

In the concluding part of this paper, the present authors draw out the broader implications of their study and its relevance to other service providers. As Barnes and Wistow (1994a) pointed out, there is a need to generalise lessons learned from successful partnerships between service users and providers. In this chapter, the present authors explore some of the meanings and experiences of what 'successful' user involvement may involve and the conditions that underpin 'success'.

CONTEXT OF THE STUDY: BARROW COMMUNITY GYM

The present study took as its focus a community-based gym in Barrow-in-Furness, Cumbria, UK, which has been developed by the Bay Community Trust's physiotherapy service and is aimed at improving the physical well-being of people with mental health problems. Jointly financed by the Regional Mental Health Partnership Fund and the Morecambe Bay Health Authority, the gym has recently moved from a hospital-based service to one that is more centrally based within the local community in Barrow-in-Furness. At the point where it was relocated to a community site, the exercise facility was renamed the Barrow Community Gym (BCG).

In addition to the direct benefits of providing an exercise facility, the gym also provides users with opportunities to gain experience and vocational qualifications in fitness training through a system of volunteering. Therefore, while other initiatives exist in the UK as part of *Active for Life* schemes (Health Education Authority 1997), which use exercise in a therapeutic capacity for people with mental health problems, BCG takes this model one step further by providing not only an exercise facility, but also a range of opportunities for users to acquire and develop experience and training within the operation of the gym. There are different means and levels of user involvement at BCG, the nature of which may vary from casual 'help' to a more formalised agreement under the auspices of the gym's volunteer scheme. In the latter stages of the present research study, some users have been involved in an 'evaluation group' to develop a user-led evaluation tool for use within the gym (see Truman and Raine 2001). The flexible and positive approach to involving service users in service delivery and development means that user involvement may potentially take place within a range of aspects of the gym, and at a variety of different levels of commitment or responsibility. Therefore, the present authors outline the extent to which user involvement is possible within a community mental health service. In order for user involvement to flourish, organisational conditions need to be right. These conditions then shape types of user involvement, which will differ in different settings. Therefore, the present findings suggest that involvement is not a straightforward prospect for all users, nor is it likely to be viable in every organisation. The authors argue that, to be successful, it requires adaptation not only on the part of the organisation, but also by service providers and non-involved users. [...]

RESULTS AND DISCUSSION

The remainder of this chapter focuses on the results of the study. It discusses involvement, barriers and sustainability for users. The broader implications of the project are considered, with the present research showing a positive effect on mental health patients.

CHARACTERISTICS AND NATURE OF USER INVOLVEMENT

User involvement in mental health services can take place on several levels:

- through campaigning groups at both national and local levels (Perkins and Repper 1998);
- in the planning, organising and managing of services; and
- in organising individual care; for example, in needs assessment procedures and the development of care plans

Differences in mental health services with a high level of user involvement at service level (our main focus) in comparison to 'traditional' services for this client group should be clearly recognisable. For example, they should be seen to be more democratic and less hierarchical in their organisation, with clear policies and established structures for users to influence the 'making and creating' of the services they receive (Barnes 1999: 84). The volunteer scheme at BCG exemplifies one way in which services can be 'opened up' to users who have traditionally been situated at the foot of the hierarchy. Therefore, the present authors took the scheme as their starting point in exploring the context of user involvement in the facility

Therefore, importantly, BCG provides the organisational conditions in which user involvement can take place, with clear means of progression from 'patient' to staff member, from work experience through training to paid work. Formal policies and procedures have been introduced to support user involvement. However equally important are the meanings attached to participation by users and service providers.

EXPLORING THE MEANINGS OF 'USER INVOLVEMENT'

Research demonstrates that problems experienced by people suffering from mental health problems, such as social isolation, finding constructive ways of spending the day, loss of status, and the lack of a sense of belonging and importance, may usefully be addressed by involvement in work-related activity (Pilling 1991; Di Mascio and Crosetto 1994; Sheid and Anderson 1995; Mitchell 1998). Service users in BCG endorse the importance of work experience and opportunities for education and training which the volunteer scheme provides. It is seen as a way of working towards personal goals, whether or not these are directly connected with the gym, or as a 'stepping stone' towards other possibilities. Volunteers explained, for example:

> *It's really changed my life, given me the chance to do something I want to do. Without this place I couldn't do that.*

> *...It gives you the chance to get your life kick started again. 'Cause coming here you can meet people, you can train, and there's also career opportunities.*

However, there are intrinsic satisfactions in the role of volunteer which are of equal importance; e.g., building confidence, feeling useful by helping others in the gym, and breaking down the perceived 'gap' between 'mental patients' and professional staff by acting as a role model to others. Feelings of achievement and increased self-confidence, for example, were typical gains described by those actively participating in BCG. This corroborates other research evidence which suggests that there are also important subjective benefits to be gained from user involvement in service delivery (Barnes and Wistow 1994a,b; Harrison *et al.* 1997).

User involvement may also be seen as a means of enabling service users to regain a sense of control over events, and increase their ability to make constructive choices and decisions (Lindow and Morris 1995). However, in the present study, only staff and referral agents stressed the importance of users gaining increased control over their lives, suggesting perhaps that users' priorities are different.

The data analysis identified social elements of participation as important to gym users; e.g., in providing opportunities to mix with others (including NHS trust staff) on an even footing. This can be a starting point for reintegration into the community for those who have felt excluded.

As one service user said, it is part of 'having a life, being normal'. Finally, becoming a volunteer is seen by some as a means of de-stigmatising mental illness, in demonstrating capabilities which they feel are often doubted by others. A user who was involved in planning a gym newsletter felt that such an initiative could help to illustrate that:

> *We are just ordinary people, people who happen to have some chemical imbalance.*

BARRIERS TO MEANINGFUL INVOLVEMENT

However, despite the perceived benefits, it became evident during the course of the present study that some gym users were reluctant to become actively involved in the BCG for a variety of reasons. While it is recognised that there may be times when the symptoms of mental illness preclude active participation (Hickey and Kipping 1998), the present data showed that there are also other factors at work. It became apparent that the presence of user involvement at any level requires adaptation on the part not only of organisations, but also users themselves, service providers and non-involved users.

As previous research has indicated, service users have clear ideas concerning the respective roles of staff and users (Mowbray *et al.* 1998). The service user can be seen to have a 'foot in both camps' as a service user and a member of staff, a role that has both advantages and tensions. For example, a number of respondents in the present study saw volunteering in the gym as crossing an 'invisible dividing line' between users and staff. A gym user commented, for example:

> *They [staff] treat you like one of them, but you're not sort of thing; you're still a user. It was a bit confusing really.*

The potential difficulty experienced in negotiating staff/service user role boundaries, and the tensions which can arise as a result, was a recurring theme in interviews with users. This is partly because the nature of fitness instruction requires staff to have a level of training and expertise which was perceived as somewhat exclusive. A gym user explained that:

> *There's such a strict line, I think, between what the staff do, and what the patients do.*

Staff responsibilities in BCG do not involve fitness instruction alone. Initial assessments for new members and ongoing monitoring of the mental health status of gym users are vital aspects of the service. For example, potential volunteers expressed concern about issues of confidentiality when dealing with potentially sensitive personal information held on file about other users. Therefore, while there are advantages in having ex-users with knowledge of mental health problems involved in service provision, there are also issues which require delicate negotiation. Moreover, encroachment on what has traditionally been a professional sphere by volunteers has been identified by research as potentially threatening to staff (Barnes *et al.* 1996; Williams and Lindley 1996). A service user interviewed in the present study made this point:

> *I don't know what the staff feel about that [user involvement]. They might think, 'Will I be required, or will they be taking over?' The users doing the whole thing, they might feel a bit threatened.*

Service users were concerned about the type of strains that could arise when dealing with others with similar mental health problems. As one user explained:

> *Actually dealing with people who have problems similar to myself and can get really upset, I wouldn't know how to deal with it with someone else.*

These data suggest that both service users and involved professionals were concerned about the potential for user participation to create undue stresses for individuals. A referral agent stated that:

> *I feel concerned sometimes if users get heavily involved in service planning and development. The pressure it creates for them.*

Participating in providing a service may also seem to users to require a level of commitment that they might find difficult to sustain, should they suffer a relapse, however temporary. Another referral agent explained the nature of the problem:

> *I get the impression that people think if they commit themselves to that, they've got to do it every week. They've got to be there every*

Wednesday, or whatever, come what may, and they can't be flexible, they can't ... and I suppose it's a little bit of responsibility, and some people don't want responsibility.

Non-involved users also voiced doubts concerning the ability of certain individuals to participate meaningfully in BCG as a result of their mental health status.

Trying to get people involved in doing stuff, when the person's depressed. They're probably just wanting to go to the gym, get home...

Obviously there'd be certain people you'd think – 'He couldn't do that, or she couldn't do that'.

Such concerns echo general perceptions in society about the competence of people with mental health problems to make decisions (cf. Department of Health 1996; Hickey and Kipping 1998), and their ability to make valuable contributions to service planning and provision.

USER INVOLVEMENT AND SUSTAINABILITY

The present findings reinforce the importance of formal structures to safeguard the well-being of users. For example, a volunteer contract drawn up by BCG clarifies roles and responsibilities, both on the part of the service user and the organisation. As some of the barriers to involvement described above have emerged, the contract has been subject to several revisions. Because of the innovative nature of BCG, it has primarily been a case of learning through experience, and responding to the needs of both users and staff in developing supportive structures.

One way in which a culture of user participation has developed in BCG is by the visible presence of volunteers in key roles. Their perceived success was encouraging to other users, helping to dispel the 'staff as expert' notion:

...It's another way of breaking that gap down [...] between patients and staff. People aren't always saying, 'Oh well, I'm a patient forever'. Ben [a volunteer] – he's a member of staff now. That could be me. You do get better. It's a great motivation.

Previous research has identified the need for continuing support for service users and monitoring of their progress to offset any stress experienced (Barnes and Wistow 1994b; Lindow and Morris 1995; Foulds *et al.* 1998). The volunteer contract includes the requirement for users to have the ongoing support of a mental health key worker (external to the gym), regular supervision, opportunities for training and periodic reviews of progress. Such elements are intended to provide a degree of protection from stress for volunteers or at least provide an 'early warning system' of difficulties.

Alongside the structured approach of the volunteer scheme, more flexible forms of user participation requiring varying degrees of responsibility have also been developed. This process was ongoing throughout the period of the present research: as certain forms of involvement (e.g. a user group that was active in the initial move from the hospital site) faded from view, others, like the gym newsletter, were initiated. It is hoped that this will help to encourage, for example, the participation of those users who are wary of the commitment involved in regular volunteering.

Encouraging service users to recognise their existing skills, and to develop new ones, at a pace that suits their particular circumstances and personal resources would appear to be an essential prerequisite for successful participation.

BROADER IMPLICATIONS OF THE BARROW COMMUNITY GYM EXPERIENCE

As user involvement becomes more and more common within service provision, and becomes an increasing feature of policy in health and social welfare, the challenges extend beyond whether or not users are involved. In this chapter, the present authors have argued that it is also important to consider:

- the conditions which enable user involvement to take place;
- the means through which user involvement occurs; and
- how involvement may be meaningfully sustained by all stakeholders.

Facilitating user involvement is more complex than simply providing the correct structures (although this is important). It is unlikely that one approach to encouraging participation by service users will, as a stand-alone feature, adequately challenge the *status quo* and bring about lasting changes. Barriers concern not only practical limitations, but also perceptions among service users (and others) as to what is possible for them to achieve in terms of influencing services. Constraining factors extend beyond the individual organisation, encompassing general social attitudes towards people with mental health problems. Typically, they may be seen as irrational, impulsive and generally lacking in the necessary attributes for sensible decision-making (Department of Health 1996; Hickey and Kipping 1998). At worst, they may be perceived as 'dangerous lunatics', from whom the public need protecting (a view not discouraged by certain sections of the media) (Philo *et al.* 1996; Godfrey and Wistow 1997). Therefore, it is suggested that:

> *...for many services (mental health in particular) the struggle for involvement may be concerned with a wider aspiration of users to participate more fully in society.*
>
> (Shaw 1997: 763)

Therefore, as the present research demonstrates, active involvement in mental health services may draw people who have felt excluded as a result of their illness back into community life, and be one means of combating the discrimination and exclusion typically experienced by this group.

ACKNOWLEDGEMENTS

The research was funded by the Research and Development Programme of the North-west NHS Executive, grant number RDO/11/11/5.

REFERENCES

Barnes, M. (1999) 'Users as citizens: collective action and the local governance of welfare', *Social Policy and Administration* 33 (1): 73–90.

Barnes, M., Harrison, S., Mort, M., Shardlow, P. and Wistow, G. (1996) 'Users, officials and citizens in health and social care', *Local Government Policy Making* 22 (4): 9–17.

Barnes, M. and Wistow, G. (1994a) 'Achieving a strategy for user involvement in community care', *Health and Social Care in the Community* 2: 347–356.

Barnes, M. and Wistow, G. (1994b) 'Learning to hear voices: listening to users of mental health services', *Journal of Mental Health* 3: 525–540.

Biehal, N. (1993) 'Changing practice: participation, rights and community care', *British Journal of Social Work* 23: 443–458.

Bowl, R. (1996) 'Legislating for user involvement in the United Kingdom: mental health services and the NHS Community Care Act 1990', *International Journal of Social Psychiatry* 42 (3): 165–180.

Campbell, P. (1996) 'The history of the user movement in the United Kingdom', in

Heller, T., Reynolds, J., Gomm, R. and Pattison, S. (eds) *Mental Health Matters*, London: Macmillan Press Ltd.

Department of Health (1989) *Caring for People: Community Care in the Next Decade and Beyond*, London: HMSO.

Department of Health (1994) *The Health of the Nation: Key Area Handbook, Mental Illness*, 2nd edn. London: HMSO.

Department of Health (1996) *Attitudes to Mental Illness: Summary Report*, London: Department of Health.

Department of Health (1999) *National Service Framework for Mental Health*, HSC 1999/223, London: HMSO.

Di Mascio, A. and Crosetto, P.G. (1994) 'Work reintegration of the mentally disabled', *International Journal of Mental Health* 23 (1): 61–70.

Forbes, J. and Sashidharan, S.P. (1997) 'User involvement in services – incorporation or challenge?' *British Journal of Social Work* 27: 481–498.

Foulds, G., Wood, H. and Bhui, K. (1998) 'Quality day care services for people with severe mental health problems', *Psychiatric Bulletin* 22: 144–147.

Godfrey, M. and Wistow, G. (1997) 'The user perspective on managing for health outcomes: the case for mental health', *Health and Social Care in the Community* 5 (5): 325–332.

Harrison, S., Barnes, M. and Mort, M. (1997) 'Praise and damnation: mental health user groups and the construction of organisational legitimacy', *Public Policy and Administration* 12 (2): 4–16.

Health Education Authority (1997) *Active for Life*, London: Health Education Authority.

Hickey, G. and Kipping, C. (1998) 'Exploring the concept of user involvement in mental health through a participation continuum', *Journal of Clinical Nursing* 7: 83–88.

Lindow, V. (1994) *Self-Help Alternatives to Mental Health Services* London: MIND.

Lindow, V. and Morris, J. (1995) *Service User Involvement: Synthesis of Findings and Experience in the Field of Community Care*, York: Joseph Rowntree Foundation.

Mitchell, D. (1998) 'Purposeful activity for people with enduring mental health problems: reflections from a case study', *Archives of Psychiatric Nursing* 12 (5): 282–287.

Morgan, D.L. (1988) *Focus Groups as Qualitative Research*, London: Sage Publications.

Mort, M., Harrison, J. and Wistow, G. (1996) 'The user card: picking through the organisational undergrowth in health and social care', *Contemporary Political Studies* 2: 1133–1140.

Mowbray, C.T., Moxley, D.P. and Collins, M.E. (1998) 'Consumers as mental health providers: first person accounts of benefits and limitations', *Journal of Behavioural Health Services and Research* 25 (4): 397–411.

Myers, F. and MacDonald, C. (1996) 'Power to the people? Involving users and carers in needs assessments and care planning – views from the practitioner', *Health and Social Care in the Community* 4 (2): 86–95.

Perkins, R. and Repper, J. (1998) *Dilemmas in Community Mental Health Practice: Choice and Control*, Abingdon: Radcliffe Medical Press Ltd.

Philo, G., Secker, J., Platt, S., Henderson, L., McLaughlin, G. and Burneside, J.

(1996) 'Media images of mental distress', in Heller, T., Reynolds, J., Gomm, R. and Pattison, S. (eds) *Mental Health Matters*, London: Macmillan Press Ltd.

Pilgrim, D. and Waldron, L. (1998) 'User involvement in mental health service development: How far can it go?' *Journal of Mental Health* 7 (1): 95–104.

Pilling, S. (1991) *Rehabilitation and Community Care*, London: Routledge.

Plumb, A. (1993) 'The challenge of self-advocacy', *Feminism and Psychology* 3 (2): 169–187.

Rogers, A. and Pilgrim, D. (1991) 'Pulling down churches: accounting for the British mental health users' movement', *Sociology of Health and Illness* 13 (2): 129–148.

Shaw, I. (1997) 'Assessing quality in mental health care: the United Kingdom experience', *Evaluation Review* 21 (3): 364–370.

Sheid, T.L. and Anderson, C.E. (1995) 'Living with chronic mental illness: understanding the role of work', *Community Mental Health Journal* 31 (2): 163–176.

Truman, C. and Raine, P. (2001) *User Participation, Mental Health and Exercise: Learning from the Experiences of Barrow Community Gym, Final Report*, Lancaster: Lancaster University.

Williams, J. and Lindley, P. (1996) 'Working with mental health service users to change mental health services', *Journal of Community and Applied Social Psychology* 6: 1–14.

Wolfensberger, W. (1972) *The Principle of Normalisation in Human Services* Toronto: *National Institute on Mental Retardation.*

CHAPTER 6

CULTURAL AND HISTORICAL ORIGINS OF COUNSELLING

John McLeod

To understand the diversity of contemporary counselling, and to appreciate the significance of the current patterns of practice ... it is necessary to look at the ways in which counselling has developed and evolved over the past 200 years. The differences and contradictions that exist within present-day counselling have their origins in the social and historical forces that have shaped modern culture as a whole.

People in all societies, at all times, have experienced emotional or psychological distress and behavioural problems. In each culture there have been well established indigenous ways of helping people to deal with these difficulties. The Iroquois Indians, for example, believed that one of the causes of ill-health was the existence of unfulfilled wishes, some of which were only revealed in dreams (Wallace 1958). When someone became ill and no other cause could be determined, diviners would discover what his or her unconscious wishes were, and arrange a 'festival of dreams' at which other members of the community would give these objects to the sick person. There seems little reason to suppose that modern-day counselling is any more valid, or effective, than the Iroquois festival of dreams. The most that can be said is that it is seen as valid, relevant or effective by people in this culture at this time.

Although counselling and psychotherapy have only become widely available to people during the second half of the twentieth century, their origins can be traced back to the beginning of the eighteenth century, which represents a turning point in the social construction of madness. Before this, the problems in living which people encountered were primarily dealt with

Source: *An Introduction to Counselling* (1998) Open University Press/McGraw-Hill.

from a religious perspective, implemented at the level of the local community (McNeill 1951; Neugebauer 1978, 1979). In Europe, the vast majority of people lived in small rural communities and were employed on the land. Within this way of life, anyone who was seriously disturbed or insane was tolerated as part of the community. Less extreme forms of emotional or interpersonal problems were dealt with by the local priest; for example, through the Catholic confessional. McNeill (1951) refers to this ancient tradition of religious healing as 'the cure of souls'. An important element in the cure of souls was confession of sins, followed by repentance. McNeill (1951) points out that in earlier times confession of sins took place in public, and was often accompanied by communal admonishment, prayer and even excommunication. The earlier Christian rituals for helping troubled souls were, like the Iroquois festival of dreams, communal affairs. Only later did individual private confession became established. McNeill (1951) gives many examples of clergy in the sixteenth and seventeenth centuries acting in a counselling role to their parishioners.

As writers such as Foucault (1967), Rothman (1971), Scull (1979, 1981b, 1989) and Porter (1985) have pointed out, all this began to change as the Industrial Revolution took effect, as capitalism began to dominate economic and political life and as the values of science began to replace those of religion. The fundamental changes in social structure and in social and economic life which took place at this point in history were accompanied by basic changes in relationships and in the ways people defined and dealt with emotional and psychological needs. Albee (1977) has written that:

> *Capitalism required the development of a high level of rationality accompanied by repression and control of pleasure seeking. This meant the strict control of impulses and the development of a work ethic in which a majority of persons derived a high degree of satisfaction from hard work. Capitalism also demanded personal efforts to achieve long-range goals, an increase in personal autonomy and independence ... The system depended on a heavy emphasis on thrift and ingenuity and, above all else, on the strong control and repression of sexuality.*
>
> (Albee 1977)

The key psychological shift that occurred, according to Albee (1977), was from a 'tradition-centred' (Riesman *et al.* 1950) society to one in which 'inner direction' was emphasised. In traditional cultures, people live in relatively small communities in which everyone knows everyone else, and behaviour is monitored and controlled by others. There is direct observation of what people do, and direct action taken to deal with social deviance through scorn or exclusion. The basis for social control is the induction of feelings of shame. In urban, industrial societies, on the other hand, life is much more anonymous, and social control must be implemented through internalised norms and regulations, which result in guilt if defied. From this analysis, it is possible to see how the central elements of urban, industrial, capitalist culture create the conditions for the development of a means of help, guidance and support which addresses confusions and dilemmas experienced in the personal, individual, inner life of the person. [...]

THE EXPANSION OF COUNSELLING IN THE LATE TWENTIETH CENTURY

[...] Counselling, as a distinct profession, came of age only in the 1950s, and so an understanding of the history of psychotherapy is necessary to make the link between counselling and earlier forms of healing and care. Although in many respects counselling can be seen as an extension of psychotherapy, a way of 'marketing' psychotherapy to new groups of consumers, there are also at least two important historical strands that differentiate counselling from psychotherapy: involvement in the educational system and the role of the voluntary sector.

Counselling of various kinds came to be offered within the school and college systems in the 1920s and 1930s, as careers guidance and also as a service for young people who were having difficulties adjusting to the demands of school or college life. Psychological testing and assessment were bound up with these activities, but there was always an element of discussion or interpretation of the student's problems or test results (Whiteley 1984).

Counselling also has very strong roots in the voluntary sector. For example, the largest single counselling agency in Britain, the National Marriage Guidance Council (RELATE), was created in the 1940s by a group of people who were concerned about the threat to marriage caused by the war (Lewis *et al.* 1992). Similarly, other groups of volunteers have set up counselling services in areas such as rape, bereavement, gay and lesbian issues and child abuse.

The existence of educational and voluntary sector traditions, alongside strong psychotherapeutic and somewhat diffuse religious traditions, has meant that there has always been a face of counselling that has kept its gaze on current social problems. Further, counselling has a life outside of the medical establishment, whereas psychotherapy is closely identified with health care provision through psychiatry, and with professions allied to medicine, such as clinical psychology and psychiatric social work. Finally, counselling has had a thriving non-professional sector which has drawn it in to local communities as a means of securing volunteer workers and funding. So, although counsellors and psychotherapists possess much the same skills, and tend to see similar groups of clients, they are culturally positioned in somewhat different territories. Unfortunately, a comprehensive cultural history of counselling remains to be written.

Why has counselling grown so rapidly in the final quarter of the twentieth century? Certainly in Britain and the USA, the number of counsellors, and the general availability of counselling, has shown a significant increase since the 1970s. There would appear to be a number of converging factors responsible for this growth:

- In a postmodern world, individuals are reflexively aware of choices open to them around identity; the self is a 'project'; counselling is a way of reflexively choosing an identity (Giddens 1991).
- Caring and 'people' professions, such as nursing, medicine, teaching and social work, which had previously performed a quasi-counselling role, were financially and managerially squeezed during the 1970s and 1980s. Members of these professions no longer have time to listen to their clients. Many of them have sought training as counsellors, and have created specialist counselling roles within their organisations, as a way of preserving their quality of contact with clients.
- There is an entrepreneurial spirit in many counsellors, who will actively sell their services to new groups of consumers. For example, any personnel director of a large company must have a filing cabinet full of brochures from counsellors and counselling agencies eager to provide employee counselling services.
- Counselling regularly receives publicity in the media, most of which is positive.
- We still live in a fragmented and alienated society, in which there are many people who lack emotional and social support systems. For example, in any major city there may be large groups of refugees. Increasing numbers of people live alone.

There is, therefore, a multiplicity of factors that would appear to be associated with the expansion of counselling. What seems clear is that counselling has grown in response to social demands and pressures, rather than because research or other evidence has proved that it is effective. [...]

THE IMAGE OF THE PERSON

At a practical level, an approach to counselling such as psychoanalysis or behaviour therapy may be seen to consist merely of a set of strategies for helping. Underneath that set of practical procedures, however, each approach represents a way of seeing people, an image of what it is to be a person, a 'moral vision' (Christopher 1996). Back in the days of the asylums, lunatics were seen as being like animals: irrational, unable to communicate, out of control. Some of these meanings were still present in the Freudian image of the person, except that in psychoanalysis the animal/id was merely one, usually hidden, part of the personality. The behaviourist image of the person has often been described as 'mechanistic': clients are seen as like machines that have broken down but can be fixed. The image of the counselling client in cognitive approaches is also mechanistic, but uses the metaphor of the modern machine, the computer: the client is seen as similar to an inappropriately programmed computer, and can be sorted out if rational commands replace irrational ones. The humanistic image is more botanical. Rogers, for example, uses many metaphors relating to the growth of plants and the conditions which either facilitate or inhibit that growth.

Each of these images of self has a history. In the main, counselling has emerged from a long historical journey in the direction of self-contained *individualism* (Baumeister 1987; Logan 1987; Cushman 1990, 1995). The profoundly individualistic nature of most (if not all) counselling limits its applicability with clients who identify with collectivist cultural traditions.

The question of the kind of world that is represented by various approaches to counselling goes beyond the mere identification of the different 'root metaphors' or images of self that lie at the heart of the different theoretical systems. There is also the question of whether the counselling model reflects the reality of the world as we experience it. For example, psychoanalytic theory was the product of an acutely male-dominated society, and many women writers and practitioners have asserted that they see in it little that they can recognise as a woman's reality. Humanistic approaches represent a positive, optimistic vision of the world, which some critics would see as denying the reality of tragedy, loss and death. It could also be said that virtually all counselling theories embody a middle-class, white, Judaeo-Christian perspective on life.

The importance for counselling of the image of the person or world view represented by a particular approach or theory lies in the realisation that we do not live in a social world that is dominated by a unitary, all-encompassing set of ideas. An essential part of the process of becoming a counsellor is to choose a version of reality that makes sense, that can be lived in. But no matter which version is selected, it needs to be understood that it is only one among several possibilities. The client, for example, may view the world in a fundamentally different way, and it may be that this kind of philosophical incompatibility is crucial. Van Deurzen (1988: 1) has suggested that

> *every approach to counselling is founded on a set of ideas and beliefs about life, about the world, and about people ... Clients can only*

> *benefit from an approach in so far as they feel able to go along with its basic assumptions.*
>
> (Van Deurzen 1988: 1)

The different root metaphors, images or basic assumptions about reality which underlie different approaches to counselling can make it difficult or impossible to reconcile or combine certain approaches, as illustrated by the debate between Rogers and Skinner on the nature of choice (Kirschenbaum and Henderson 1990). Historically, the development of counselling theory can be seen as being driven at least in part by the tensions between competing ideologies or images of the person. The contrast between a biological conception of the person and a social/existential one is, for example, apparent in many theoretical debates in the field. Bakan (1966) has argued that psychological theories, and the therapies derived from them, can be separated into two groups. The first group encompasses those theories which are fundamentally concerned with the task of understanding the mystery of life. The second group includes theories that aim to achieve a mastery of life. Bakan (1966) views the 'mystery–mastery complex' as underlying many debates and issues in psychology and therapy.

Finally, there is the question of the way the image of the person is used in the therapeutic relationship, whether the image held by the counsellor is imposed on the client, as a rigid structure into which the client's life is forced, or, as Friedman (1982) would prefer, the 'revelation of the human image ... takes place *between* the therapist and his or her client or *among* the members of a group'.

CONCLUSIONS

This chapter began by noting the diversity of counselling theory and practice. To understand this diversity requires an appreciation of the history of counselling and its role in contemporary society. Members of the public, or clients arriving for their first appointment, generally have very little idea of what to expect. Few people can tell the difference between a psychiatrist psychologist, counsellor and psychotherapist, never mind differentiate between alternative approaches to counselling that might be on offer. But behind that lack of specific information, there resonates a set of cultural images which may include a fear of insanity, shame at asking for help, the ritual of the confessional and the image of doctor as healer. In a multicultural society, the range of images may be very wide indeed. The counsellor is also immersed in these cultural images, as well as being socialised into the language and ideology of a particular counselling approach or into the implicit norms and values of a counselling agency. To understand counselling requires moving the horizon beyond the walls of the interview room, to take in the wider social environment within which the interview room has its own special place.

REFERENCES

Albee, G.W. (1977) 'The Protestant ethic, sex and psychotherapy', *American Psychologist* 32: 150–161.

Bakan, D. (1966) *Against Method*, New York: Basic Books.

Baumeister, R.F. (1987) 'How the self became a problem: a psychological review of historical research', *Journal of Personality and Social Psychology* 52 (1): 163–176.

Christopher, J.C. (1996) 'Counseling's inescapable moral visions', *Journal of Counseling and Development* 75: 17–25.

Cushman, P. (1990) 'Why the self is empty: toward a historically-situated psychology', *American Psychologist* 45: 599–611.

Cushman, P. (1995) *Constructing the Self, Constructing America: a Cultural History of Psychotherapy*, New York: Addison-Wesley.

Foucault, M. (1967) *Madness and Civilization: a History of Insanity in the Age of Reason*, London: Tavistock.

Friedman, M. (1982) 'Psychotherapy and the human image', in Sharkey, P.W. (ed.) *Philosophy, Religion and Psychotherapy: Essays in the Philosophical Foundations of Psychotherapy*, Washington, DC: University Press of America.

Giddens, A. (1991) *Modernity and Self-Identity: Self and Society in the Late Modern Age*, Cambridge: Polity Press.

Kirschenbaum, H. and Henderson, V.L. (eds) (1990) *Carl Rogers: Dialogues*, London: Constable.

Lewis, J., Clark, D. and Morgan, D. (1992) *Whom God Hath Joined Together: the Work of Marriage Guidance*, London: Routledge.

Logan, R.D. (1987) 'Historical change in prevailing sense of self', in Yardley, K. and Honess, T. (eds) *Self and Identity: Psychosocial Perspectives*, Chichester: Wiley.

McLeod, J. (1997) *Narrative and Psychotherapy*, London: Sage.

McNeill, J.T. (1951) *A History of the Cure of Souls*, New York: Harper and Row.

Neugebauer, R. (1978) 'Treatment of the mentally ill in medieval and early modern England: a reappraisal', *Journal of the History of the Behavioral Sciences* 14: 158–169.

Neugebauer, R. (1979) 'Early and modern theories of mental illness', *Archives of General Psychiatry*, 36: 477–483.

Pilgrim, D. (1990) 'British psychotherapy in context', in Dryden, W. (ed.) *Individual Therapy: a Handbook*, Milton Keynes: Open University Press.

Pilgrim, D. (1992) 'Psychotherapy and political evasions', in Dryden, W. and Feltham, C. (eds) *Psychotherapy and Its Discontents*, Buckingham: Open University Press.

Porter, R. (ed.) (1985) *The Anatomy of Madness, Volumes 1 and 2*, London: Tavistock.

Riesman, D., Glazer, N. and Denny, R. (1950) *The Lonely Crowd*, New Haven, CT: Yale University Press.

Rothman, D. (1971) *The Discovery of the Asylum: Social Order and Disorder in the New Republic*, Boston: Little Brown.

Scull, A. (1979) *Museums of Madness: the Social Organization of Insanity in Nineteenth Century England*, London: Allen Lane.

Scull, A. (ed.) (1981) *Mad-houses, Mad-doctors and Madmen*, Pennsylvania: University of Pennsylvania Press.

Scull, A. (1989) *Social Order/Disorder: Anglo-American Psychiatry in Historical Perspective*, London: Routledge.

Van Deurzen, E. (1988) *Existential Counselling in Practice*, London: Sage.

Wallace, A.F.C. (1958) 'Dreams and the wishes of the soul: a type of psychoanalytic theory among the seventeenth century Iroquois', *American Anthropologist* 60: 234–248.

Whiteley, J.M. (1984) 'A historical perspective on the development of counseling psychology as a profession', in Brown, S.D. and Lent, R.W. (eds) *Handbook of Counseling Psychology*, New York: Wiley.

CHAPTER 7

COMMUNICATION CULTURE: ISSUES FOR HEALTH AND SOCIAL CARE

Deborah Cameron

INTRODUCTION

In 1994, applicants for a vacant position in a National Health Service hospital were sent a 'person specification' describing the ideal candidate as someone who could:

- demonstrate sound interpersonal relationships and an awareness of the individual client's psychological and emotional needs;
- understand the need for effective verbal and nonverbal communication; and
- support clients and relatives in the care environment by demonstrating empathy and understanding.

These might seem unremarkable requirements for a caring professional – a nurse, psychologist, counsellor or social worker, but in fact, the hospital was advertising for a cleaner. Although cleaners do talk to patients and relatives, this is not usually thought of as their core function, nor is it a kind of talk that requires specialist expertise. Some commentators suggested that the person specification was a 'politically correct' attempt to boost cleaners' status by describing the ordinary ability to converse with other people as if it were an arcane professional skill.

But this cannot be the whole story, for similar language can be found in job and person specifications across the occupational spectrum. Institutions not often suspected of political correctness, from engineering firms to banks, all routinely inform job applicants – whether they aspire to be the receptionist or the chief executive – that they 'must have excellent communication skills'. If we substituted 'customer' for 'client' and took out the reference to 'the care environment', the text quoted above would not be out of place in a specification for an estate agent, hotel manager or insurance broker.

Concern about communication is not confined to the sphere of employment. Communication is one of the 'key skills' that are now emphasised in the national school curriculum and in higher education. Self-help books and television talk shows preach that fulfilling relationships depend on our ability to communicate with partners, family and friends. All kinds of problems, from marital breakdown to teenage suicide, are blamed on inadequate communication. In short, we live in a 'communication culture': a culture obsessed with communication and the skills that it supposedly demands. Here I want to explore critically what lies behind that obsession. Where did it come from and what are its effects? I will begin by examining these questions in general terms, then move on to consider the implications for the field of health and social care specifically.

WHAT IS COMMUNICATION CULTURE AND WHERE DID IT COME FROM?

According to the sociologist Anthony Giddens (1991), it is characteristic of modern societies that traditional ways of knowing and acting are progressively displaced by 'expert systems', specialised and technical knowledge produced and regulated by professionals. The displacement of traditional healing practices by modern medicine is an obvious instance. A more recent example offered by Giddens is 'parenting'. The skills involved in child-rearing were once acquired informally, through practice, experience and advice from older relatives. Today, by contrast, 'parenting' is a set of skills which experts define. Parents may still take informal advice, but they are also likely to turn to books, magazines and classes for more authoritative guidance. In Britain, parents who are judged inadequate can be compelled to receive training in parenting.

'Communication' is an analogous case. The mundane social activity of talking to others has been redefined as a set of skills requiring effort and expert guidance to master. As with parenting, the message of experts on communication is that there's a right way and a wrong way. All kinds of sources, ranging from training courses to radio phone-ins to popular self-help books, explain what the 'right way' is. Many people who have not sought it out voluntarily will encounter this body of expert knowledge through education or workplace training.

So, the rise of 'communication skills' is an example of a much more general trend. But why has communication, specifically, become such a prominent concern in recent years? There are a number of reasons, but two are particularly important.

One has to do with economic change. In a 'post-industrial' age, fewer jobs are about manufacturing things, while more are about providing services to customers and clients. Whereas a traditional assembly-line worker's communication skills were of marginal relevance, service jobs inherently involve communication. There has been a growing tendency for businesses to regulate and standardise the language in which employees interact with customers, treating their speech as part of the corporate 'brand'. In addition, global competition has spurred many businesses, in both the service and manufacturing sectors, to restructure their operations and introduce new management approaches emphasising quality, flexibility and teamwork. This means that talking, in settings like team meetings, 'quality circles' or appraisal interviews, has come to play a more significant 'behind the scenes' role at work.

The second key factor underlying the rise of communication culture has to do with shifts in the way we think about our identities and personal relationships. Giddens (1991) points out that modernity loosens the traditional ties people have to their kinfolk and local communities. Few people now spend their whole lives in the same place, among others who have known them from birth: they are continually having to reinvent themselves. Under these conditions, Giddens argues, 'the self becomes a *reflexive project*' (1991: 32) – something to be worked on, perfected. Just as dieting and exercise can reshape our physical bodies, so other technologies of self-improvement can reshape our inner selves. Working on one's 'communication skills' has a particular significance, because communication is seen as vital to the ability to form and maintain intimate relationships with others. In modern conditions, these relationships often do not have the external supports they would have had in traditional society (for instance, couples no longer stay together because of inviolable religious and moral codes). Maintaining intimacy depends on a continuous process of mutual self-disclosure, so that parties to a relationship remain in touch with one another's activities, feelings, needs and desires.

It might seem as if these two sets of developments are unrelated: one set affects individuals in their lives as workers and consumers, while the other affects them in their personal lives. But in fact there is a relationship. Communication was a central concern of what is often loosely referred to as the 'personal growth' movement of the 1960s and 1970s, when significant numbers of people turned to the ideas and techniques of psychology and therapy – to approaches such as transactional analysis (Berne 1966) and assertiveness training (Rakos 1991) – as part of a quest for personal fulfilment. While this began as a counter-cultural movement, with 'personal growth' being seen as a form of resistance to mainstream corporate culture, the same ideas were soon taken up by the corporate sector itself.

If training in assertiveness or transactional analysis could help people lead happier lives outside the workplace, then perhaps it could also help them to function better inside it. Organisations managed and staffed by effective communicators would be more efficient, more harmonious and ultimately more successful economically.

Because of their shared roots, communication training materials designed for professional contexts have much in common with those that focus on personal growth and relationships. In both types we find the same recommendations – for instance, speak directly using 'I' statements, use open rather than closed questions, listen without judging, use verbal acknowledgement tokens like 'yes', 'I see', don't interrupt. The expertise being drawn on, whether or not this is made explicit, is that of psychiatrists, psychologists, therapists and counsellors. Almost invariably, the rules and recommendations can be traced to some practice that originated in a therapeutic setting. Assertiveness training, for instance, began as a behavioural therapy for psychiatric patients who had become passive and withdrawn. Transactional analysis emerged out of the practice of group therapy. Non-judgemental listening is a central technique of counselling.

The linguist, Norman Fairclough (1992), uses the term 'technologisation of discourse' to theorise the process whereby a way of talking designed for one context gets transferred to a wide range of others, as if it were part of an ideologically neutral 'toolkit'. He regards the language of therapy as a particularly important contemporary 'discourse technology', and argues that there is nothing neutral about its use in non-therapeutic contexts. Consider workplace appraisal, a discourse practice which uses many of the conventions of a counselling session. The appraisee talks about her or his achievements and problems while the appraiser listens and supports. But the goals of appraisal, and the power relations that are operative in an appraisal interview, are quite different from the goals and relationships involved in counselling. The appraiser is not there primarily to help the appraisee meet his or her own goals, but to judge how well the organisation's goals are met – a judgement that may have consequences for the appraisee's job prospects. In Fairclough's view, the 'therapeutic' frame obscures what is really going on.

To summarise, 'communication culture' has developed along with changing economic conditions and ideas about 'personal growth' which have influenced both organisations and individuals. In communication cultures we find the following general characteristics:

- A widely shared belief in the importance of communication and a perception that many problems (and their solutions) are linked to it.
- An acceptance that there is a 'right way' and a 'wrong way' to communicate, and a proliferation of expert discourse about the 'skills' required to do it right.

- A growth in specific training in communication, and an increasing desire to assess or evaluate individuals' performance as communicators.
- A tendency to regulate and standardise communication practices within particular institutions.

COMMUNICATION CULTURE AND THE FIELD OF HEALTH AND SOCIAL CARE

Few people would dispute that in the context of health and social care, interaction between service providers and users is important. The question is not whether it deserves attention, but about the helpfulness or otherwise of the approaches characteristic of communication culture. In the remainder of this chapter I examine some cases where versions of these approaches used in health and social care might be deemed unhelpful or problematic. These cases illustrate more general problems with the discourse and practice of 'communication skills'.

CASE 1

Problems of knowledge: rules for 'effective communication' are typically formulated without reference to what is normal sociolinguistic behaviour.

One defining feature of communication culture is its reliance on expert knowledge about the 'right way' to perform particular communicative acts. But this is a particular kind of expert knowledge, originating mainly in therapeutic fields where the prevailing approach to language-use is normative rather than descriptive. Expert recommendations on how speakers ought to communicate are rarely informed by any knowledge of the patterns uncovered by empirical research on naturally-occurring talk. Consequently the experts may end up exhorting people to behave in ways that are linguistically unnatural and socially bizarre.

Assertiveness training (AT), for instance, is the source of many prescriptions about 'effective communication', but its recommendations have been criticised for their marked divergence from 'normal' practice. In everyday non-therapeutic contexts, 'assertive' strategies like making 'I-statements' or repeating a point until it is acknowledged may be interpreted as rude and egocentric (Cameron 1995; Gervasio and Crawford 1989).

One piece of AT-derived advice which is common in health education and care work with young people who are thought to be at risk of sexual exploitation and violence is encapsulated in the slogan 'just say no': in other words, be direct in refusing unwanted sexual advances. Assertiveness training teaches that everyone has the right to refuse without apologising or giving reasons; rape prevention programmes also teach that a direct 'no' is preferable to alternative strategies because it leaves no room for misunderstanding.

However, this line of argument overlooks a large body of empirical work in conversation analysis (CA), which shows that successful refusals in naturally-occurring talk are virtually never performed in such a bald, unmitigated way. Acceptance and refusal form what CA calls a 'preference system' in relation to invitations, propositions and requests: the 'preferred' move, acceptance, is simple and brief, whereas the 'dispreferred' move, refusal, is much more elaborate. Thus if I ask, 'd'you want to meet for a drink after work?' you can accept by simply saying 'OK'. Refusals, by contrast, are usually prefaced by a pause or hesitation marker (um, er), often accompanied by 'well', and they include an explanation or excuse. So in the drink-invitation case, a typical refusal might go: 'er, sorry, I'd love to, but I've got to work late tonight'.

For obvious reasons, there is little natural data available specifically on sexual refusals, but the feminist researchers Celia Kitzinger and Hannah Frith (1999) conducted a study with focus groups of young heterosexual women who were asked what they said if they wished to refuse a sexual invitation. Only two out of 58 claimed to feel comfortable saying 'No'. The rest favoured the strategies described above for making dispreferred conversational moves: hesitating, giving reasons which would not offend (e.g. 'I'm really knackered'), and sometimes inserting a 'softener' like 'I'm really flattered, but ...'. They also reported that in their own experience, men correctly interpreted these strategies as refusals.

Rape prevention advice to 'just say no' is flawed in two ways. First, it is based on the assumption that less direct ways of refusing carry a high risk of misinterpretation. If, as empirical research suggests, this assumption is false, then the advice is unnecessary: other strategies will work equally well (or badly). That leads on to the second point, that the recommended strategy of saying 'No' without elaboration is in conflict with the norms of ordinary interaction. Kitzinger and Frith's informants were familiar with advice to 'just say no', but most unequivocally rejected that advice. Initiatives like rape prevention (or safer sex advice or drugs education) will usually be less effective where they do not take account of the target group's beliefs, values, and habitual ways of behaving. The knowledge-base for interventions in communicative practice thus needs to include a knowledge of what is 'normal' behaviour for particular groups of people communicating in particular contexts.

CASE 2

Problems of power: norms for communication may gloss over conflicts and asymmetrical power relations.

In communication culture it is commonly believed that many problems are most effectively addressed by adjusting the way people communicate. This belief underpins a therapy called 'Reality Orientation' (RO) which is widely used with confused elderly people in institutional care. RO's goal is to put patients back in touch with reality, by way of 'a continual process whereby staff present current information ... in every interaction, reminding the patient of time, place and person, and providing a commentary on events' (Holden and Woods 1982: 51).

The sociolinguist Karen Grainger (1998) carried out ethnographic fieldwork in a number of hospitals where RO was practised. Her analysis focuses on the problems and conflicts that the prescribed ways of communicating created for both patients and staff. In practice, she observed that staff did not observe the rules of RO consistently. Sometimes, for instance, they would enter into patients' 'confused' fantasies (e.g. that they were someone else or somewhere else) because this made it easier to secure co-operation with routines like washing or dressing. Conversely, there were occasions when patients made coherent factual statements about current events, and carers denied that these corresponded to reality. One patient who complained that the bath water was too cold was informed that it was really 'nice and warm'; another who referred to being 'alone' was reminded that she was surrounded by other patients.

Grainger relates her observations to the conflicting realities and asymmetries of power that exist in care institutions. The 'official' reality of the institution, as represented in its mission statement or the literature given to relatives, does not coincide with reality as perceived by front-line care workers, and that in turn differs from the reality experienced by elderly patients. Power differences are highly relevant in these circumstances. Though carers are not a powerful group, one power they do have is the power to present their own definition of reality as more valid than that of a confused elderly patient. They also have a motive to do this, precisely because their working conditions disempower them. Acknowledging and dealing with the reality of patients' discomfort or distress is emotionally challenging and makes it more difficult for hard-pressed carers to get through their daily routine.

Grainger also points out that the external realities emphasised in RO are unlikely to resonate with patients' perceptions, because of their remoteness from institutional life:

> *For many residents ... their entire world consisted of spending night-times in the dormitory ... and day-times sitting in a chair in the dayroom. Heat was kept at a constant level, the same group of uniformed staff came and went around them, there was rarely a chance to go outside the room, let alone outside the hospital ... It is my view that external reality (i.e. the date, day, time, year, address) can have had little significance for these people.*
>
> (Grainger 1998: 52)

Grainger wonders how far the confusion of elderly patients is produced by the regime of the institution itself, as opposed to by clinical conditions like dementia. Patients' 'confused' relationship to the external world is not simply a linguistic or cognitive problem, but reflects their social isolation, the monotony of their routine and their powerless position in the institutional hierarchy. RO does not address these problems, and may even exacerbate them by imposing on elderly patients a definition of 'reality' that denies their lived experience.

CASE 3

Problems of 'skill': criteria for defining and assessing 'communication skills' are often vague, subjective or simply vacuous, and there is little critical reflection on underlying principles.

An important characteristic of communication culture is its concern with the explicit teaching and assessment of communication skills. This requires the activity of 'communication' to be broken down into discrete elements which can be taught and assessed; assessment also requires that criteria be devised to distinguish various levels of performance. But the highly contextualised nature of social interaction makes this enterprise highly problematic. To illustrate the problem, let us examine the level 2 NVQ (National Vocational Qualification) in Social Care, a nationally accredited course in the UK designed for trainees who work, for instance, as assistants in residential care homes.

Assessment for NVQ courses is 'competence based' – assessors consider portfolios of evidence compiled by the learner to show s/he has demonstrated the particular skills and compentencies that are required for the level of award s/he is seeking. 'Communication' is a category for assessment in all NVQ courses, though the required skills and competencies vary with the area of work as well as the level of the award. Below I reproduce seven criteria on which Social Care trainees' communication skills are assessed at level 2.

1 Effective communication is promoted in ways consistent with the worker's role.
2 Communication with an individual is consistent with her/his understanding, preferred form of communication and manner of expression.
3 The manner, level and pace of communication is appropriate to the individual's abilities and personal beliefs and preferences.
4 Any obstacles which may make communication difficult are minimised.
5 Effective communication is encouraged by appropriate facial expression, body language, sensory contact, position and environment.
6 Where the initial form of communication is not effective, different approaches are used or sought.
7 Information given by an individual is checked with her/him for accuracy.

(source: NVQ Assessment Specification and Record Sheet, Element O.e)

This list illustrates how difficult it is to break communication down into a set of discrete skills, and to produce meaningful criteria for assessing its quality. One noticeable feature of the list is the overlap between supposedly different criteria (what is the difference between 2. and 3., or 4. and 6.? Does 1. not just subsume all the others?). Another is the lack of clarity about what key terms mean. The words 'appropriate' and 'effective' appear in several criteria, begging the question of what will count as 'appropriate' or 'effective'. (If we take criterion 5., for instance, what is an 'appropriate facial expression'?) 'Appropriate' and 'effective' are terms whose meanings are inherently context-dependent. But if context is all, if good communication means neither more nor less than a way of interacting that is appropriate and effective in the context of a particular interaction, then it might be argued that general performance criteria for communication are vacuous.

In practice, assessors will fill the vacuum with their own judgements. But judging what is appropriate communication in care settings is not like judging whether, say, a trainee electrician has followed appropriate safety procedures. There is little argument about what constitutes safe practice when dealing with electricity, for this is fundamentally a technical issue. But the question of what constitutes appropriate behaviour to clients inevitably has a moral and ideological dimension. Therefore, it is important to give trainees the opportunity to discuss – and reflect critically upon – the beliefs and values that underpin judgements on communication in care settings. If these are presented as simply common sense, there is no way to resolve the problems and contradictions which may arise in real-world situations.

For example, criterion 3. in the NVQ list, which states that communication in care settings should be 'appropriate to the individual [client]'s ... personal beliefs', might look like an uncontroversial statement of the obvious. But what are the implications for black or gay carers dealing with clients whose personal beliefs are racist or homophobic? Does meeting the

NVQ standard require them to abdicate their own right to respectful treatment? If not, how should they deal with interactions where a client's prejudices become overt? This is not some abstruse philosophical problem with no place in a vocational training programme, but a matter of immediate practical relevance for many care workers. But the competence-based schemes that are typical of communication training leave little space for reflection on issues of this kind. That might prompt questions about the ability of such schemes to produce 'skilled' workers; for skill is not just a matter of being able to act in certain ways, it also requires a principled understanding of why you do what you do.

CONCLUSION

I have suggested that there are problems with the application of currently favoured approaches to communication in the field of health and social care. Am I saying then that communication skills training is useless? Not entirely: the mere fact of drawing attention to questions of communication may have a useful awareness-raising function. Some genres of care-talk (such as counselling and medical history taking) are founded on principles that do require explicit teaching; many benefit from practice in 'safe' situations where poor performance will not do serious harm.

Yet a lot of what goes on under the heading of communication skills training is of unproven value. In research carried out in commercial service organisations (Cameron 2000), I asked managers whether training had any measurable impact on recipients' subsequent performance. Though they all had an opinion, not one was able to produce any non-anecdotal evidence to support it: they did not carry out systematic evaluations. Responses to my follow-up question – a diplomatically-worded version of 'why do you spend money on training when you don't know if it works?' – were generally along the lines of 'our competitors do it'. I detected, however, two other factors at work.

One was the need managers felt to regulate the behaviour of individual employees, subordinating their individual styles to a centrally-designed corporate style or brand. They cared less whether training produced 'skilled' communicators than whether it produced 'standard' communicators who all followed the same rules. The second factor was a belief in the almost magical power of messages to determine the behaviour of the recipient. Words, phrases or gestures, used in just the right way, were credited by many of my informants with the ability to clinch the sale, defuse the argument, win the customer's lifelong loyalty. This magical thinking is overt in magazine articles and adverts for 'inspirational' business seminars, which are full of the 'seven secrets of X' and the 'ten top tips about Y'. But miracle solutions rarely hold up when put to the test in a real-life situation.

I once chaired a panel interviewing candidates for an administrative position in my University department. The last candidate, when asked 'do you have any questions for us?', replied: 'where is your organisation going and where does it want to be in five years' time?' Afterwards, a panellist remarked that this candidate must have been on a course where the question was presented as an example of effective interview technique. But we all agreed that in this case it had not been effective at all. For one thing it came across as glib and formulaic. For another, it assumed an attitude to change and a collective commitment to corporate objectives at odds with academic culture. The candidate's 'magic words' did not fit the context, and their effect on us was negative.

Attempts to promote 'better communication' will not succeed unless they are based on an understanding that all human communication is necessarily embedded in social contexts and relationships. Since these are complex and variable, there is no single 'right way' to communicate, no universally applicable 'magic words', and no quick fix for every problem. 'Skilled' communicators are those with the resources (linguistic, intellectual and experiential) to reflect on the context and the relationships involved in a particular communicative event, and in the light of that reflection, gauge the effects of different ways of interacting. Without this deeper dimension, communication skills training becomes a superficial exercise, of little benefit either to trainees themselves or to the recipients of their professional attentions.

REFERENCES

Berne, E. (1966) *The Games People Play*, New York: Grove Books.

Cameron, D. (1995) *Verbal Hygiene*, London: Routledge.

Cameron, D. (2000) *Good To Talk? Living and Working in a Communication Culture*, London: Sage Publications

Fairclough, N. (1992) *Discourse and Social Change*, Cambridge: Polity Press.

Gervasio, A. and Crawford, M. (1989) 'Evaluations of assertiveness: a critique and speech act reformulation', *Psychology of Women Quarterly* 13: 1–25.

Giddens, A. (1991) *Modernity and Self-Identity: Self and Society in the Late Modern Age*, Cambridge: Polity Press.

Grainger, K. (1998) 'Reality Orientation in institutions for the elderly: the view from interactional sociolinguistics', *Journal of Aging Studies* 12 (1): 39–56.

Holden U.P. and Woods, R.T. (1982) *Reality Orientation: Psychological Approaches to the 'Confused' Elderly*, Edinburgh: Churchill Livingston.

Kitzinger, C. and Frith, H. (1999) 'Just say no? The use of conversation analysis in developing a feminist perspective on sexual refusal', *Discourse and Society* 10: 293–316.

Rakos, R. (1991) *Assertiveness Training: Theory, Training and Research*, London: Routledge.

CHAPTER 8

POSTMODERNISM AND THE TEACHING AND PRACTICE OF INTERPERSONAL SKILLS

Helen Jessup and Steve Rogerson

INTRODUCTION

Interpersonal communication is the primary medium for the practice of social work. Yet social work has long borrowed the tools of other disciplines, specifically psychology, in the arena of micro skills, producing a dissonance for practitioners. Our belief is that social work is a separate discipline and as such requires a specific form of interpersonal communication practice as a vehicle for its particular concern: the interface between the personal and socio-structural.

We have designed a process for both teaching and practising interpersonal communication which produces an educational rather than a therapeutic landscape. This offers critical emancipatory skills which express contemporary postmodernist ideas. As a device for assisting access to some of these ideas, we have invented an imaginary respondent to ask us questions about our approach. This enables us to ground our explanations in a more accessible conversational style and breaks the monological tone of one voice.

Source: Pease, B. and Fook, J. (1999) *Transforming Social Work Practice: Postmodern Critical Perspectives*, London: Routledge.

WHY DEVELOP A POSTMODERN APPROACH TO TEACHING AND PRACTISING INTERPERSONAL COMMUNICATION SKILLS?

As qualified social workers and teachers of welfare workers, our experience was that the training courses on which we taught, and had ourselves been taught, included a critical structuralist approach to practice. Yet the teaching and practice of interpersonal communication (microskills) produced a dichotomy because they were not integrated with this critical approach. Students and teachers were often confused, being taught incongruent theoretical approaches which resulted in the situation that practitioners either 'did' social change or they 'do' interpersonal work.

We say this because interpersonal communication appears to represent a void in the development of a social work practice which is concerned with dismantling those forms of power relations which place individuals, groups, communities – whole cultures – in situations of oppression and distress. As social workers, we were well versed in the so-called 'radical' practice of social work, including community work, advocacy and political action. Yet casework, including interpersonal communication, was regarded as suspect by many because it remained determined by a therapeutic explanation of human difficulty grounded in humanistic ideas.

In other words, what distinguishes social work from other corollary disciplines – psychology, psychiatry, even primary health care – was omitted from interpersonal communication. On the one hand, we were teaching students critical social change through political practice – locating individual difficulty within a socio-structural context – with modules such as 'Social and Economic Issues' and 'Social Processes'. Yet, at the same time, students would be taught to interview a 'client' or other interviewee by listening, following, responding empathically and so forth. They would explore problems, current/past relationships, childhood, behavioural patterns, motivation, intent, responsibility, honesty. We were teaching technical skills within humanist principles, without reference to any political context. Students themselves identified this dissonance. At that stage, we did not have the means to apply comparative political analysis to interpersonal communication skills theorists and their practice skills, as we did with other aspects of the course.

The risk in teaching in that way was to produce a social work response to oppressive social structures which remained largely a theoretical exercise, since the practice of critical strategies relied on the most basic of skills (talking to one another). These 'different' modes of practice were located within paradoxical theories of social change. We were searching for new knowledge which would bridge this divide.

WHAT DOES POSTMODERNISM OFFER?

Fundamentally, the poststructuralism of Foucault and the educational strategy of Freire provide the theoretical framework for teaching and practising critical emancipatory interpersonal communication skills. Foucault's poststructuralism is particularly useful because it offers a political approach to social construction rather than the often nihilistic deconstruction of some other postmodernist writers. This distinction between poststructuralism and postmodernism is important. Peters (1995: 10) reminds us about the latter that:

> *postmodernism signifies a change in people's relation to … meaning … the conditions of existence of meaning(s) can no longer be taken for granted or blithely assumed. Meaning must be understood as implicated in power relations … meaning/knowledge/truth has lost its innocence and so have we.*
>
> (Peters 1995: 10)

To borrow a concept of Calinescu (1987), poststructuralism can be conceptualised as a 'face' of postmodernism. It has grown out of the ideas and practices of postmodernism, but deals with the implications of language as a producer of the social and cultural world. Its focus is around disclosing the implications of cultural and social discourse as a production of the interaction of people whose very subjectivity is a product of that discourse. Most importantly, it is a site for realising the critical potential for change within the postmodern world. Lonsdale (1991: 11) comments:

> *Poststructuralism can be understood as that theoretical 'stream' within the broader umbrella of postmodernism which radically subverts and problematises taken for granted assumptions about language.*
>
> (Lonsdale 1991: 11)

Poststructuralism considers language to be the producer of meaning. This is in contradistinction to the notion which has dominated previous interpersonal communication theory and practice: that language is a reflector of reality.

LANGUAGE IS IMPORTANT HERE?

The interpersonal communication processes we use as social beings primarily involve language in its many forms. Among poststructural theorists, language is a collective concern. As Chris Weedon (1987: 21) puts it:

> *Language is the place where actual and possible forms of social organisation and their likely social and political consequences are defined and contested. Yet it is also the place where our sense of ourselves, or subjectivity, is constructed.*
>
> (Weedon 1987: 21)

Immediately, then, the site for change appears in the many forms of language and their 'signified' meanings. This suggests a powerful strategy for change: discourse analysis.

In this sense, the Foucauldian conceptualisation of 'discourse' challenges the concept of 'paradigm'. Deconstruction of the text reveals the politics inherent in both theory and methodology. The nature of the inquiry becomes the focus of inquiry. It is a strategy which transgresses the limitations of Marxist practice, where it is assumed that 'language bears a fixed and definite relationship with reality ... language is regarded as a mere tool for communication' (Rojek *et al.* 1988: 118).

Foucault's discourse analysis reveals the objective construction of the person for the purpose of subjugation through 'dividing practices', including scientific classification. The range of social control has been extended since the seventeenth century through normalising knowledge systems which produce ascribed personal and social identities – such identities determining levels of social power and attracting disciplinary processes: violence, incarceration, poverty and so forth. However, Foucault is not limiting his approach to revealing symbols or signifying structures:

> *Here I believe one's point of reference should not be to the great model of language (langue) and signs, but to that of war and battle. The history which bears and determines us has the form of a war rather than that of language: relations of power, not relations of meaning.*
>
> (cited in Gordon 1980: 114)

As social workers, we needed to consider how our own practice might be divisive and how we could make it less so. Discourse analysis could unlock the power/knowledge nexus through an examination of the organisation of social institutions – specifically the production of heterogeneous textual positions which construct the basis of social relationships. The professional institution of social work can be included in these organisations.

FOUCAULT'S MAJOR CONTRIBUTION IS DISCOURSE ANALYSIS?

Discursive practices establish power relations. Power is produced historically through knowledge systems. Thus Foucault determines the historical construction of madness, sexuality and the prison – inquiring into the formulation of truths and the subsequent disciplining of people. He calls this a *genealogical* inquiry (Foucault 1979: 23).

It is a subjective process with objective outcomes. This disciplining process necessarily recruits people into maintaining their own subjugation – in actively participating in operations which shape their lives according to norms, even though those operations appear to be against their interests. For Foucault, power is productive. It subjects persons to normalising truths which shape their lives and relationships. It produces realities. As Billington (1991: 42) comments:

> *concepts of normality apply to all sorts of ideas we have about ourselves and for which we set standards: 'a healthy body', 'a stable personality', 'sanity', 'a normal family', 'a proper man and woman' and so on. Moreover they institute new ways of exercising power through disciplinary mechanisms ... psychological in character ... through school rooms, welfare offices, hospitals, mental institutions, prisons, families and workplaces, through the cultural practices of welfare workers and others.*
>
> (Billington 1991: 42)

For Foucault, then, knowledge is power and subject positions are constructed through discourse. 'The individual which power has constituted is at the same time its vehicle' (Foucault, in Gordon 1980: 98). Foucault thus offers an adequate account of people's toleration of, and participation in, oppressive power structures. This is often missing from other social theoretical analyses – liberal to radical.

WHAT IS FREIRE'S CONTRIBUTION?

The educational strategy of Freire provides the methodological framework for the teaching of interpersonal communication skills. While there are differences between Foucault and Freire – for example, understandings of ideology – both involve transgressing the boundaries of positivism and both have inspired a tradition of writers from philosophy, psychology and education – and at last social work – who challenge the restraints imposed by science and humanism.

Foucault and Freire would concur on the notion of power and its social construction. They would also agree that poststructural ideas are a bridge between theory and practice, between a theory of social oppression and the practice of subjective change. Where Foucault uses discourse, Freire uses dialogue: the former is an analysis, the latter is an exchange to promote change. However, they both involve critical questioning. Freire uses the educational dialogical process to explore another person's subjective view 'communicating with each other not as objects being used by anyone ... but in equality' (cited in Shor 1987: 223). Foucault uses discourse analysis to unsilence the process of 'use' and thus allow the construction of alternative social worlds.

The philosophy of Foucault complements the practice of Freire. Freire has developed the critical dialogical techniques which can engage people in discovering the process suggested by Foucault. Freire is thus an educational bridge between Foucault and social work practice. Both integrate knowledge and power through the practice of criticism.

SO CRITICAL QUESTIONING IS INTRINSIC TO DISCOURSE ANALYSIS?

For Freire, critical education is part of the process of social change and this process is subjective and political: it is concerned with identifying who has power over whom and how it is maintained – with disclosing hegemony.

Without critical questioning, people continue to hold cultural meanings about the way their lives ought to be, even when their situations are oppressive. They may say: 'I'm not alright because I'm not like that', or 'I'm mad because the rest of the world act although they are not mad'. People tolerate these ideas, accepting what is called *doxa* in discourse analysis. This is:

> *the prevailing view of things, which very often prevails to the extent that people are unaware that it is only one of several possible alternative views.*
>
> (Sturrock 1979: 143)

For Freire, liberation from such a construction involves critically questioning the ideas which inform such an understanding – or model. He says:

> *Intellectuals need ideas in order to understand the world but if these ideas become models ... if they are not applied creatively ... we run the risk of regarding them as reality ... so concrete reality has to be made to fit in with our ideas and not the other way round.*
>
> (Freire and Faundez 1990: 29)

For Foucault, the production of 'models' or 'truths' is discovered through a genealogical process:

> *One has to dispense with the constituent subject, to get rid of the subject itself, that's to say, to arrive at an analysis which can account for the constitution of the subject within a historical framework. And this is what I would call genealogy, that is a form of history which can account for the constitution of knowledges, discourses, domains of objects, etc.*
>
> (cited in Gordon 1980: 117)

Foucault's work critically targets the many forms of institutional technologies (for example, the Gulag, monarchy and prisons) through which disciplinary power systems are established.

Our experience was that social workers develop and use uncritical interpersonal communication models. In doing so, they are both discipliners and disciplined, conducting the interpersonal communication intervention process through a myriad of linguistic constructions including 'contracting', 'deprofessionalisation', 'help', 'support', 'problem solving', listening and empathy. This could well construct the subject of their own investigation, participating in the continual renewal of oppressive power and discrimination.

A formative text for us, which analysed this productive process in relation to education, was Walkerdine (1984). She examines a number of texts, including nursery record cards and teacher training content, within the context of conventional developmental psychology, medicalisation and normalisation. Walkerdine demonstrates that it is not that there is a 'pre-existent real object' (1984: 188) – in this case the developing child – which developmental psychology has 'distorted'. Rather, this is a decentred subject and it is:

> *developmental psychology itself which produces the particular form of naturalised capacities as its object. The practices of production can, therefore, be understood as the production of subject-positions themselves.*
>
> (1984: 164)

It is through such processes that educational powerlessness and its many material forms may be constructed. Those processes do not have within them the means of producing alternative ideas about the social world and consequent subject-positions. However, linguistically grounded social work (see Rojek *et al.* 1988) sees interpersonal communication become a primary focus for the process of critical questioning and social change. Here's Freire again:

> *In communicating among ourselves, in the process of knowing the reality which we transform, we communicate and know socially even though the process of communicating, knowing, changing, has an individual dimension ... Knowing is a social event with nevertheless an individual dimension.*
>
> (Freire and Shor 1987: 99)

WHAT ARE THE MAJOR THEORETICAL DIFFERENCES BETWEEN THIS POSTSTRUCTURAL APPROACH AND THE HUMANIST APPROACH?

It is important to distinguish theoretically between different approaches to interpersonal communication. From the theoretical difference flows distinctive practice. For convenience, examine Table 8.1, which categorises difference while not implying exclusivity.

Humanist interpersonal communication practice is generally about exploring an individual problem, finding the psychosocial cause and identifying a solution which enables the client to operate more effectively and eventually achieve self-actualisation. It is therefore linear in its historical construction, developmental in conception and therapeutic and reformative in intent. Genealogically, this discursive position has its roots both in the secular confession and the cathartic psychoanalytical talking cure of Freud. This is the common discursive base to the various forms of casework, problem-solving and other strategies engaged by the social worker and mediated through the interpersonal communication process in the interview.

Table 8.1 Features of humanist and poststructural interpersonal communication approaches

Humanist	*Poststructural*
Linear	Lateral
Developmental	Genealogical
Centred subject	Decentred subject
Individual	Cultural
Therapeutic	Educational
Reformative	Diverse
Disciplining	Emancipatory
Normative	Critical
Causal	Archaeological
Reduction	Deconstruction
Self-actualise	Re-author

Prevailing humanist approaches are based on the notion of a self-contained unified subject. The intervention strategy utilised sees language as a reflection of the rational unified world to which we all belong. The goal is to find a way for the individual to 'self-actualise' within this given reality. This applies not only to Gerard Egan (1982) or Bolton (1987), but also to radical structuralist (as distinct from poststructuralist) feminist and Marxist approaches which often seek to liberate people from a 'false consciousness'. Communication skills including listening, empathy, following and so on are seen as technical devices which enable a shared understanding of their purpose and impact. For this to occur, it is assumed that both the worker and the skills used are largely objective, neutral and facilitative.

A poststructural approach reconstructs the 'individual' as a 'vehicle and site' of cultural meaning. Language is the means of our subjectivity; it constructs multiple cultural meanings (including the very notion of one 'reality'). Subjectivity is at the same time constructed and producing meanings itself, primarily through discourses. This is the genealogy of Foucauldian philosophy applied to social work's interpersonal methodology.

A poststructural approach is therefore a decentred and discursive approach to theory and practice where history moves from a causal, binarist and linear past and present to a lateral archaeological critique of ideas and practices. The poststructural process deconstructs the genealogy of meaning, the process of subjectification, through a discourse analysis generating an archaeology of knowledge. Behaviours and their meanings are externalised, action is purposive rather than reactive and, as we shall see, technical interpersonal communication skills themselves are subject to this 'gaze'. [...]

CONCLUSION

In this chapter, we invited our anonymous interlocutor to ask questions which would allow us to deconstruct the dominant humanist discursive position that had informed our teaching and practice of interpersonal communication skills. This brief genealogy disclosed how certain concepts have been constructed to produce an oppressive, rather than liberating, social work practice. We then argued that an alternative discourse and practice are possible, which coherently address the primary concern of our profession: personal and social change.

We have developed an approach which integrates poststructural Foucauldian discourse analysis and Freirean educational practice. This produces a distinctly postmodern and decentred dimension to social work, which retains the importance of individual material conditions in its interpersonal context, while seeking genuine radical change in society.

REFERENCES

Billington, R. (1991) *Culture and Society: A Sociology for Culture*, London: Macmillan Education.

Bolton, R. (1987) *People Skills*, Brookvale: Simon & Schuster.

Calinescu, M. (1987) *Five Faces of Modernity*, Durham: Duke University Press.

Egan, G. (1982) *The Skilled Helper*, Monterey: Brooks & Cole.

Foucault, M. (1979) *Discipline and Punish*, Harmondsworth: Penguin.

Freire, P. and Faundez, A. (1990) *Learning to Question: A Pedagogy of Liberation*, Geneva: WCC Publications.

Freire, P. and Shor, I. (1987) *A Pedagogy for Liberation: Dialogues on Transforming Education*, Cambridge: Macmillan.

Gordon, C. (1980) *Power/Knowledge: Selected Interviews and Other Writings 1972–1977: Michel Foucault*, Brighton: Harvester.

Lonsdale, M. (1991) Postmodernism and the Study of History, unpublished MEd thesis, Melbourne: La Trobe University.

Peters, M. (ed.) (1995) *Education and the Postmodern Condition*, Westwood: Bergin and Garvey.

Rojek, C., Peacock, G. and Collins, S. (1988) *Social Work and Received Ideas*, London: Routledge.

Shor, I. (1987) *Freire for the Classroom*, Portsmouth: Boynton/Cook Publishing, Heinemann.

Sturrock, J. (ed.) (1979) *Structuralism and Since*, Oxford: Oxford University Press.

Walkerdine, V. (1984) 'Developmental psychology and the child centred pedagogy: The insertion of Piaget into early education', Henriques, J., Holloway, W., Urwin, C., Venn, C. and Walkerdine, V. (eds), *Changing the Subject: Psychology, Social Regulation and Subjectivity*, London: Methuen.

Weedon, C. (1987) *Feminist Practice and Poststructural Theory*, Oxford: Blackwell.

CHAPTER 9

PRACTISING REFLEXIVITY

Carolyn Taylor and Susan White

[...] Evidence-based and reflective practice have their place in health and welfare (HW) practice, but they are not sufficient. Our argument is that we need to go further and practise reflexively, but this begs the questions what is reflexivity and how is it an improvement on evidence-based and reflective practice?

WHAT IS REFLEXIVITY?

Reflexivity is a curiously elusive term. It is widely used in the social sciences, but often in passing and without clear definition. It is used in different ways which makes its meaning quite difficult to fix. Indeed, some characterisations of it render it interchangeable with reflection. Its origins lie in the Latin word *reflectere* which means to bend back. So, a reflexive analysis:

> *interrogates the process by which interpretation has been fabricated: reflexivity requires any effort to describe or represent to consider how that process of description was achieved, what claims to 'presence' were made, what authority was used to claim knowledge.*
>
> (Fox 1999: 220)

This may help us to mark a distinction between reflection and reflexivity. In our view, reflection is the process of thinking about our practice at

Source: *Practising Reflexivity in Health and Welfare: Making Knowledge* (2000) Maidenhead: Open University Press/McGraw Hill.

the time (reflection-in-action) or after the event (reflection-on-action). For example, as a practitioner you will be 'thinking on your feet' as you go about your daily work and responding to whatever comes up. Given the nature of the work and its people orientation, it can never be entirely predictable. You will constantly be called on to work out what to do next to defuse conflict, to manage deep distress, to convey bad news, to ask awkward and difficult questions and so forth. You will also be subjecting your work to reflection after the event, working out what went well or badly, whether you said and did the appropriate thing at the appropriate time, how you might do things differently next time. You will thus be acknowledging your impact on the situation for good or ill. The primary focus of reflection is on process issues and how the worker handled their practice. Its focus on knowledge is primarily confined to the application of 'theory to practice'.

Reflexivity includes these forms of reflection but takes things further. Specifically, it problematises issues that reflection takes for granted. Reflection tends to accept the client/worker relationship and concerns itself with how to improve it. It also takes propositional and process knowledge at face value. For example, it assumes that through reflection the worker can become more adept at applying child development and attachment theory to childcare practice or that workers can apply intervention theories more effectively. Reflexivity suggests that we interrogate these previously taken-for-granted assumptions (Ixer 1999).

The 'bending back' of reflexivity is not simply the individualised action of separate practitioners in the manner suggested by reflective practice. Rather it is the collective action of an academic discipline or occupational group. In the case of HW-practitioners, it implies that they subject their own knowledge claims and practices to analysis. In other words, knowledge is not simply a resource to deploy in practice. It is a topic worthy of scrutiny. We need to question the Discourses within which social workers, nurses, doctors and others work, and indeed compare them. How does attachment theory shape our thinking about childhood, children's 'needs' and the roles of mothers and fathers? How does biological psychiatry shape our thinking about mental illness and its treatment? We also need to think about how the client/practitioner relationship and the concept of needs are constituted within HW practice. Authors such as Fraser (1989) and Rojek *et al.* (1988) argue that concepts of need are socially constructed, as the latter indicate:

> *discourse analysis reverses the accepted priority of need in humanist social work ... [which] portrays the social worker as the servant of needs which spread out from the client ... Among the most prominent are the needs for compassion, respect, dignity, and trust. Social work, the humanists say, is about fulfilling these needs through the provision*

> *of care with responsibility. Yet, from the perspective of discourse analysis, this puts the cart before the horse. Compassion, respect, dignity etc., do not arise spontaneously from the client. Rather they are constructed through discourse and the client is required to fit in with them.*
>
> (Rojek *et al.* 1988: 131)

This in turn can lead us to unpick some of the concepts that are regarded as unproblematic and inherently positive within HW. Empowerment and autonomy are two obvious candidates here. It is not a question of applying these principles better in practice, as reflective practice suggests, but exploring *how* they are deployed in practice and to what end. We are also led into a more fine-grained analysis of power relations between HW practitioners and clients. On the one hand, we do not assume that power exists as an entity which is brought into all such encounters (or that social factors such as race, class or gender offer straightforward causal explanations of events and situations). Alternatively, we do not deny that power relations exist. This is a tendency with reflective practice (and with Evidence based practice (EBP) which assumes the neutrality of technical expertise) where it is implicitly assumed that there is a harmony of goals and perspectives between worker and client and that workers may speak for clients. This means that we are subjecting to scrutiny both the Discourse and the discourses which both shape our practice and are constituted within it.

Knowledge does not have fixed, stable meanings. It is made rather than revealed. Embedded within the conception of reflexivity is the notion that, as Hall argues, 'By considering the constructedness of social reality we accept the constructedness of all claims, including our own' (1997: 240). This also applies to our own writing. We cannot escape the constraints of language and within this text we have employed particular devices in order to convince you of the 'truth' of our approach. Usually these have been of the standard academic variety and you may have noticed that we have used empiricist discourse to make claims in such a way that their 'constructedness' is disguised. In order to make this knowledge making process more obvious some authors have chosen to write using alternative forms. Hall (1997), for example, has included dialogues between himself and various interested parties (a social worker, a researcher and so forth) to emphasise that his is but one (contestable) version and to introduce other voices into the text (although it is arguable that he retains control over these alternative voices). We have adopted a more conventional style; however, our conventional approach does not make it immune to scrutiny. Nor do we forget that, although authored by us, you will make your own reading of this text and produce other versions of it.

REFLEXIVITY AND UNCERTAINTY

One of the principal objections to practising reflexively is the uncertainty it is said to produce. It can seem much more straightforward to work with the certainties of evidence-based research and the technical problems of applying it to practice; or so it may seem. However, the fit between 'objective theory' and 'practice' may not be so easy to manage in daily work routines where formal propositional knowledge may seem to have little bearing on how to manage the client/worker relationship. Herein lies the appeal of reflective practice because it switches focus from the application of technical knowledge to managing the (often painful and difficult) minutiae of day-to-day practice. It offers the comfort of dealing with 'the real issues' and focusing on the subjective elements of practice. However, while reflective practice opens up the possibility of a more uncertain, ambiguous and complex world, it tends to close much of this down again by obscuring clients' perspectives and freezing practitioners' confessional accounts as true representations of what happened.

Our overriding message is that unexamined forms of realism, whether objectivist or subjectivist, are problematic foundations on which to build professional practice. Moreover, the debate between the 'high ground' of research and the 'swampy lowlands' of practice (Schön 1983, 1987) is misplaced. There is no high ground; rather there are swampy lowlands in (scientific and social science) research as there are in practice. Difficulty, ambiguity and complexity characterise the making of technical/rational knowledge just as they do HW work. We cannot eliminate uncertainty simply by denying its existence. It is something which has to be confronted in all professional work. We have therefore to work out better ways to deal with it, and the refinement of objectivist, technical rationality in the form of evidence-based practice or an individualised focus on practitioners' thought, feelings and actions are insufficient.

We need to produce better understandings of HW practice in an overarching sense (Discourse) and at a micro level (discourse). Other writers, notably Foucauldians, have produced analyses which examine Discourse (see, for example, Armstrong 1983; Rojek *et al.* 1988; Rose 1989; Petersen and Brunton 1997; Chambon *et al.* 1999). Our suggestion is that microanalyses of talk and text can further contribute to this process of sense making. Do such analyses inhibit the capacity to practise? We would argue not. In relation to charges of political quietism, Herrnstein Smith contends that:

> *Those ... persuaded ... of the political necessity of objectivism, commonly cannot imagine themselves – or by extension – anyone else making judgements, taking sides, or working actively for political causes without objectivist convictions and justifications. Consequently they resist – indeed cannot grasp – the idea that the reason other*

> *people reject objectivism is not only that its claims seem, to them, conceptually problematic, but that such claims are, for them, otherwise ('practically' or 'politically') unnecessary. Contrary to the charge of quietism, non-objectivists need not and characteristically do not refuse to* judge. *Nor, also contrary to that charge, must they or do they characteristically refuse to* act. *Nor must they be, or are they characteristically, incapable of acting* effectively. *Nor are they incapable of* justifying *– in the sense of explaining, defending, and promoting – their judgements and actions to other people…*
>
> (Smith 1994: 291)

A similar argument can be applied to HW practice. We are not asking you to abandon action, but we are asking you to approach your practice differently. Our suggestion is that practising reflexively is essential for good practice and that it entails analysing how practitioners make knowledge in their daily work routines. […]. Since we cannot escape these processes of knowledge making, it is important to understand them better.

REFERENCES

Armstrong, D. (1983) *The Political Anatomy of the Body*, Cambridge: Cambridge University Press.

Chambon, A.S., Irving, A. and Epstein, L. (1999) *Reading Foucault for Social Work*, New York: Columbia University Press.

Fox, N. (1999) *Beyond Health: Postmodernism and Embodiment*, London: Free Association Books.

Fraser, N. (1989) *Unruly Practices: Power. Discourse and Gender in Contemporary Society*, Cambridge: Polity Press.

Hall, C. (1997) *Social Work as Narrative: Storytelling and Persuasion in Professional Texts*, Aldershot: Ashgate.

Ixer, G. (1999) 'There is no such thing as reflection', *British Journal of Social Work* 29 (4): 513–528.

Petersen, A. and Brunton, R. (eds) (1997) *Foucault, Health and Medicine*, London: Routledge.

Rojek, C., Peacock, G. and Collins, S. (1988) *Social Work and Received Ideas*, London: Routledge.

Rose, N. (1989) *Governing the Soul: The Shaping of the Private Self*, London: Routledge.

Schön, D.A. (1983) *The Reflective Practitioner*, New York: Free Press.

Schön, D.A. (1987) *Educating the Reflective Practitioner: Towards a New Design for Teaching and Learning in the Professions*, San Francisco, CA: Jossey-Bass.

Smith, B. Herrnstein (1994) 'The unquiet judge: activism without objectivism in law and politics', in Megill, A. (ed.) *Rethinking Objectivity*, London: Duke University Press.

PART II

ANALYSING ASPECTS OF COMMUNICATION

Carol Komaromy

Part Two takes as its focus aspects of communication that lie within everyday experience and relationships in health and social care. The chapters here explore the way that communication is experienced and played out at the sharp end of practice by frontline service providers and users. The key aspects of power, diversity, language and the body are all brought into profile as equally important facets of communication within relationships. Deconstructing these aspects reveals some of their complexity. In this way these chapters provide challenges to simple taken-for-granted notions about communication and raise questions about the extent to which these understandings can be maintained. For example, is it possible to 'empower' service users through developing and enhancing communication skills? Is it enough to understand cultural differences in communication, or are there wider implications? In what ways does language carry meaning and how does it help to construct both understanding and identity? Finally, what role do bodies play in communication and to what extent do they communicate in their own right and not simply non-verbally? These are just some of the aspects of communication that this section of the Reader addresses.

Chapter 10 'The smoke and mirrors of empowerment: a critique of user-professional partnership' is written by Christine Descombes, a researcher in the area of medical ethics. It is based on her study of the everyday practice of medical ethics which explored the concept of a profession's ethos and its influence on the application of ethical principles. Not only was the rhetoric of 'partnership' not matched by the reality, but more than that, the author's findings show that the reality of empowerment was more complex. For example, while doctors 'permit' and sometimes encourage patients to take part in consultations, those patients who try to take control are strongly resisted by doctors. The nurse-patient relationship tends to reflect more their own position of, or lack of power. So this suggests that power is treated as if it is something that can be given to patients. Linda Finlay, an Open University consultant author who is also a psychologist and occupational therapist, would challenge this notion. Chapter 11 'Feeling powerless: therapists battle for control' draws upon her professional background and is based on data from a qualitative study of the way that occupational therapists experience feelings of power and powerlessness. As the title suggests, professionals also have to negotiate, challenge and resist power.

This sets the scene for the following three chapters that focus upon difference and diversity in communication. Are there structural issues in society that continue to disadvantage particular groups? To what extent is diversity between individuals and groups in society something that is 'celebrated', as poststructuralists would suggest? The first of this trio, Chapter 12 'Beliefs, values and interethnic communication', is written by Lena Robinson, an academic and social work educator who has a special interest in racial identity and whose chapter explores intercultural communication in health and social care settings. In particular she asks, what are the values that communications are based upon? She extends this to discuss the way that values dictate not only the nature of communication but also the way that people judge each other. Chapter 13 'Men talking about fatherhood: discourse and identities' by Martin Robb, an Open University lecturer, draws upon critical discursive psychology and highlights some of the complexity that is associated with notions of men's caring relationships. The chapter draws on the author's own research and reveals how, rather than being fixed, fatherhood is relational, contextual and discursively produced. Beverley Burke and Philomena Harrison in Chapter 14, 'Anti-oppressive Practice' write from a social work perspective. As the title suggests, the authors explore the way that anti-oppressive approaches can allow professionals to work more effectively and dynamically with disadvantaged and oppressed groups in society.

The role of language in identity and communication in the context of care is the focus of the next two chapters. The first is written by Richard Gwyn, an academic and writer on health and communication, who discusses the role of narratives in Chapter 15 'Narrative analysis and illness experience'. The author argues that stories not only convey information about people's lives and experiences, but also construct their identities. In Chapter 16 'Preparing for linguistically sensitive practice', social work educator Richard Pugh continues this theme, discussing the ways that power, identity and culture in care settings are constructed through language.

Gender and identity play a significant role in communication and this is also played out through the 'body'. The final two chapters of this section focus upon the role of the body as communication in two distinct ways. Chapter 17 'Embarrassment, social rules and the context of body care' by Jocalyn Lawler, a professor of nursing, is taken from a much wider ethnographic account of the role of bodies in health care. Here she explores the way that nurses and patients manage the embarrassment that is an inevitable part of the task of nursing which involves intimate personal care. This form of 'non-verbal communication' is a powerful reminder that we communicate with our bodies and not just in place of language. Chapter 18 'Technology, selfhood and physical disability', which concludes Part II, is written by sociologists Deborah Lupton and Wendy Seymour. The authors argue that technology is both normalising and stigmatising to disabled people. Certainly technologies can replace the functions of disabled parts of the body or can help to overcome disability in different ways, but they also mark the body as 'different'. Of course, this form of difference is not necessarily negative, but as the authors argue, technology makes a qualitative difference to relationships.

CHAPTER 10

THE SMOKE AND MIRRORS OF EMPOWERMENT: A CRITIQUE OF USER-PROFESSIONAL PARTNERSHIP

Christine Descombes

In company with many similar ideas that sound not only simple but also 'right', empowerment is quite a complex notion that requires us to think across a broad perspective rather than along the narrow lines of a superficial judgement. In critiquing it we are looking to explore the significance of the concept to the reality of everyday practice. In this Chapter I will focus on empowerment in relation to health care interactions, patient empowerment, as that is my research field. However, the arguments apply across the range of empowerment environments.

> *To move empowerment from rhetoric to reality requires leaping some well established hurdles, among the most significant of which are: the credibility and legitimacy of the power exercised by health care professionals, the needs and career aspirations of many professionals, and the bureaucracy of the health service.*
>
> (Lamont 1999)

The core of empowerment is power and control. The first questions this chapter addresses is: whose power? The answer, according to the professionals who now espouse the notion, is the client, the patient, the service user. Thus, for example, many doctors speak positively of patient empowerment (BMJ 18 Sept. 1999: 319), as do nurses (RCN June 2000, October 2001), the leaders of patient groups (BMJ 17 June 2000: 320; Rethink Policy Statement 50, Sept. 2002), and the politicians who hold the purse strings of the NHS (DoH 2002). They all agree that patient empowerment is the way ahead for the moden health service.

However, empowerment is not just about a group such as patients gaining power. As Parker (1999: 9–10) observed, albeit somewhat caustically, empowerment carries within it a power relationship. He refers to the powerful experts who condescend to grant a little power to their lessers. Empowerment can mean no more than actions that reinforce existing and established power imbalances.

Sinclair, in his study of medical training, offers an example. In response to the emphasis on empowerment, medical schools' curricula now include courses in 'Doctor-Patient communication' and 'Communication Skills' in which the students doctors learn new ways of listening and talking to patients. (Sinclair 1997: 220) The rhetoric is positive yet in reality these courses are not given high status within the teaching hospitals and, in Sinclair's considered assessment, have little significant impact on actual practice. They are merely grafted onto, and absorbed into, traditional medical practice. Thus, one consultant reportedly tells his students 'Patients think they are being listened to more if you look them in the eye ... So you have the opportunity to examine the iris closely while you take a history' (Sinclair 1997: 220, 325)

Nevertheless, there is a new openness in the medical consultation that suggests doctors are taking patient empowerment seriously. Within the NHS today the emphasis is on Patient-Centred medicine with patient and practitioner working together to explore the illness experience and identify common ground for the management of the disease/illness (Stewart 1995). Whereas doctors used to consider it their right, even a moral duty, not only to routinely and actively withhold information but to lie to patients (Bok 1989: 222–226) now transparency is the watchword and patients are given full information relating to their condition and the pros and cons of the treatment options (Gawande 2002: 210, 212). It is then for the patient, rather than the doctor, to decide what course to follow. Patient empowerment in action. Or is it? Note the comment of the Associate Professor and Director at the Centre for Research and Clinical Policy in Sydney, Australia in a BMJ debate on empowerment:

> *Although much has changed over the last 20 years in moving away from a paternalistic medical model of care, many service providers of health, particularly medical practitioners still feel uncomfortable with sharing information, knowledge, or decision making with their patients.*
>
> (Boyages 1999)

In the same debate a GP observed that 'Medical Training (sic) encourages us to think that decision making should be doctor-centred'. Later he referred to 'an absolute paranoia about any form of transference taking place between doctor and patient' (Manning 1999). From another practitioner came the comment 'Many doctors practice "Don't ask! Don't tell!"' (Andrews 1999). A medical professor writing in support of empowerment recognised that asking professionals to view 'the patient as expert is often an affront to our self-image as experts, (Selby 1999). Finally, a Clinical Fellow in primary care noted that is not unusual for patients, even those 'armed with some medical knowledge', to find a consultation with their doctor 'disempowering' (Slowie 1999).

It is still the doctor who controls the whole patient-practitioner encounter. It is the doctor who decides just what information will be given and how much use can be made of it. A person might be given no information at all, carefully edited information, or a barrage of technical language and statistics. Any of these presentations can leave the individual consulting the doctor overwhelmed and feeling powerless.

And what happens when a patient decides to take a course of action with which the doctor disagrees? One doctor answers in the following terms:

> *Our contemporary medical credo has made us exquisitely attuned to the requirements of patient autonomy. But there are still times – and they are more frequent than we readily admit – when a doctor has to steer patients to do what is right for themselves.*
>
> (Gawande 2002: 216)

Indeed, the idea that patients would want to ignore the commonly called doctors' orders 'is widely construed as irrational' (Lupton 1994: 116 quoting Ehrenreich and Ehrenreich). So patients who choose to pursue a course contrary to current medical thinking must be persuaded or cajoled into compliance. As Gawande observes, 'before a thoughtful, concerned and, yes, sometimes, crafty doctor, few patients will not eventually "choose" what the doctor recommends' (Gawande 2002: 219). The same result is no doubt achieved by, in the words of one GP, the 'supercilious, arrogant, haughty, opinionated ... and unhelpful' medical men and women whom he recognises that patients all too often meet (Manning 1999).

All this appears to support the view that in practice, in the reality of the everyday encounter between doctor and patient, empowerment goes only as far as the individual doctor is prepared to let it go. The doctor might, as in Parker's description, condescend to raise the lesser patient up a little, but there is no sharing of power; power remains firmly in the hands of the professional. The patient may be allowed a voice, however, it is 'heard but not heeded' (Lamont 1999). Empowerment itself becomes another tool of control. This may strike the reader as cynical and manipulative on the part of the professional. Yet, in the context of the sociocultural environment within which the medical profession traditionally operates it is no more than we should expect.

In her discussion on 'Power relations and the medical encounter' Lupton (1994) explores from a number of different perspectives the influence of the sociocultural context on the formation and maintenance of the continuing doctor-patient power differential. Among these is the functionalist perspective. This sees the power of the medical practitioner as granted by general consensus, and accepted by the community as legitimately exercised for the good of the wider society. On an individual level, the authority of the doctor allows the patient to hand over the burden of decision-making to one who society recognises as a trusted and respected expert (Lupton 1994: 105, 106).

If patient empowerment has any meaning it is exercised in the decision to consult a doctor and, in so doing, to abrogate further decision-making power to the professional expert. Once an individual has made that decision the doctor, in turn, has the duty to take control of the interaction, make a diagnosis, and implement appropriate treatment (ibid. 118). This is the perspective that still dominates in the training of new doctors. Students are taught to see patients who reject the authority of the doctor as difficult and they 'intensely resent' such a lack of respect; 'good' patients are those who co-operate with the doctor (Sinclair 1997: 34).

The doctor's role is to 'tend their [patients'] physical and emotional needs, to nurture and protect them and take control of a frightening and anxiety-provoking situation' (Lupton 1994: 106). Or, as one GP put it, 'taking patients by the hand and leading them through the system until they come out at the other end cured' (Descombes 2001). The idea of equal partnership sits uneasily within this frame of thinking (Carvel 1999).

> *The trend of passing the decision making to the patient and his family appears politically correct, and as such is supported by many laws in many countries. However, not all patients feel comfortable with this new burden put on them ... but medical training emphasizes (sic) decision-making. We are experts in making decisions. We have the background and the tools that make difficult decisions possible.*
>
> (Rabinovich 1999)

And this understanding seems to be borne out in the experience of those confronting an illness crisis. Thus, a 'highly intelligent and well motivated' academic who was determined to control her illness experience, nevertheless found that the authority of the doctor was particularly important in helping her accept difficult decisions regarding aspects of the treatment programme (DiGiacomo, quoted by Lupton 1994: 116). Another, himself a doctor, describes the anguish of trying to decide on the best treatment for his very sick baby. 'In many ways', he writes, 'I was the ideal candidate to decide what was best ... And yet when the team of doctors came to talk to me ... I wanted them to decide – doctors I had never met before ... The uncertainties were savage and I could not bear the possibility of making the wrong call ... I could not live with the guilt if something went wrong' (Gawande 2002: 221).

But, of course, not all patients feel the need to hand over decision making to a health professional. They are not waiting on a doctor to empower them, they are actively taking control. The response to such individuals suggests that health professionals 'are still far from comfortable with empowerment that moves beyond the lowest rungs on the ladder of participation' (Lamont 1999), beyond their own control. The medical professional appears reasonably happy to 'allow' or 'permit' or even 'encourage' patients to take part in the consultation process but patients who try to shift the power imbalance to the point where they are taking control will often meet with highly effective resistance.

However, it is not just the medical profession that finds it difficult to cope with real patient involvement. Lamont (1999) offered the observation that 'the needs and career aspirations of many professionals tends to prevent the shift in power needed if patients and the general public are to take some control over their health care, and become real partners'. The role and status of the nurse presents an example of this challenge to the reality of empowerment.

'Nursing relations are constitutively structured by the vulnerability of inequalities and dependency at many different levels' (Bowden 1997: 116). Thus, on the one hand there is the relationship with the patient which has 'significant areas of overlap ... with aspects of maternal caring ... A continuity with the vulnerability of childhood and the mothering it elicits (Bowden 1997: 101, 112, 116b). In this relationship the professional nurse enjoys power and respect. On the other hand, there is the relationship with other professionals, and particularly with members of the most senior profession, medicine, wherein the nurse has a traditionally lower status. 'In keeping with the dominant [socio-cultural] norms ... nursing care is encumbered with much of the social apparatus that operates to undermine the value both of women's practices in general and the social possibilities of their practitioners' (ibid.: 104). Here the nursing profession itself is disempowered, traditionally lacking recognition and the nurse is left without a real voice in decision making (ibid.: 20, 121).

All this suggests that nurses will find it as difficult as doctors to accept patient empowerment beyond low-level profession-controlled participation. The need of the professional to maintain their status as the experts works against patients exercising anything other than minimum control over their own health care.

In a paper on the rhetoric and reality of empowerment written by a group of people with disabilities, the authors identified as disempowering a range of professional attitudes and practices common in the everyday hospital routine. These included a number of standard nursing practices such as how patients are addressed, questions of privacy, continence and pressure relieving care, and writing up care plans. They referred specifically to the 'we know best' attitude of staff as 'adversely controlling', voicing particular concern at the lack of respect shown by staff to the disabled persons' own expertise, or that of their non-professional long-standing carers and supporters (DCDP 1992).

The Royal College of Nursing (RCN) in its statements on empowerment shows up the profession's equivocal position. It has committed itself to the principle of patients as equal partners in their own health care with honesty and respect as core values of this partnership (RCN 2001: 5). It acknowledges the need for health professionals to 'modify their position to ensure that power rebalance is effectively achieved' (RCN 2000: 25). In practice this apparently requires more nurse experts. Thus, in the field of care of the elderly and chronically sick the main need is for a 'specialist' nurse with 'authority' who would 'provide leadership' to a cross-disciplinary team caring for the elderly patient cum client (RCN 2000: 5–7). One is led to suggest that this emphasis on enhancing the power of the nurse sits rather uncomfortably with the profession's commitment to 'partnership with the elderly person', 'collaboration' and 'patient and professional as equals'.

Patient empowerment meets another obstacle in the structures of the NHS itself and the will of its political masters. Though the political rhetoric since the early 1990s has endorsed and, indeed, encouraged, patients to think in terms of active partnership and choice in their health care, the structure of the NHS made that virtually impossible. The reality is of a system that was and is not designed to give patients real choices as equal partners in meeting their health care needs (Klein 1995: 232). Once again the historical context has dictated this reality. The NHS reflected the sociocultural position at the time of its creation. Fifty years ago there was no place for patients, the vast majority of whom were working class, to be anything other than passive and grateful to the system manned and managed by their social superiors. And they complied. There was no need to consider 'the patients' voice', they didn't have one. The accepted wisdom was that patients didn't need a voice as all their needs would be identified and met by the twins of administrative technology and professional expertise (Allsop 1995: 240). Much has changed since those early days but patient power still cannot find a real foothold in the highly bureaucratised NHS.

Similarly, the political emphasis on empowerment has been identified not with real power passing to patients, but rather as a means by which government 'could justify policies of cost containment, of restriction of medical autonomy and a focus on lower cost forms of health provision' (Benidge 1999: 57). No matter that the political rhetoric is empowerment, the reality of increasingly centralised decision-making and local cost containment leaves the patient more disempowered.

Everyone is, indeed, talking about empowering patients. However, the established systems involved in providing health care to the majority, including attitudes and practices taught in medical school and reinforced in the ward and consulting room, the place of the nurse in the hierarchy of professions, the demands of politicians for greater and greater control, not only limit that empowerment but have often become tools for disempowering patients, for reducing their choices and the opportunities for partnership. It is for society, and not just individuals, to decide if that is an acceptable situation or whether it is time to pursue more effective power sharing relationships (Sinclair 1997: 327; cf. Descombes 1999: 152–161).

REFERENCES

Allsop, J. (1995) *Health Policy and the NHS*, London: Longman.

Andrews, A. (1999) 'The times of "Don't Ask! Don't Tell" are gone', *BMJ* 319: 783.

Benidge, V. (1999) *Health and Society in Britain since 1939*, Cambridge: Cambridge University Press.

BMJ (2000) 18 September, 320: 1660–1664.

BMJ (1999) 17 June, 319: 780.

Bok, S. (1989) *Lying. Moral Choice in Public and Private Life*, New York: Vintage Books.

Bowden, P. (1997) *Caring. Gender-Sensitive Ethics*, London: Routledge.

Boyages, S.C. (1999) 'Revealing the magician's secrets: patients as partners and doctors as navigators', *BMJ* 319: 783.

Carvel, D. (1999) 'Political correctness going too far', *BMJ* 319: 783.

DCDP (1992) *'Patient' Empowerment with Specific Reference to Disabled People A reponse to the Department of Health 'Patient Charter' 1992*, produced by the Derbyshire Coalition of Disabled People.

Descombes C. (1999) 'Passive patient or responsible consumer: market values and the normative ideal', in Norman, Richard (ed.) *Ethics and the Market*, Aldershot: Ashgate Publishing Company.

Descombes, C. (2001) *Before Ethics? A Study of the Ethos of the Medical Profession*, unpublished thesis, Milton Keynes: Open University.

DoH (2002) 'New era in patient and public involvement in NHS', Department of Health Press release: reference 200210533.

Gawande, A. (2002) *Complications: A Surgeon's Notes on an Imperfect Science*, London: Profile Books.

Klein, R. (1995) *The New Politics of the NHS*, Harlow: Longman.

Lamont, S.S. (1999) 'Participating in theory', *BMJ* 319: 783.
Lupton, D. (1994) *Medical Culture*, London: Sage Publications.
Manning, C. (1999) 'Partnership – the best option', *BMJ* 319: 783.
Parker, (1999) *Deconstructing Psychotherapy*, London: Sage, 9–10.
Rabinovich, Y. (1999) 'The patient's right to sound decision', *BMJ* 319: 783.
RCN (2000) *Developing a National Plan for the New NHS June 2000*, London: Royal College of Nursing.
RCN (2001) *Learning the Lessons: The RCN Response to the Bristol Royal Infirmary Inquiry*, London: Royal College of Nursing.
Selby, P. (1999) 'All the solutions lie with patients – we need to listen', *BMJ* 1999; 319: 783ff.
Sinclair, S. (1997) *Making Doctors: an Institutional Apprenticeship*, Oxford: Berg.
Slowie, D.F. (1999) 'Our duty is firstly to help patients improve their communication with doctors', *BMJ* 319: 783.
Stewart, M. *et al.* (1995) *Patient-Centered Medicine: Transforming the Clinical Method*, London: Sage Publications.

CHAPTER 11

FEELING POWERLESS: THERAPISTS BATTLE FOR CONTROL

Linda Finlay

INTRODUCTION

> *'If you would just listen to me!' Paula didn't say it to her patient, but she wished she could.*
>
> (extract from observation notes)

Much of the literature devoted to examining the power dimension embedded in therapeutic relationships suggests that professionals wield considerable power. Such findings do not, however, reflect the subjective sense of powerlessness that seems to be experienced by many therapists in their day-to-day work. The sentiment expressed in the above extract is a common, if largely unexpressed, lament from therapists struggling to retain control over resistant or recalcitrant patients/clients. This gap between literature and experience provided impetus for further research.

Twelve occupational therapists from a range of contexts (physical and psychiatric hospitals, social services and community mental health) were studied (Finlay 1999). I used qualitative methodology in the form of in-depth interviews and participant observation. I chose this methodology in order to capture something of the meanings and subjective experiences of each individual. I adopted a phenomenological approach to *describe* the individual's life world, as opposed to *explaining* how or why particular meanings arise. Analysis of the interviews and observations involved repeated and systematic readings of the individual transcripts to identify common themes in line with the analytic method suggested by Giorgi (1985).

FINDINGS

The occupational therapists' narratives revealed, both implicitly and explicitly, how therapists struggle with power in practice. Three themes are discernible:

- the battle for control;
- coping with threat; and
- feeling powerless within the system.

THE BATTLE FOR CONTROL

All the occupational therapists who participated in the study seem to find control an issue within their relationships. While the therapists all acknowledge they have a degree of control, it is interesting to explore when and how they exercise that control.

Jane, for example, expresses feeling in control at the same time as wanting to ensure her clients feel empowered themselves. She believes this is best achieved by giving clients choices and adopting a non-assertive approach – an approach she uses routinely and strategically:

> *I wouldn't use the assertive approach, I'd backtrack and come at them from an unassertive position, because quite often I think it's a control thing. People are terrified of losing control and if you could sort of go in from a less dominant position and make them feel as though they've got control of the situation and have got control of yourself, then I think you get further.*

Stephen is more accepting of the authority conferred upon him by his status and professional expertise. He is conscious of the point where he stops negotiating with patients. He gives his instructions (particularly regarding safety precautions) and expects his patients to be rational and follow the advice:

INTERVIEWER: So there isn't ... lots of negotiation with the patient?

STEPHEN: Not really, because the type of injury they've got is quite dictative of what they must do. I mean you can negotiate with the patient for a while on it, but at the end of the day they mustn't flex beyond 90°, they mustn't internally rotate; they mustn't adduct or the hip will dislocate and they'll go back into hospital.

Karen similarly feels she needs to be directive though she is mixed about how she is received by patients when she pushes them against their will:

> *Sometimes it's almost like a battle, trying to show the patient's what they are doing to themselves by doing too much ... We're like a firing squad! It makes us sound awful! ... I think the patients might view it like that.*

On occasions when therapists' control is wrested away from them, the therapy relationship can feel like a battleground. Paula, for instance, struggles to control her angry, defensive feelings and accept that her clients ultimately have the last say:

PAULA: You got all the flack from the daughters, 'we don't want a stair lift, we don't want this, we don't want that' ... I thought 'Oh no' ... you can deal with one person going ... mad at you, but I find it hard when it's all at you, and you think, 'I didn't ask for this, you know, this defensive attitude!' But you learn to deal with it ... because it's so easy to become on the defensive yourself, when you're getting a lot from people. I've learnt to literally just to sort of state my situation, and state where I'm coming from, and leave it at that, really...

INTERVIEWER: When you say it would be easy to become defensive, do you mean to kind of get angry yourself, and say, 'Right, well, stuff you'?

PAULA: Well yes, because in some situations you just think 'God! You know, I wish you'd listen to what I was saying. You're not ... actually listening and taking it on board'.

Stephen similarly can feel aggressive but he knows he has to turn away. He has learned to distance himself, accepting he cannot control every situation:

> *I get quite aggressive sometimes ... it's a bit of a power thing ... I've had words with the patient to try and persuade them ... It certainly makes the job easier now that I've accepted the fact that patients sometimes don't do things. Whereas as a basic grade the patients had to do things or else it was my fault.*

Underlying the more overt issues of control, therapists negotiate a minefield of emotional dynamics. Jenny, for instance, sees some of her patients as demanding and dependent. She likens them to children; they get jealous, have tantrums and need her attention. She struggles not to act like an authoritarian parent in response and she has to remind herself to be empathetic. Speaking about a particularly demanding patient she explains:

JENNY: She is still very, very dependent on people…

INTERVIEWER: … What does it feel like to have somebody like that be so dependent on you?

JENNY: It's very weird at times … If I'm stood talking to my colleague, she doesn't like it, especially if it's one of the younger, more attractive nursing staff. She doesn't like it and woe betide me … I get messages like … 'you were talking to so and so and you didn't acknowledge me'. … What she reminds me of, very much in the way she handles things and the way she behaves, is a child. And having a four-year-old daughter, the comparisons are quite similar, in that if things don't go her way, you can almost see the tantrum arriving. And sometimes it's very difficult for me not to treat her in the same manner as I do a four-year-old in the supermarket … And she is extremely trying and she's extremely wearing because it's like one step forward, ten steps back…

INTERVIEWER: … She's clearly a difficult person, but it also sounds like you've got a fondness for her(?)

JENNY: Oh, most definitely.

Therapists see their intense emotional relationships with clients as something they have to negotiate over time. Resisting 'transferences' of the patient/client as a dependent child is part of the therapy process (whether done explicitly in a psychodynamic treatment context or less self-consciously outside of particular theoretical frames). However, as 'weary parents' they feel guilty about not giving enough or feeling angry. At the same time they also experience a tension of not wanting to give too much as that mitigates against aims of enabling independence.

Mary sees some of her clients as demanding and constantly needing her reassurance. They grab at her – suck her dry. Sometimes it feels she will have to give endlessly and she feels tired. She views the process of treatment as weaning these clients off her and therapy:

> *It just kinda makes you feel a bit uneasy, because it's almost like she's setting you up, that you have to be there every time she needs you and be there forever and a day … she needs constant reassurance about this, and gets very anxious … And she wants you to make a decision on her behalf the whole time … she sort of sits the chairs so close together, you're always within touching range, and she sort of grabs*

your hand ... Sometimes you sort of think, 'Well, God, you know, get a grip!' ... it's things we've been over before, and we've talked through ... and then you can go next time and there's all this drama again ... it's like going over old ground again ... If I'm feeling tired when I go ... it's very difficult to concentrate and be constructive and positive, when it's like somebody's whittering. You think, 'I've heard all this before'.

COPING WITH THREAT

The therapists are aware of an ever-present threat of violence. This feeling is experienced most acutely by those working in mental health where they seek constantly to manoeuvre to avoid abuse. Sometimes, there is nothing they can do and this is unnerving.

In the context of her forensic unit, Jenny recognises her particular risk of being attacked both physically and sexually:

You always have to be very assertive with him, but it's got to the point where no matter how I deal with him, it makes no difference, because he still insists on doing it. And it is very much about me ... as a woman and you know. The women who can ... control him if you like, he doesn't have a problem with them. They are a lot older than I am. And yes, they're able to set their boundaries, but then he's obviously neither as attracted or as, you know having fantasies about or whatever. He even does things like, there's a large observation window from the other ward, and even if he can't physically get to you, he'll stand there and rub his groin and drool ... at the window and things like that. It's those invidious bits of behaviour. He'll crawl across the floor to get to you.

Speaking of another patient, Jenny describes her defensive manoeuvres in the face of such a threat:

He fantasises an awful lot and ... it got to the point where his boundaries were breaking down and ... in the corridor, and you'd have to pass, he would actually come into the office, which they know they are not really supposed to do, and he would interrupt phone calls ... But he is much more covert about it really. But again I am very much aware of what's going on in his head. I don't isolate myself with him. I have very little to do with him. I knew him when I worked in local services ... I think because of that connection, he's then twisted it round in his head that most of what's happened to him subsequently is my fault. And so again I just had to keep a very wide berth from him.

Dealing with patients who have violent sexual histories is experienced as both distasteful and threatening. For women like Jenny, somehow the threat of being sexually assaulted or 'invaded' is more frightening and distressing than the threat of straightforward physical violence.

Julie and Jenny both understand that as therapists they run a risk of being hit and abused. They are more frightened about being sexually attacked. They feel this threat more personally – as women, not just as therapists:

JENNY: I have never, touch wood, been hit and never been threatened. But you accept that a thump is a thump, with him it's not going to be a thump, its going to be something sexual. Now any woman can put their hand on their heart and say that's their worst nightmare, is to actually get attacked in that way, whether they are working in a secure unit or not. Um, and that's the way that he would attack. He would not attack in a physical way. So it's a very different feeling and it's a very different, um, fear if you like, in terms of somebody wanting to hit you ... One of the patients, his offence was rape and he is very inappropriate with females. You know, if you met him now he would be totally inappropriate with you. You are a very new female and he always sort of tries it on with new females.

JULIE: I could not work as this guy's key therapist. I couldn't tell you what it was about him, because he was superficially quite pleasant, but he just made my skin creep. He used to have serious problems with proximity in that he would get too close and he would position himself so that he trapped you at your desk or in your room. If he was in the doorway he would be standing with his hand across the frame, so you couldn't get out ... I wasn't actually alone. None of the female members of staff here or on the ward felt comfortable with him.

INTERVIEWER: Were you threatened by him like it was a sexual thing?

JULIE: There was a sexual element to it because none of us felt physically threatened. I could have ... over my knees, he was only little! He was probably verging on having emphysema or something, so – it was a psychological threat rather than a physical one ... There was something unwholesome about him.

FEELING POWERLESS IN THE SYSTEM

All the therapists express feeling assaulted by the demands of the health care system. There are too many patients to see, too much to do, and not enough resources to get them done. Therapists also feel insecure in their jobs: threatened by, and powerless against, management priorities.

Paula feels swamped by the numbers of people referred. She is constantly aware of waiting list numbers and the need to keep ploughing through her growing case load. She struggles with her time management, juggling her hours, trying to squeeze more in. She works hard to prioritise her cases and save time by not getting too involved.

> *I may get 9–10 referrals a day, and ... I don't get any extra time to do the referrals. It's part and parcel of my morning, and I literally need to look at them and decide there and then ... I'd love to ... find out more, but I just do not have the time.*

Stephen concurs:

> *It is frustrating. And it makes me angry sometimes, because there's things you want to do but you just can't fit them in. There's too many patients needing the bog standard things.*

Jenny is under pressure from the Trust's management to produce reports to deadlines. She doesn't have enough hours in the day. She sees the demands on her as being so excessive they are a 'farce'.

> *Because of the way the Trust works we had to produce that information very quickly ... I can work anything up to a 14 to 15 hour day, and still do, because of the deadlines ... On top of all that we are supposed to carry a clinical load which is an absolute farce!*

The therapists (particularly in physical practice) live with the ever present threat of litigation. They always have to watch their step and minimise risk. With management watching, a lot of their practice is defensive, 'to cover themselves'. Peter and Anne are constantly alert to the threat of litigation and the need to ensure the safety of their patients and practice. On home visits, for instance, they are focused solely on minimising physical risks on discharge, rather than quality of life.

Stephen feels disempowered by the role required from him by management, which he perceives is largely to rubber-stamp doctors' discharge decisions.

STEPHEN: In general surgery we're often called in just to, 'somebody's going home this afternoon and we want to cover ourselves'. So you do a quick assessment, tell them they're fine ... The person would go home anyway, so what's the point, apart from legally ... it can be frustrating ...

INTERVIEWER: You'd want to do it properly rather than rubber stamp?

STEPHEN: Yeah, so that my assessment had a meaning...

INTERVIEWER: So it's quite disempowering then when the consultants ask you to rubber stamp it. How do you handle that?...

STEPHEN: Yeah. I don't think we've really got a choice in it. The pressure ... they're pushing through I think three or four thousand patients in a quarter, that you've actually got to fit in with that. The organisation wouldn't accept, you know, an individual saying, 'Well, that's not how I think it should be done'. It can be difficult, but you just do it because it means that the next patient can get in and have a bed ... It's the way we are treated from above. But the Chief Executive said that there would be no jobs at risk for people who are involved in discharge planning, discharge facilitating. So I think that typifies what the value, what the important part is for them. It's not the actual rehabilitation.

Other therapists similarly feel insecure, living with a threat of redundancy if they cannot demonstrate their value. Cathy, for instance, wonders if there is a point to continuing to battle at work if she is going to lose her job anyway.

> *I think we've got jobs for another year ... but meanwhile we've got out of 14 CPNs they're going to probably be making two redundant ... next year it will be likely the OTs ... It makes life very difficult, not knowing whether on one hand to fight the battle, or not ... you think, 'Well what's the point if there's no job anyway?'*

SUMMARY

The above findings have shown therapists routinely confront a power dimension embedded in all their relationships. This is evidenced in the way they constantly compromise their role decisions in the face of management priorities and in the way they control their patients/clients. Although the therapists seem to want to minimise the negative effects of their power, they also recognise they are in a position of authority and they act on this by giving directive instruction and expert advice. However, sometimes this authority is challenged and the therapists and patients/clients battle for the upper hand. In extreme cases, where clients become abusive, the power balance shifts.

The findings expose a distinction, made by Jarman *et al.* (1997), between *being in control* and *feeling in control*. The participant's narratives suggests that therapists can sometimes feel anything but powerful. Rather, as Lyons (1997) among others have noted, the therapists seem to manoeuvre to retain control with manipulative clients who resist their advice. All the participants in my research routinely battled with complaining, dependent or resistant clients and some had to handle more overt violence and sexual harassment noted by Schneider *et al.* (1999). These therapists find themselves engaged in power battles while defensively attempting to keep safe in the face of emotional assault and physical threat. That power can work in both directions should not be forgotten. That this power operates within what is often a demanding and disempowering system is also pertinent.

Just highlighting therapists' use of power is too simplistic, serving only to demonise the professional and thus ignore more complex social dynamics. Not only is power negotiated within the context of particular relationships and settings, it occurs in a broader social context. In particular, professional power can be seen to be cross-cut by structures of gender, class, race (Hugman 1991), for instance, as revealed in the way male patients can threaten female therapists. Further, therapists in this study expressed feeling pressured and assaulted by their own institutional system. In the face of job insecurity the therapists feel powerless in their relationships with management. More exploration is needed of how power emerges through on-going relationships and out of these wider social contexts.

REFERENCES

Finlay, L. (1999) 'The life world of the occupational therapist: meaning and motive in an uncertain world', unpublished PhD thesis, Milton Keynes: The Open University.

Giorgi, A. (ed.) (1985) *Phenomenology and Psychological Research*, Pittsburgh: Duquesne University Press.

Hugman, R. (1991) *Power in the Caring Professions*, Basingstoke: Macmillan Press.

Jarman, M., Smith, J.A. and Walsh, S (1997) 'The psychological battle for control: a qualitative study of health-care professionals' understandings of treatment of anorexia nervosa', *Journal of Community and Applied Social Psychology* 7: 137–152.

Lyons, M. (1997) 'Understanding professional behaviour: experiences of occupational therapy students in mental health settings', *American Journal of Occupational Therapy* 51: 686–692.

Schneider, J., Weerakoon, P. and Heard, B. (1999) 'Inappropriate client sexual behaviour in occupational therapy', *Occupational Therapy International* 6: 176–194.

CHAPTER 12

BELIEFS, VALUES AND INTERCULTURAL COMMUNICATION

Lena Robinson

INTRODUCTION

This chapter explores intercultural communication in the health and social care setting. It is written from a psychological perspective and explores some of the variables that are central to the topic of intercultural communication. Little of the current health and social care literature in Britain has addressed the issue of intercultural communication. This chapter argues that understanding minority communication styles and patterns is indispensable for health care workers working with ethnic minority groups. Euro-American cultural values have dominated the social sciences and have been accepted as universal. It attempts to articulate from a cross-cultural perspective, a precise framework in which to view and define the diverse factors at work during intercultural communication. It focuses on the concepts of belief and value and the impact they have on the communicator's behaviour in intercultural communication.

BELIEFS

According to Rokeach (1973: 2), 'Beliefs are inferences made by an observer about underlying states of expectancy'. A belief is any simple proposition, conscious or unconscious, inferred from what a person says or does, capable of being preceded by the phrase 'I believe that' (Rokeach

1973: 113). The content of a belief cannot be directly observed by others but must be inferred by an observer on the basis of the overt behaviour of the believer. What the believer says or does becomes the clue to his or her belief system. A white man who publicly states that he believes black people are equal to him but who resists black people moving into his neighbourhood demonstrates that expressed beliefs are very poor predictors of behaviour (Fishbein and Ajzen 1975).

Beliefs among black groups and the white majority can differ. For instance, a black person and a white person may share the same value of equality. The white person who has never been refused employment or promotion may believe that equality of opportunity exists – after all he/she never had any trouble. However, the black person who has always been relegated to menial tasks with no possibility for advancement perceives the situation differently. He or she believes that he or she has been discriminated against, and that equality of opportunity in employment does not exist.

BELIEFS AND INTERETHNIC COMMUNICATION

Conflict arising from differences in core beliefs among communicators can result in the disruption of interethnic communication. Core beliefs are based on an individual's direct personal experience with reality. They are held firmly and are resistant to change. White practitioners and black clients experience different realities. Such a divergence in experience will consequently result in a different set of core beliefs. Understanding this variation in core beliefs between white and black people points to the enormous distance between interethnic communicators and the problems they must overcome in order to engage in effective interaction.

Given the different realities of majority and minority people living in Britain, conflicts in beliefs serve as a persistent obstacle to interethnic communication.

In interethnic communication, there are no rights or wrongs as far as beliefs are concerned. White social and health care workers must be able to recognise and to deal with their black clients' beliefs if they wish to obtain satisfactory and successful communication.

ATTITUDES

Attitudes are generally conceptualised as having three components: cognitive, affective and conative (Baron and Byrne 2002). The cognitive component involves our beliefs about the attitude object. The affective component involves our emotional or evaluative reaction to the attitude object. Finally, the conative component of an attitude involves our behavioural intentions toward the attitude object – for example, an intention to avoid black people.

One of the most disruptive attitudes that can emerge in interracial/ethnic communication is racial prejudice. Allport (1979: 7) defined prejudice as 'a judgement based on previous decisions and experiences'. While prejudice can be positive or negative, there is a tendency for most of us to think of it as negative. Allport (1979: 9) defined negative ethnic prejudice as 'an antipathy based on a faulty and inflexible generalisation. It may be felt or expressed. It may be directed toward a group as a whole, or toward an individual because he [or she] is a member of that group'.

Prejudice differs from its behavioural counterpart, discrimination. Prejudice 'includes internal beliefs and attitudes that are not necessarily expressed or acted upon' (Ponterotto and Pedersen 1993: 11). An individual who discriminates 'takes active steps to exclude or deny members of another group entrance or participation in a desired activity' (Ponterotto and Pedersen 1993: 34). Discrimination may exist in the absence of prejudice due to social pressures to conform or as a consequence of routine institutional practices.

VALUES

Values are influential in dictating the behaviour of a communicator in interethnic settings. Rokeach (1979: 2) defines a value 'as a type of belief that is centrally located within one's total belief system'. Values tell us of how we should behave. Values may be explicit (stated overtly in a value judgement) or implicit (inferred from nonverbal behaviour), and they may be individually held or seen as part of a cultural pattern or system. In addition to our unique set of personal values, individuals hold cultural values. Culture-bound values are especially relevant for intercultural communication. These include power-distance, uncertainty avoidance, individualism versus collectivism, and masculinity (Hofstede 1983); low and high context communication, immediacy and expressiveness (Hall 1966); emotional and behavioural expressiveness, and self disclosure.

There are several different conceptualisations of how cultures differ. Hofstede's work represents the best available attempt to measure empirically the nature and strength of value differences among cultures. He published the results of his study of over 100 000 employees of a large multinational in 40 countries (Hofstede 1983) and identified four dimensions that he labelled power-distance, uncertainty avoidance, individualism and masculinity.

POWER-DISTANCE

Each culture, and all people within cultures, develop ways of interacting with different people according to the status differential that exists between the individual and the person with whom he or she is interacting. Power-distance (PD) refers to the degree to which different cultures encourage or maintain power and status differences between interactants. Cultures high on PD develop rules, mechanisms and rituals that serve to maintain and strengthen the status relationships among their members. Cultures low on PD, however, minimise those rules and customs, eliminating, if not ignoring, the status differences that exist between people.

UNCERTAINTY AVOIDANCE

Uncertainty avoidance (UA) is a dimension observed in Hofstede's (1983) study that described the degree to which different cultures develop ways to deal with the anxiety and stress of uncertainty. It refers to 'how well people in a particular culture tolerate ambiguity and uncertainty' (Hofstede 1983: 65). Sex differences in 'uncertainty avoidance are negligible ... [and] the most important correlations are with national anxiety level' (Hofstede 1983: 110).

Differences in the level of uncertainty avoidance can result in unexpected problems in intercultural communication. For instance, when white British social workers communicate with a client from Pakistan, they are likely to be perceived as too non-confirming and unconventional by the client, and the social workers may view their client as rigid and overly controlled. Social and health workers need to have an understanding of the consequences of uncertainty avoidance for intercultural communication.

INDIVIDUALISM VERSUS COLLECTIVISM

Individualism and collectivism have been two of the most extensively studied concepts in the field of intercultural communication (e.g. Hofstede 1983; Triandis 1986) and is the major dimension of cultural variability used to explain intercultural differences in behaviour. Individualism refers to 'the subordination of the goals of the collectivities to individual goals, and a sense of independence and lack of concern for others', and collectivism refers to 'the subordination of individual goals to the goals of a collective and a sense of harmony, interdependence, and concern for others' (Hui and Triandis 1986: 244–245).

While cultures tend to be predominantly either individualistic or collectivistic, both exist in all cultures. Individualism has been central to the life of Western industrialised societies such as the US and Britain (Hofstede 1983). Collectivism is particularly high among Asian and African societies. However, diversity within each country is very possible. In the US, for instance, Hispanics and Asians tend to be more collectivist than other ethnic groups (Triandis 1990), and in Britain, Asians and African Caribbeans tend to be more collectivistic than white people.

To summarise, the individualism–collectivism dimension allows for similarities and differences in communication to be identified and explained across cultures.

MASCULINITY

The masculinity dimension refers to the degree to which cultures foster or maintain differences between the sexes in work-related values. Cultures high on masculinity such as Japan, Austria and Italy, were found to be associated with the greatest degree of sex differences in work-related values. Cultures low on masculinity – such as Denmark, Netherlands, Norway and Sweden – had the fewest differences between the sexes.

LOW AND HIGH CONTEXT COMMUNICATION

A high context communication or message is one in which 'most of the information is either in the physical context or internalised in the person, while very little is in the coded, explicit, transmitted part of the message' (Hall 1976: 79). High context cultures pay great attention to the surrounding circumstances or context of an event; thus, a high context communication relies heavily on nonverbals and the group identification/understanding shared by those communicating. It therefore follows that in interethnic communication the elements of phrasing, tone, gestures, posture, social status, history and social setting are all crucial to the meaning of the message.

As with individualism–collectivism, low and high context communication exists in all cultures, but one tends to predominate. Understanding that a client is from a high or low context culture, and the form of communication that predominates in these cultures, will make the black client's behaviour less confusing and more interpretable to the practitioner.

IMMEDIACY AND EXPRESSIVENESS

The 'immediacy dimension is anchored on one extreme by actions that simultaneously communicate closeness, approach, accessibility, and at the other extreme by behaviours expressing avoidance and distance' (Hecht *et al.* 1989: 167). Immediacy is the degree of perceived physical or psychological closeness between people (Richmond and McCroskey 1988). Immediacy behaviours communicate warmth, closeness and availability for communication. Examples of these behaviours are smiling, touching, eye contact, close personal distance and vocal animation. Cultures that reflect immediacy behaviours or expressiveness are often called 'high contact cultures' (Hall 1966).

EMOTIONAL AND BEHAVIOURAL EXPRESSIVENESS

Emotional expressiveness refers to the communication of feelings and thoughts. It 'can refer to both one's own and one's partner's expression, with lack of expressiveness on either one's part seen as dissatisfying'(Hecht *et al.* 1989: 392).

Hecht *et al.* (1989) report that African Americans perceive emotional expressiveness as important to their communication satisfaction with whites (European Americans). Other independent variables – related to communication satisfaction – identified by black people include: acceptance, authenticity, negative stereotyping, understanding, goal attainment and powerlessness (see Hecht *et al.* 1989 for a detailed review). Africans and African Caribbeans tend to be emotionally expressive, while whites have a more emotionally self-restrained style and often attempt to understate, avoid, ignore, or defuse intense or unpleasant situations. One of the dominant stereotypes of African Caribbeans in British society is that of the hostile, angry, prone-to-violence black male. It is not unusual for white practitioners to describe their black clients as being 'hostile and angry' (for example, see Fernando 2002).

SELF-DISCLOSURE

Self-disclosure refers to the client's willingness to tell the practitioner what she/he feels, believes or thinks. Interethnic comparisons of self-disclosure patterns show that European Americans are more disclosive than African Americans (Diamond and Hellcamp 1969) and Asians (Segal 1991).

Indeed, Segal (1991: 239) describes Indians as being 'reserved and reluctant to discuss their problems outside the family'. Most forms of counselling tend to value one's ability to self-disclose and to talk about the most intimate aspects of one's life. Indeed, self-disclosure has often been discussed as a primary characteristic of the healthy personality. The converse of this is that people who do not self-disclose readily in counselling are seen as possessing negative traits such as being guarded, mistrustful and/or paranoid. Intimate revelations of personal or social problems may not be acceptable to many Asians, since such difficulties reflect not only on the individual, but also on the whole family.

Social and health care workers unfamiliar with these cultural ramifications may perceive their clients in a very negative light. They may erroneously conclude that the client is repressed, inhibited, shy or passive. On the other hand, Asian clients may perceive the 'direct and confrontative techniques [of white practitioners] in communication as "lacking in respect for the client", and a reflection of insensitivity' (Sue and Sue 2002: 51).

Black people may also be reluctant to disclose to white practitioners because of hardships they have experienced via racism (Vontress 1981). For black people, 'race is a significant part of history and personal identity' (Vontress 1981: 16). Thus, the reality of racism in British society needs to be acknowledged in any counselling or social work relationship involving a black client (Phung 1995).

IMPLICATIONS FOR SOCIAL AND HEALTH CARE SERVICES

Each of Hofstede's four dimensions provides insights into the influence of culture on the communication process. As frames of reference, Hofstede's dimensions provide mechanisms to understand interethnic communication events. For instance, the consequences of the degree of power–distance that a culture prefers are evident in the relationship between the client and social worker. Clients raised in high power–distance cultures are expected to comply with the wishes and requests of their social workers and doctors, and conformity is regarded very favourably. Even the language systems (for example the Korean language) in high power–distance cultures emphasise distinctions based on a social hierarchy. Witte and Morrison (1995: 227) note that 'in many cultures [for example Asian], authority figures cannot be disagreed with, challenged, or contradicted'. Thus, 'differences in communication styles between healers and patients, especially in terms of politeness behaviour, may lead to miscommunication and misunderstandings' (Witte and Morrison 1995: 227).

A white practitioner with a monocultural perspective will view any behaviours, values and lifestyles that differed from the Euro-American norm as deficient (cultural racism). He or she will, for example, view certain nonverbal behaviours (lack of eye contact) as deviant behaviour. Eye contact during verbal communication is expected in Western culture because it implies attention and respect toward others. Among Asians, however, eye contact is considered a sign of lack of respect and attention, particularly to authority and older people. Cultures differ in their values on individualism versus collectivism; low and high context communication; immediacy and expressiveness; uncertainty avoidance; emotional and behavioural expressiveness; and self-disclosure. People from different cultures have different patterns of communication. Asians, coming from a high context culture, often rely on nonverbal communication, while Euro-Americans rely more on words. Asians' oral messages frequently are more implicit and depend more on context (people and situations), while Euro-Americans' verbal messages are explicit and less concerned with context. Members of Asian cultures are more likely to be offended by direct and explicit messages and prefer indirect and implicit messages (Witte and Morrison 1995). There may be clear rules regarding how older members of the family should be addressed by the younger members. This attitude will influence the doctor–patient or social worker–client relationship, because if the patient or client is not used to challenging authority figures they will conform to everything suggested by the doctor or social worker. Problems with medical regimens may occur unintentionally or intentionally due to these politeness norms.

Many social and health care practitioners are not aware of their own value biases (Sue and Sue 2002). Katz (1985: 616) points out that 'because White culture is the dominant cultural norm in the United States [and Britain], it acts as an invisible veil that limits many people from seeing it as a cultural system'. There is an identifiable 'dominant' value system in Britain that is associated with the majority (white middle class) group, and which pervades most social work courses (Dominelli 1997). Practitioners need to understand the value bases of the power–dominant cultural system that forms the basis of training and practice. White people in Britain are raised to believe that their value system is the most appropriate, 'the best', and that people possessing non-middle class white values should try their best to assimilate and adapt to the majority culture system. This ethnocentric bias serves as a barrier to effective interethnic communication. Social and health care workers who have little understanding of black (Asian and African Caribbean) culture tend to look upon the black client's values and culture as inherently inferior to their own. For example, as noted earlier, black people come from cultures that value group affiliation and collectivism. Practitioners from a Eurocentric perspective – where individualism is valued – may misinterpret the behaviour of these clients as codependency.

Most major theories of social work, counselling and psychotherapy originated in Eurocentric ideology. To use traditional counselling theories beneficially with black people, counsellors need to evaluate them for cultural bias. Some assumptions identified by Pedersen (1988) reflecting cultural bias in counselling are:

- a common measure of 'normal behaviour';
- emphasis on individualism;
- overemphasis on independence; and
- cultural encapsulation.

Traditionally trained counsellors and social workers are so caught up in their own belief system that they are unaware of their specific values, and they neglect to realise that there are alternative, equally justifiable cultural value systems.

CONCLUSION

Some disparity does exist in beliefs and values between communicators of different racial and cultural backgrounds. There is no simple effective solution to the problem of interethnic belief and value conflict. However, social and health care workers must try in interethnic settings to step outside themselves in order to gain an understanding of the reality of others.

Social and health care workers should be aware both of their own attitudes and behaviour and those communication situations in which they are likely to display negative behaviours. Such an awareness is at least a first step in mitigating problems in black and white verbal and nonverbal communication. Practitioners need to be conscious that racist attitudes, even when expressed in a subtle or unconscious fashion, can disrupt the interethnic communication process.

Social and health care workers need to have an understanding of the taxonomies that can be used to describe cultural variations. These taxonomies include Hall's high and low context cultural patterns and Hofstede's four dimensions – power–distance, uncertainty, avoidance, individualism–collectivism, and masculinity–femininity, along which the dominant patterns of a culture can be ordered. Taken together, these taxonomies provide multiple frames of reference that can be used to understand intercultural communication. Other culture-bound values discussed in this chapter were emotional/behavioural expressiveness and self-disclosure patterns.

The practitioner's values will lead them to communicate in certain ways, because values will determine which ways of communicating are deemed more desirable than others. Conflict in value systems is a major cause of communication breakdown in interethnic settings. As noted earlier, the problem that arises with the difference in values is that we tend to use our own values as the standard when judging others. We tend to assume that our value system is best, an assumption that causes us to make value judgements of others. White practitioners need to become more aware of their own values and beliefs and should be encouraged to share these in interethnic communication. Practitioners should consciously examine the bases of their values and beliefs and the actual role served by them in their own life as well as in their culture. Workers can then determine whether any of their values and beliefs are serving as deterrents to good interethnic communication.

This chapter is based on Robinson, L. (1998) *'Race', Communication and the Caring Professions*, Buckingham: Open University Press.

REFERENCES

Allport, G.W. (1979) *The Nature of Prejudice*, Reading, MA: Addison-Wesley.

Baron, R.A. and Byrne, D. (2002) *Social Psychology*, London: Allyn and Bacon.

Diamond, R. and Hellcamp, D. (1969) 'Race, sex, ordinal position of birth, and self-disclosure in high school', *Psychological Reports* 35: 235–238.

Dominelli, L. (1997) *Anti-racist Social Work*, London: Macmillan.

Fernando, S. (2002) *Mental Health, Race and Culture*, London: Macmillan.

Fishbein, M. and Ajzen, I. (1975) *Belief, Attitude, Intention, and Behavior: An Introduction to Theory and Research*, Reading, MA: Addison-Wesley.

Hall, E.T. (1966) *The Hidden Dimension*, New York: Doubleday.

Hall, E.T. (1976) *Beyond Culture*, New York: Anchor Press/Doubleday.

Hecht, L.M., Ribeau, S. and Alberts, J.K. (1989) *An Afro-American Perspective on Interethnic Communication*, Communication Monographs, 56: 385–410.

Hofstede, G. (1983) 'Dimensions of national cultures in fifty countries and three regions', in Deregowski, J.B., Dziurawiec, S. and Annis, R.C. (eds) *Explanations in Cross-cultural Psychology*, Lisse: Swets and Zeitlinger.

Hui, H.C. and Triandis, H.C. (1986) 'Individualism-collectivism: a study of cross-cultural researchers', *Journal of Cross-cultural Psychology* 17: 225–248.

Katz, J.H. (1985) 'The sociopolitical nature of counseling', *The Counseling Psychologist* 13: 615–624.

Pedersen, P.B. (1988) *A Handbook for Developing Multicultural Awareness. Alexandria*, VA: American Counseling Association.

Phung, T. (1995) 'An experience of inter-cultural counseling: views from a black client', *Counselling* February, 61–62.

Ponterotto, J.G. and Pedersen, P.B. (1993) *Preventing Prejudice: A Guide for Counselors and Educators*, London: Sage.

Richmond, V.P. and McCroskey, J.C. (1988) *Communication: Apprehension, Avoidance and Effectiveness*, Scottsdale, AZ: Goorsuch Scarisbrick.

Rokeach, M. (1973) *The Nature of Human Values*, New York: The Free Press.

Segal, U.A. (1991) 'Cultural variables in Asian Indian families', *The Journal of Contemporary Human Services* 11: 233–241.

Sue, D.W. and Sue, D. (2002) *Counseling the Culturally Different*, New York: John Wiley and Sons.

Triandis, H. (1986) 'Collectivism vs. individualism: A reconceptualization of a basic concept in cross-cultural psychology', in Bagley, C. and Verma, G. (eds) *Personality, Cognition, and Values: Cross-cultural Perspectives of Childhood and Adolescence*, London: Macmillan.

Triandis, H.C. (1990) 'Toward cross-cultural studies of individualism and collectivism in Latin America', *Interamerican Journal of Psychology* 24: 199–210.

Vontress, C. (1981) 'Racial and ethical barriers in Counseling', in Pederson, P., Draguns, J.G., Lanner, W.J. and Trimble J.E. (eds) Counseling Across Cultures, Honolulu: University of Hawaii Press.

Witte, K. and Morrison, K. (1995) 'Intercultural and cross-cultural health communication', in Wiseman, R.L. (ed.) *Intercultural Communication Theory*, London: Sage.

CHAPTER 13

MEN TALKING ABOUT FATHERHOOD: DISCOURSE AND IDENTITIES

Martin Robb

Fathers and fatherhood have become an important topic of public interest and debate in recent years, with autobiographical accounts by fathers and explorations of the state of contemporary fatherhood a staple of the news media and popular culture (Lupton and Barclay 1997). This concern has been reflected at the level of public policy, particularly since the election of the first New Labour government in 1997. Encouraging fathers' active involvement in family life has been a consistent strand in a range of Labour initiatives (Home Office 1998; Toynbee and Walker 2001), which in turn has led to a greater emphasis on involving fathers in health and social care services, for example, in the work of family centres and in child protection (Ghate 2000; Ryan 2000).

This new focus on fatherhood reflects a number of diverse ideological strands, including an egalitarian agenda that is concerned with promoting gender equality (Cameron *et al.* 1999; Robb 2001), as well as the influence of New Right thinking on the supposed link between fathers' absence and family and community breakdown (Murray 1990; Dennis and Erdos 1993). What these different discourses have in common is an emphasis on promoting the active involvement of fathers in family life, as something that is seen to be good both for children and for men themselves.

Despite this increasing focus on fatherhood, comparatively little is known about men's experience as fathers, particularly at a time when ideas about fathers' roles are undergoing such dramatic change. This is not to say that research on fatherhood has been lacking. However, until quite recently the main focus was on fathers' influence on their children (Lamb

1997; Warin *et al.* 1999). Although some recent studies have begun to explore the subjective experience of fatherhood (for example, Plantin *et al.* 2003), there is a need for more detailed exploration of what fatherhood means to men, and of the ways in which personal meanings intersect with wider and changing public discourses.

FATHERS, IDENTITIES AND DISCOURSE

This chapter reports the findings of a research study that used a discourse analytic approach to explore the meanings that men attach to their experience as fathers. The research involved in-depth interviews with a random sample of British fathers of young children and made use of methods drawn from critical discursive psychology. The study was rooted in a poststructuralist understanding of identities as constituted in and through discourse. In Stuart Hall's words:

> *identities are never unified and, in late modern times, increasingly fragmented and fractured; never singular but multiply constructed across different, often intersecting discourses, practices and positions.*
>
> (Hall 1996: 17)

This applies to gender identities, including masculinities, which need to be understood as plural and dynamic, rather than as fixed and immutable (Connell 1995).

Critical discursive psychology, while sharing these basic poststructuralist assumptions, provides a methodological approach that enables an examination of the specific mechanisms whereby individuals produce their identities in discourse. Discussing the ways in which masculinities are discursively constructed, Nigel Edley makes the claim that:

> *when people talk, they do so using a lexicon or repertoire of terms which has been provided for them by history.*
>
> (Edley 2001: 190)

From this perspective, understanding the meanings that fatherhood holds for men involves paying attention to the ways in which they talk about their experience as fathers, analysing the frameworks and strategies that they utilise to make sense of their experience. Edley describes three distinctive concepts offered by discursive psychology as tools for analysing spoken discourse:

- interpretative repertoires;
- ideological dilemmas; and
- subject positions.

In what follows, I will use these concepts as a framework for summarising the findings of my own research with fathers.

INTERPRETATIVE REPERTOIRES: FATHERHOOD AS PRESENCE AND INVOLVEMENT

The concept of interpretative repertoires was imported into social psychology from the sociology of scientific knowledge by Jonathan Potter and Margaret Wetherell, who have defined them as:

> *basically a lexicon or register of terms and metaphors drawn upon to characterise and evaluate actions and events.*
>
> (Potter and Wetherell 1987: 138)

Interpretative repertoires can be described as culturally-available frameworks that enable individuals to make sense of their experience. As such they have something in common with the Foucauldian concept of discourses, though according to Edley:

> *compared to discourses, interpretative repertoires are seen as less monolithic ... they are viewed as much smaller and more fragmented, offering speakers a whole range of different rhetorical opportunities.*
>
> (Edley 2001: 202)

In describing their experience as fathers, the participants in this study drew on a number of shared meaning–making frameworks. Perhaps the dominant framework was one that saw the essence of fatherhood as simply spending time with one's children:

> *I see a lot of fathers who are, they come home from work, the kids are there, 'Hi, how are you doing, blah blah', and then down the pub and, you know, to me, giving your kids everything, I mean you can give your kids everything, Playstation, you can give them bikes, you can give them everything, but what they need, what they want is your time*

> *and well, it's time with you and for you to show them, you know, what you think about them. They want to be with you.*
>
> (Paul, Mauritian, 37)[1]

Tony (white, 48) also distanced himself from fathers who are 'absent a lot of the time, you know, they leave the house at seven in the morning, or whatever, and don't get back until seven at night'. By comparison, he says: 'I do feel that, most of the time, I'm there for them'.

Building on this underlying sense of fatherhood as 'presence', participants echoed public rhetoric on fatherhood in their repeated use of the word 'involved' to describe their role. Involvement tended to be both practical and emotional. When asked to describe their experiences of fatherhood, interviewees often began with a list of the practical tasks that they regularly undertook. As for emotional involvement, Paul claimed: 'I think there's a strong bond, a strong relationship between us', while Sean said:

> *I don't think there's anything wrong, and I think on the contrary it's good for men like myself to try and have this meaningful emotional relationship with their children, and that we also try and do the practical domestic tasks.*
>
> (Sean, white, 33)

Sean talked about the 'emotional adjustments' required by fatherhood, 'having to put your children's needs over your own feelings'.

All of the participants in this study described their own fathers as emotionally distant:

> *I don't think he had much time to be a loving father, if you see what I mean. He was a father figure and that was it, yeah, he was the head of the family, and it was his responsibility to bring up the family.*
>
> (Paul)

Comparing himself with his father, Gordon (white, 42) said: 'My own father wasn't really affectionate towards me, but I would see that element in the relationship with Charlie [his son]'. Sean stated that his aim as a father 'is to be close to my children, closer than my dad was, on an emotional level, that kind of thing'.

These responses demonstrate that, in developing their own personal meanings of fatherhood experience, the men in this study drew heavily on the dominant ideal of the actively involved and emotionally engaged father.

IDEOLOGICAL DILEMMAS: FATHERHOOD AND AMBIVALENCE

The concept of ideological dilemmas was first developed by Billig *et al.* (1988) as a way of capturing the fragmentary and contradictory nature of everyday common sense. In this view, lived ideologies are inherently dilemmatic, or structured around contradictions. Everyday discourse tends to revolve around sets of oppositions that have to be worked through and resolved. The ways in which the participants in this study discussed their experience as fathers reflected at least two shared ideological dilemmas.

The most obvious tension was between responsibility and freedom. Paul claimed that becoming a father had made him 'grow up' and 'become a lot more responsible than I used to be', and he described himself as being 'responsible for two children that I've brought into the world'. At the same time he admitted to being envious of men who were not fathers and confessed: 'I'd just like to be able to be my own person every now and then and just be free enough to, you know, do whatever I want to do, whatever I have to do'. Tony's talk, too, was balanced between an acceptance of responsibility and keen regret at the loss of personal freedom:

> *Well, it's completely changed my life, actually. Um, because before, yeah, I had the time to do anything I wanted, virtually. Um, yeah, it's just not having the time, I mean you just have to switch your commitment to the family, really, and I actually resented the loss of my leisure time a lot [...] You know, it's quite good fun, really, picking them up from school, you feel that, the responsibility, I think weighs quite heavily. You do feel very responsible for them and very scared that something might go wrong for them, you want to protect them.*
>
> (Tony)

Gordon's ambivalence was neatly encapsulated in this response: 'I enjoy being with Charlie. You have less personal time, you have less personal space'. Sean repeatedly described fatherhood in terms of 'responsibilities', commenting:

> *I think it's an enormous change to your lifestyle in the sense that without children, whether you're single or in a partnership, you have enormous amounts of sort of freedom, freedom of your time, freedom of the structure of the day. Freedom in social life and so on.*
>
> (Sean)

The other main tension in these men's talk was between a sense of fatherhood as struggle, and a contrasting sense of the pleasures of being a father. For Tony, the sense of fatherhood as a difficult experience was especially keen: 'I've just found it more of a strain than I thought it was going to be, to be quite honest [...] I have struggled with aspects of it, really'. Sean mentioned the 'difficult adjustments' involved in becoming a father, but added: 'I really enjoy my children ... It's enjoyable just looking after them doing simple things'.

These dilemmas point to a fundamental ambivalence in men's experience of fatherhood, and to the importance of discourse (in this case the research interview) as a means of working through these perceived tensions.

POSITIONING: OTHER MEN AS POINTS OF REFERENCE

Interpretative repertoires offer individuals subject positions from which to view themselves and make sense of their experience (Edley 2001: 209). The negotiation of personal identities involves positioning oneself in relation both to external discourses and to other people, whether real or imagined (Davies and Harré 1990). The men interviewed for this study frequently defined themselves as fathers by comparing and contrasting themselves with others. Sometimes the 'other' was the man's partner, but often it was other men who were the point of reference:

> *I've never been a stereotypical man, I mean, I'm not into football, I'm not into going to the pub all the time, every now and then I do, but I'm not the stereotypical type of man.*
>
> (Paul)

Interestingly, the most significant 'other' in relation to whom all of these men positioned themselves was their own fathers, despite an almost universal sense of their fathers' emotional distance:

> *My father's dead, he died about ten years ago. He wasn't an affectionate person, because he didn't know how to be. He never touched me [...] Well, I'm not saying ever, but probably the only memories I've got of him touching me is probably hitting me.*
>
> (Gordon)

The accounts presented by other participants were more ambivalent. Paul told the story of his Mauritian father's migration to Britain and his aspirations for his children: 'Dad knew what he wanted for us [...] he put us through different schools'. Paul added, more negatively: 'I don't think he had much time to be a loving father'. Despite this, Paul clearly admired his father for other qualities: 'but considering the way that my father was, he never discouraged me in doing things [...] my dad always said I can do whatever I think I can do'.

This kind of complex relationship was replicated in the responses of other participants, including Tony who stated: 'My father was very strict, very strict, he came from a Catholic, working-class background'. Although he was frightened of his father, Tony also claimed that to he 'enjoyed' him as a father. Sean's account of his father articulated a similar ambivalence. On the one hand 'he was very much a get up and go to work, come home, tea on the table, didn't have a lot to do with us, type father', but at the same time he remembered his father as joking and humorous. While describing him as absent both physically and emotionally, Sean admired his father's 'responsibility' as a breadwinner:

> *So, in that sense, he was doing his job and given the choice of being like my father, being like I am, or being like a young man now with no responsibilities, I think I'd rather be like my dad, than be like a dad who shirked both sets of responsibilities.*
>
> (Sean)

For all of these men, their own fathers were crucial but ambivalent points of reference in their own construction of fatherhood identities, neither completely disowned nor unequivocally admired.

NARRATIVES OF FATHERHOOD EXPERIENCE

According to Davies and Harré, 'conceptions people have about themselves are disjointed unless they are located in a story' (Davies and Harré 1990: 270). Although not featuring in Edley's outline, narrative is a concept that has become increasingly important within social psychology and in the social sciences more generally. Kenneth Gergen proposes a 'relational view of self-conception, one that views self-conception not as an individual's personal and private cognitive structure but as *discourse* about the self' (Gergen 1994: 247). Individuals do not produce narratives out of thin air, but using resources from the wider culture: 'To possess an intelligible self – a recognisable being with both a past and a future – requires a borrowing from the cultural repository' (Gergen 1994: 257).

It is possible to identify a number of shared narrative strategies, as well as some significant variations, in the talk of the fathers interviewed for this study. While drawing on shared frameworks reflecting dominant discourses of fatherhood, each participant did so in a distinctive way. The men interviewed interwove their individual narratives of fatherhood with other kinds of personal narrative, which in turn drew on wider cultural resources. Thus, Paul's story of his experience as a father was closely bound up with, and influenced by, narratives of class mobility and cultural migration. Paul's sense of what it means to be a good father was grounded in a story in which he saw myself moving away from the activities that he associated with working-class masculinity (going to the pub, 'spoiling' his children with material things) and towards a more middle-class lifestyle, which involved spending more time at home and finding 'good' schools for the children. Paul also contrasted his memory of the way Mauritian men shared in domestic tasks with the lack of such involvement among men whom he knew in Britain. In other words, Paul's fatherhood identity was closely interwoven with his class and cultural identities. A very different kind of narrative was developed by James (white, 38), a part-time Christian minister, whose account of his experience as a father was woven into a story of spiritual development, in which the struggles and challenges of fatherhood were viewed in part as a means to personal growth.

The variability in fathers' narratives is a reminder of the diversity of meanings that fatherhood can attract to itself, while making use of a shared pool of cultural meanings. It demonstrates, too, that notions of what it means to be a 'good' father are never culturally neutral, but are bound up with factors of class, ethnicity and culture. The examples quoted here raise questions as to whether the ideal of the practically and emotionally 'involved' father currently being promoted by public policy, in fact reflects a particular kind of white, middle-class experience.

CONCLUSION

The research findings discussed in this chapter suggest that, in attempting to make sense of their experience of fathers, men draw on some common frameworks that reflect the influence of dominant public discourses about fatherhood. In negotiating their identities as fathers, men appear to face similar sets of dilemmas and to articulate a shared ambivalence about their roles. Other men, and especially their own fathers, play a complex but powerful role as points of reference in the construction of individual fatherhood identities. Finally, men's narratives of fatherhood experience, while drawing on shared resources, are variable and diverse, reflecting differences of class and culture. More generally, the findings of this study demonstrate the complex ways in which men's identities as fathers are produced in and through discourse and the complex interaction between personal narratives and public discourses.

ACKNOWLEDGEMENTS

The research discussed in this chapter was made possible by a grant from the research committee of the School of Health and Social Welfare, The Open University.

NOTE

1 All names used in this chapter are pseudonyms. Details of ethnicity are drawn from participants' self-descriptions.

REFERENCES

Billig, M., Condor, S., Edwards, D., Gane, M., Middleton, D. and Radley, A. (1988) *Ideological Dilemmas: A Social Psychology of Everyday Thinking*, London: Sage.

Cameron, C., Moss, P. and Owen, C. (1999) *Men in the Nursery: Gender and Caring Work*, London: Paul Chapman.

Connell, R. (1995) *Masculinities*, Sydney: Allen & Unwin.

Davies, B. and Harré, R. (1990) 'Positioning: the *discursive* production of selves', *Journal for the Theory of Social Behaviour* 20: 43–65.

Dennis, N. and Erdos, G. (1993) *Families without Fatherhood*, London: Institute of Economic Affairs, Health and Welfare Unit.

Edley, N. (2001) 'Analysing masculinity: interpretative repertoires, ideological dilemmas and subject positions', in Wetherell, M., Taylor, S. and Yates, S.J. *Discourse as Data: A Guide for Analysis*. London: Sage/The Open University.

Gergen, K.J. (1994) *Realities and Relationships: Soundings in Social Construction*, Cambridge, MA: Harvard University Press.

Ghate, D. (2000) *Fathers and Family Centres*, London: Family Policy Research Bureau/Joseph Rowntree Foundation.

Hall, S. (1996) 'Introduction: who needs identity?' in Hall, S. and du Gay, P. (eds) *Questions of Cultural Identity*, London: Sage.

Home Office (1998) *Supporting Families. A Consultation Document*, London: HMSO.

Lamb, M. (ed.) (1997) *The Role of the Father in Child Development*, New York: Wiley.

Lupton, D. and Barclay, L. (1997) *Constructing Fatherhood: Discourses and Experiences*, London: Sage.

Murray, C. (1990) *The Emerging British Underclass*, London, Institute of Economic Affairs.

Plantin, L., Mansson, S.-A. and Kearney, J. (2003) 'Talking and doing fatherhood: on fatherhood and masculinity in Sweden and England', *Fathering: A Journal of Theory, Research and Pratice About Men as Fathers* 1: 1.

Potter, J. and Wetherell, M. (1987) *Discourse and Social Psychology: Beyond Attitudes and Behaviour*, London: Sage.

Robb, M. (2001) 'Men working in childcare', in Foley, P., Roche, J. and Tucker, S. *Children in Society: Contemporary Theory, Policy and Practice*, Basingstoke: Palgrave/The Open University.

Ryan, M. (2000) *Working with Fathers*, Department of Health/Radcliffe Medical Press.

Toynbee, P. and Walker, D. (2001) *Did Things Get Better? An Audit of Labour's Successes and Failures*, London: Penguin.

Warin, J., Salomon, Y., Lewis, C. and Langford W. (1999) *Fathers, Work and Family Life*, London Family Policy Study Centre/Joseph Rowntree Foundation.

CHAPTER 14

ANTI-OPPRESSIVE PRACTICE

Beverley Burke and Philomena Harrison

INTRODUCTION

The complex nature of oppression is witnessed in the lives of people who are marginalised in this society. As social work practitioners, we have a moral, ethical and legal responsibility to challenge inequality and disadvantage. Historically, the profession, in attempting to understand, explain and offer solutions to the difficulties experienced by groups and individuals, has drawn from, among others, the disciplines of sociology, psychology, history, philosophy and politics. This multidisciplined theoretical framework, informed by anti-oppressive principles, provides social workers with a tool to understand and respond to the complexity of the experience of oppression.

This chapter explores how a theorised social work practice informed by anti-oppressive principles can be sensitively and effectively used to address the inequalities of oppression that determine the life chances of service users. [...]

Black feminist thought is a dynamic perspective, derived from 'diverse lived experiences', that not only analyses human interactions based on principles of equality, but also considers the interconnections that exist between the major social divisions of class, race, gender, disability, sexuality and age as they impact on the individual, family and community. [...]

We hold the view that personal experiences are inextricably linked to and determined by social, cultural, political and economic relationships within specific geographical and historical situations. This process of location allows us to challenge those who see only our race, gender or class,

Source: Adams, R., Dominelli, L. and Payne, M. (2002) *Anti-Oppressive Practice*, Basingstoke: Palgrave MacMillan Ltd: 227–236.

failing to understand that it is the interconnections between the social divisions to which we belong that defines who we are (Lorde 1984).

The finding of solutions to and explanations of oppressive situations and practices poses a real challenge for those committed to making a difference. A starting point would, therefore, have to be a clear understanding of what is meant by anti-oppressive practice.

WHAT IS ANTI-OPPRESSIVE PRACTICE?

[. . .]

Anti-oppressive practice is a dynamic process based on the changing complex patterns of social relations. It is, therefore, important that a definition is informed by research within academic institutions, practitioner research and the views of service users. For the purposes of this chapter, we provide below a 'definition' (with all the attendant problems of defining) which incorporates points already discussed providing a framework to clarify and inform practice.

Clifford (1995: 65) uses the term 'anti-oppressive':

> *to indicate an explicit evaluative position that constructs social divisions (especially 'race', class, gender, disability, sexual orientation and age) as matters of broad social structure, at the same time as being personal and organisational issues. It looks at the use and abuse of power not only in relation to individual or organisational behaviour, which may be overtly, covertly or indirectly racist, classist, sexist and so on, but also in relation to broader social structures for example, the health, educational, political and economic, media and cultural systems and their routine provision of services and rewards for powerful groups at local as well as national and international levels. These factors impinge on people's life stories in unique ways that have to be understood in their socio-historical complexity.*
>
> (Clifford 1995: 65)

Within this definition, there is a clear understanding of the use and abuse of power within relationships on personal, family, community, organisational and structural levels. These levels are not mutually exclusive – they are interconnected, shaping and determining social reality. Clifford, informed by the writings of black feminist and other 'non-dominant perspectives' (Clifford 1995), has formulated the following anti-oppressive principles, which provide the foundation for a social work assessment that is theorised and empowering:

- *Social difference.* Social differences arise because of disparities of power between the dominant and dominated social groups. The major divisions are described in terms of race, gender, class, sexual preference, disability and age. Other differences, such as those of religion, region, mental health and single parenthood, exist and interact with the major divisions, making the understanding and experience of oppression a complex matter.
- *Linking personal and political.* Personal biographies are placed within a wider social context and the individual's life situation is viewed in relation to social systems such as the family, peer groups, organisations and communities. For example, the problems associated with ageing are not solely due to the individual but should be understood in relation to the ageist ideologies, policies and practices that exist within the social environment in which the individual is located.
- *Power.* Power is a social concept which can be used to explore the public and private spheres of life (Barker and Roberts 1993). In practice, power can be seen to operate at the personal and structural levels. It is influenced by social, cultural, economic and psychological factors. All these factors need to be taken into account in any analysis of how individuals or groups gain differential access to resources and positions of power.
- *Historical and geographical location.* Individual life experiences and events are placed within a specific time and place, so that these experiences are given meaning within the context of prevailing ideas, social facts and cultural differences.
- *Reflexivity/mutual involvement.* Reflexivity is the continual consideration of how values, social difference and power affect the interactions between individuals. These interactions are to be understood not only in psychological terms, but also as a matter of sociology, history, ethics and politics.

The above principles relate to each other, interconnecting and overlapping at all times. Working from a perspective that is informed by anti-oppressive principles provides an approach that begins to match the complex issues of power, oppression and powerlessness that determine the lives of the people who are recipients of social care services. An understanding of these principles brings with it a fundamental transformation in the relationship that exists between the assessment of a situation and the nature of the action that is required to change the existing state of affairs.

The driving force of anti-oppressive practice is *the act of challenging inequalities*. Opportunities for change are created by the process of the challenge. Challenges are not always successful and are often painful for the person or group being challenged or challenging. A challenge, at its best, involves changes at macro- and micro-levels. If anti-oppressive practice is to provide appropriate and sensitive services that are needs-led rather than resource-driven, it has to embody:

> *a person centred philosophy; and egalitarian value system concerned with reducing the deleterious effects of structural inequalities upon people's lives; a methodology focusing on both process and outcome; and a way of structuring relationships between individuals that aims to empower users by reducing the negative effects of social hierarchies on their interaction and the work they do together.*
>
> (Dominelli 1994: 3)

Work in welfare organisations is constrained by financial, social, legislative and organisational policies. Social workers operating within such an environment will inevitably face conflicting and competing demands on their personal and professional resources. The use of anti-oppressive principles offers the worker a way of responding to and managing these sometimes hostile and disempowering situations which affect both worker and user. [...]

A decision was made by a social services department that changed the life of a family. A young, single, 19-year-old black woman was told that the care plan regarding her 20-month-old son was that of adoption. The decision was based on evidence from extended social work involvement, which was ultimately influenced by information obtained from reports written by a white male psychologist and a white female psychiatrist. [...]

AMELIA'S STORY

Amelia had left home at the age of sixteen and a year later began living with a man who became violent towards her when she was pregnant. Going into a hostel for mothers with children, Amelia experienced racial abuse and began taking heroin which was freely available there. She gave birth to her son three months prematurely and spent a stressful time visiting him during his recovery. Her appeals for financial support for travelling to the hospital went unheard.

After her son's discharge from hospital Amelia felt overwhelmed when her son became ill. She started taking drugs to cope and he was taken into care again. To get him back Amelia had to be assessed as a fit carer. Meantime non-black foster parents, despite her objections to this, fostered her son.

Amelia's son was returned to her under a supervision order. The combination of feeling unable to cope with living alone; the lack of any nursery placement, and her disclosure (as a request for help) that she had attempted to harm her son – culminated in him being taken back into care. After 'keeping' her son following a visit, Amelia's access to him was restricted.

She was afraid to display the strong emotions that she felt about her loss – in case this harmed her case to get her son back. The threat of him being adopted left Amelia in a state of uncertainty about how to fight to keep him.

THEORY INTO PRACTICE

[...]
The anti-oppressive principle of *reflexivity* demands that workers continually consider the ways in which their own social identity and values affect the information they gather. This includes their understanding of the social world as experienced by themselves and those with whom they work. The remainder of this chapter focuses on Amelia's story.

Involvement in Amelia's life is not a neutral event. It is determined by the interaction between the personal biographies of the worker and Amelia, and will be expressed in the power relationships that arise from their membership of differing social divisions.

For example, a white male social worker brings to the situation a dynamic that will reproduce the patterns of oppression to which black women are subjected in the wider society. In this scenario, Amelia feels she is silenced. Her plea for 'someone to talk to', to be listened to and taken seriously, is neither understood nor acted upon. This is highlighted in the powerlessness expressed in the telling of her story.

The challenge to you, the worker, is to reflect on your social division membership, your personal and professional biography and the impact that this will have on your involvement with Amelia. Are you the right worker for her? If the answer is no, the challenge is not only to find a more appropriate worker but to look to ways in which you may minimise the potential for oppressive practice at the point of referral. In and through this process of thinking and reflecting, which should take place in supervision, team discussions and interactions with service users, you will begin to work in an anti-oppressive way.

Society is divided along the major divisions of race, class, gender, sexual preference, disability and age. There are also other divisions which occur as a result of inequality and discrimination, such as poverty, geographical location, mental distress and employment status. The *social difference* principle is based on an understanding of how the divisions interconnect and shape the lives of people.

Amelia is young, black, unemployed, female, of a particular class background, living in poverty and a single parent. Yet in the scenario, she is seen merely as a young woman suffering domestic violence and in need of accommodation. Her needs as a black woman from a particular background with a specific history are not fully considered. Amelia's experience of racism in the hostel compounded her overall experience of oppression, forcing her into independence before she was ready.

The challenge for you, the worker, is to understand both the specific and general nature of social division membership and how it may contribute to the individual's experience of oppression. As a worker, you must make a systematic analysis of the social division membership of all the individuals involved in Amelia's life and understand the relevance of this for your intervention.

It is important to locate both Amelia's and her son's life experiences and events within a *historical and geographical context*. Those experiences need to be chronologically charted and their relevance clearly understood and applied to Amelia's story. In doing that, you, the worker, will get an accurate picture of how events within the family, community and society have influenced Amelia's current situation. Amelia's story will have been influenced by previous specific historical and geographical factors.

As the worker, you need to be aware of how prevailing ideologies have influenced legislation, agency policy and practice relating to childcare, homelessness and parenting by single mothers. The challenge is to use that analysis to inform your assessment and decision-making. You need to question the agency's policies on work with homeless young women. Amelia's needs as a homeless, black young woman were never assessed with reference to research evidence which documents the oppression and lack of services faced by this specific user group.

The principle of historical and geographic context directs the worker to consider not only the individual worker's relationship with the service user, but also the team and agency practice. The following are some of the questions that need to be considered: 'How does a prevailing ideology of a mixed economy of care affect practice within the team?'; 'How does the team prioritise work with homeless young people?'; and 'How far has the historical development of service provision in the area determined current practices?' Such questions will help workers to understand what is constraining their practice. Anti-oppressive thinking moves the worker beyond the confines of agency policy and practice and directs the challenge more appropriately.

In understanding the *personal* as *political*, the everyday life experiences of individuals need to be located within social, cultural, political and economic structures which are historically and geographically specific. This process of location ensures that, in practice, the individual is not pathologised, and weight is given to the interconnections and interactions between that individual's story and the social systems they encounter.

Amelia is defined in terms of the domestic violence she has experienced. The assessment is not placed in a wider context, failing to make sense of Amelia's whole life experience. You, the worker, need to take into account the structural factors that contribute to womens' experience of violence and how, for Amelia, the dimension of race and her membership of other social divisions added other layers to her experience of oppression.

The social workers' decision in the scenario to formulate a care plan which put forward adoption as a solution to Amelia's problems needs to be analysed. Their decision appears to be highly influenced by the expert evidence which focused on Amelia's psychiatric and psychological functioning. How did these assessments inform the workers' analysis of Amelia's ability to parent adequately? Here, we see a failure to locate assessment evidence within a framework that takes into account all aspects of Amelia's existence – her gender, her race, her poverty, her single parenthood – as well as making reference to assessment evidence from other professionals.

The challenge to the worker is to examine the range of evidence used in decision-making, asking questions about why any one piece of evidence is given more weight than another. Does that weighting pathologise the individual by not taking into account the assessments made by other professionals, such as the health visitor and the foster carers. For example, was the support offered by the extended family and informal community support networks considered? By ignoring the impact of oppressive social values and policies in the decision-making process, the worker can further devalue the service user's capacity to function.

In addressing *power* and *powerlessness*, it is essential to understand how the differential access to power shapes and determines relationships on an individual, group, community, organisational and societal level. We get a glimpse of Amelia's feelings of powerlessness when she says, 'I do not know how I can fight any of this'. Central to her powerlessness is the lack of access to many social resources. There is evidence in Amelia's story of her being denied access to the resources she feels will help her to parent effectively.

You, as the worker, need to take into account the professional and personal power (based on your particular social division membership) you hold. What power does the service user have from her previous life experiences?

How do you, as a worker, ensure that your assessment and intervention includes an analysis of power? The worker in this situation could have advocated on behalf of Amelia, working creatively to explore other options which would have supported her in her parenting. It appears that the workers ignored the personal strengths of Amelia, gained from her experiences of oppression, leading to practice which compounded her feelings of powerlessness. They failed to listen and work in partnership with Amelia.

The misuse of power by the worker culminates in a situation in which decisions can be made where the outcome labels Amelia as a non-deserving case. Amelia, however, is not alone in her powerlessness. There are clear differences of the power ascribed to the opinions of one professional group over another. It appears that extended social work practice had little impact on the overall decision regarding the future of the family. Explanations of Amelia's behaviour are reduced to the opinions of one professional group who are seen as 'expert', reducing complex explanations of her behaviour to psychology and psychiatry.

Social workers are well placed to make assessments that are theoretically informed, holistic, empowering and challenging. Anti-oppressive practice should not negate the risks posed to the child. Intervention based on anti-oppressive practice incorporates a risk and needs analysis of both mother and child.

To work effectively, it is important to have a perspective that:

- is flexible without losing focus;
- includes the views of oppressed individuals and groups;
- is theoretically informed;
- challenges and changes existing ideas and practice;
- can analyse the oppressive nature of organisational culture and its impact on practice;
- includes continuous reflection and evaluation of practice;
- has multidimensional change strategies which incorporate the concepts of networking, user involvement, partnership and participation;
- has a critical analysis of the issues of power, both personal and structural.

[...] Service users, practitioners, students and academics continue to try to find ways of dealing with issues of oppression in the delivery of health and social care services. [...]

Anti-oppressive practice then moves beyond descriptions of the nature of oppression to dynamic and creative ways of working.

The principles of reflexivity, social difference, historical and geographical location, the personal as political, power and powerlessness, and the act of challenging provide a framework which can be used to inform work with people in need.

REFERENCES

Barker, R. and Roberts, H. (1993) 'The uses of the concept of power', in Morgan, D. and Stanley, L. (eds) *Debates in Sociology*, Manchester. Manchester University Press.

Clifford, D.J. (1995) 'Methods in oral history and social work', *Journal of the Oral History Society* 23 (2).

Dominelli, L. (1994) 'Anti-racist social work education', Paper given at the 27th Congress of the International Association of Schools of Social Work, Amsterdam, July.

Lorde, A. (1984) *Sister Outsider*, New York: The Crossing Press.

CHAPTER 15

NARRATIVE ANALYSIS AND ILLNESS EXPERIENCE

Richard Gwyn

Story telling is a quintessential human activity. In recent years the appeal of narratives has taken a substantive turn towards the pathologised body, and the recounting of chronic illness experience. It is likely that this fascination with self-related decrement and self-disclosure on themes relating to mortality and death is the logical progression of an increasing tendency towards self-reflexivity in western culture generally, a tendency echoed in the social sciences. Over the past 15 years we have witnessed a sudden deluge of biographical accounts of illness experience written by media celebrities, journalists, academics and members of the general public.

A narrative account involves a sequence of two or more bits of information (concerning happenings, mental states, people, or whatever) which are presented in such a way that if the order of the sequence were changed, the meaning of the account would alter. It is this sequentiality which differentiates narrative from other forms of conveying and apprehending information. Narrative can therefore be regarded as depending upon a specific construction of temporality, in which events occur within and across time. *Narrative is the form of human representation concerned with expressing coherence through time: it helps to provide human lives with a sense of order and meaning.* By imposing an orderly sequence of events upon an inchoate mass of experience, expanses of time can be *retrospectively structured*, and in the process, made meaningful; an ambiguity which did not escape the philosopher Kierkegaard, who observed that we lead our lives facing forward, but account for them looking backward (Kierkegaard 1987: 260). Ensuring sequentiality between events, imposing a beginning, a middle and an end, can serve to assure human lives of direction and growth: at the very least, as Barthes put it, what is narrated is 'hemmed in' (Barthes 1993).

A narrative account of illness reproduces what the psychologist James Hillman has called an individual's 'sustaining fiction' (1983: 17). We are, he says, constantly in the process of adding new stories to the sustaining fictions of our own biographies. With time these fictions become embroidered and adapted to suit different tellings, or to serve distinct explanatory purposes. For Hillman this is largely a creative or 'imaginal' enterprise, that is, the teller's imaginative resources have time to 'go to work on' their experience, resulting in a story which is meaningful to them personally. It needs to be stated that Hillman is not using the term fiction in a deprecatory fashion as indicating that what a person believes is fundamentally or in any other way 'untrue' (1983: 48). A sustaining fiction represents a model of the 'way things are' (or 'the way things were') to the individual's subjective understanding and its 'truth value', for what it is worth, is not under investigation.

The people with whom I have spoken in my own research experience often seem to be seeking to establish the meaning of an illness through their talk. For this reason, I see the purpose of narrative research in a medical context as identifying individual grains of meaning that together might constitute, for any individual, their sustaining fiction, or their subjective understanding of illness.

Recent writings by medical scholars have seen a turn towards narrative as a means of developing a more holistic approach to patient care and as a potent reserve to be explored in the formulation of new therapies. Thus a 'narrative based medicine' (Greenhalgh and Hurwitz 1999) has arisen in counterpoint to the equally peculiar-sounding 'evidence-based medicine' (Sackett *et al.* 1997) (what, one wonders, did doctors base their treatments on before this strain of practice emerged?). Although it might be contended that narrative-based medicine is simply a case of re-inventing the wheel, there is considerable interest being generated in medical circles, and in the pages of medical journals, by the phenomenon of narrative.

However, the researcher who seeks to elicit conversational narratives (Wolfson 1976) from a group of patients is in an advantageous position compared to the medical professional wishing to practise a narrative-based medicine. There is a simple reason for this. However well-intentioned, health care professionals are surrounded by the paraphernalia of the medical institution in which they work (Williams 1990). They are lodged within their own professional domain, with all the connotations of power asymmetry and specialised knowledge that accompanies the 'consulting room', the 'surgery' or the 'hospital'. Patients are far more likely to talk extensively to a sympathetic listener within the comfort of their own home, where they will feel less daunted, or threatened, and where the researcher, or interviewer, is not constrained by the kinds of time limits facing most care providers. These are the circumstances that are perhaps best suited to the eliciting of illness narratives, and can provide an invaluable resource for students and practitioners of health care who wish to practice a narrative-based medicine. We shall consider just such a case shortly.

While there is considerably more to narrative than merely iterating a series of events in sequence, the 'progressive' nature of much illness lends itself to 'storied' form, that is, a sequencing of events in chronological order (Labov and Waletsky 1967; Labov 1972; Mishler 1986; Cortazzi 1993; Riessman 1993). Most people construct a narrative around their experiences of illness, and it is the *process* of reconstruction, this telling and re-telling that I wish to examine in this chapter. We will therefore be investigating the explanatory basis of narrative while at the same time analysing a short text according to the narrative principles laid down by Labov (1972), which helps demonstrate the sequential basis of narrative form. This model of narrative, sometimes referred to as the *Labovian* model, can be a useful tool in breaking a story down into its component parts. At the same time, however, we might attempt to extrapolate the storied nuances and asides that make such a model a starting point for deeper narrative analysis rather than an end in itself.

Labov's model of narrative suggests that stories are typically presented in four stages, although there may be a degree of overlap between these, and the categories do not always follow a straightforward pattern. These are: the *orientation*, which informs the listener of the time, the place and the players involved in the story; the *complicating action*, which contains the essential plot of events, telling the listener 'what happened'; the *evaluation*, which informs us either directly or indirectly why the story was worth telling, and the *result*, which tells what happened in the end. In addition, one or both of two optional phases might flank the main story: the *abstract*, which gives an introductory précis of the gist or purpose of the story in one or two clauses, and the *coda*, which serves as a 'bridge' between the end of the story and current time.

Let's consider how this structure might be applied to an illness narrative. The interviewee is an eighty-one-year-old man whom I will call Ben Coates. The opening question of the interview is aimed towards eliciting a narrative response. What in fact emerges is a fully-formed narrative which might be designated labels according to Labov's terminology as follows:

01	INT	what is your own experience of (.) of illness?	
02	BC	uh (.) overseas I nearly died (.) uh (.)	A
03	INT	is this during the war?	
04	BC	before the war uh I was in India before the war (3.0)	O
05		I got um (.) apart from malaria and things like that	O
06		that was the only illness I got out there	O
07		I got um (.) *heat* stroke uh first I got sand fly fever	CA
08		and doped myself and carried on (.)	CA
09		in the end I collapsed with a temperature of	CA/R
10		a hundred and seven point five (.)	CA/R

11		they wheeled me off into hospital	CA
12		there was a nursing sister there (.) [clean] under canvas	CA
13		they had nursing sisters there like hospital staff here	O
14		you know (.) and um (.) she worked at me eight hours	CA
15		(.) give up after eight hours covered me with a sheet	CA
16		this is what I was told I wasn't (.) compos mentis [laughs]	E
17		uh (.) this nursing orderly he you used to get	CA/O
18		nursing orderlies from different battalions of (.) infantry	O
19		would supply nursing orderlies for the hospital and the	O
20		Q Q Queen Alexandra's used to supply the sisters and the	O
21		doctors I suppose [mumbles]	O
22		um (2.0) and he says she lifted up the sheet again and said	CA/R
23		uh bugger's still fighting come on [laughs]	CA/R
24	INT	yeah so they'd given up on you?	E
25	BC	well (.) when you've got a hundred and seven point five	E
26		you you=	
27	INT	=you should be dead	E
		[	
28	BC	getting a bit close to it but then you wouldn't	E
29		know about it cos they bury you the same day out there you	E
30		know (.) no (.) they don't keep you very long (.) um	E
31		(.) so that's my first *real* illness	C

Key
(.) = pause of less than 0.5 seconds; (2.0) = pause of two seconds etc.
[clean] = unclear utterance
[laughs] = non-verbal utterance
[= overlapping speech
heat = word or words spoken with emphasis
A = abstract; O = orientation; CA = complicating action; E = evaluation; R = result; C = coda.

Ben takes the opening question as a cue to tell his first story of illness in its entirety. After line 24, he does not return to this episode in the interview, but goes on to move through his life in a more or less chronological order to the present day. His opening is typical of the kind of short pithy introductions that Labov defines as an *abstract*:

02	BC	uh (.) overseas I nearly died (.) uh (.)

where 'I nearly died' is the focal event, and is followed by two short pauses that perhaps invite the interviewer to press for details. The fact that there has been no previous mention of 'overseas' is no deterrent since the predominant landscape in Ben Coates' interview is to be one of 'wartime' where the particularities of geography are rendered temporarily redundant. 'The war' along with 'the army' was, throughout the conversation, Ben's dominant sustaining fiction. Hence this episode is placed 'before the war' and, specifically 'in India'.

Locating the narrative in space ('in India'), and time ('before the war') serve the basic function of *orientation* according to Labov's definition. The minimal information on other illnesses can also be seen as orientation, acting to accentuate the importance of the episode about to be described:

04	BC	before the war uh I was in India before the war (3.0)
05		I got um (.) apart from malaria and things like that
06		that was the only illness I got out there
07		I got um (.) *heat* stroke

The emphasis given to the word 'heat' suggests the arrival of important new material, which marks the beginning of the complicating action of the narrative:

uh first I got sand fly fever and doped myself and carried on (.) (ll. 07–8)

Not 'allowing oneself' to succumb to illness is a cultural phenomenon that has been remarked upon at length in the sociology of health and illness (Herzlich 1973; Blaxter 1983; Williams 1990). The *struggle with illness* is seen in western culture as heroic, a role compounded perhaps by Ben's position as a professional soldier, where the accusation of 'malingering' might be particularly face-threatening or otherwise problematic.

in the end I collapsed with a temperature of a hundred and seven point five (ll. 09–10)

The prepositional phrase 'in the end' aids the temporal sequencing of the narrative just as the question 'what happened next?' requires an answer. The crucial event ('I collapsed') is presented alongside its justification, which is precisely articulated as a numeral plus decimal point ('a hundred and seven point five'). This, I would argue, constitutes a 'mini-result' as well as a part of the continuing complicating action. The shared knowledge that Ben assumes with this utterance is that such a temperature is exceedingly high for a human being. This is followed by a pause ('what happened next?') before we are told:

they wheeled me off into hospital (l. 11)

We are not told who 'they' are, but from the context are no doubt expected to infer his fellow-soldiers or the medical orderlies attached to the regiment. The complicating action continues with details about the staffing of the makeshift hospital:

12	BC	there was a nursing sister there (.) [clean] under canvas they had
13		nursing sisters there like hospital staff here you know (.)

We have already been assured of the severity of Ben's condition by two pieces of information, firstly that his temperature was 107.5 degrees Fahrenheit, and secondly that he had to be 'wheeled' into hospital, presumably because he was unconscious, and/or unable to walk. We are now presented with further information that allows the narrative to progress from being a 'near to death' story to being a 'left for dead' story. Again pauses are made in the appropriate 'what happened next?' slots:

14–15	BC	she worked at me eight hours (.) give up after eight hours covered me
15–16		with a sheet this is what I was told I wasn't (.) compos mentis [laughs]

Ben Coates would have been unable to ascertain that the nursing sister had 'worked at' him for eight hours or covered him with a sheet: this is reported narrative relayed to him after the event by a nursing orderly. He evidently needs to explain this detail, thus validating the authenticity of his account (it comes from an identified other, not himself), and while so doing explains the presence of the orderly in the hospital. But the orderly fulfils another criterion of Labov's: by introducing a 'third party' to the narrative, the narrator is able to provide a *neutral evaluation*, which will carry more dramatic force than his own uncorroborated one (Labov 1972: 373).

16 this is what I was told I wasn't (.) compos mentis [laughs]
17 uh (.) this nursing orderly he you used to *get*
18 nursing orderlies from different battalions of (.) infantry
19 would supply nursing orderlies for the hospital and the
20 Q Q Queen Alexandra's used to supply the sisters and the
21 doctors I suppose [mumbles] um

This amount of orientation does not assist the forward flow of the narrative, but it contextualises the presence of the orderly, without whose account Ben might have been denied knowledge of certain crucial details (the nurse 'working eight hours at him'; the sheet covering his head) and is therefore provided in full. It thus provides an explanatory link between the two stages of the split *evaluation*.

We are then told:

22 and he says she lifted up the sheet again and said
23 uh bugger's still fighting come on [laughs]

The *result* of a narrative in Labovian analysis provides an answer to the question 'what finally happened' (Toolan 1988: 152). Here we are given the result, which paves the way for the second part of the *evaluation*. In Ben's account the denouément is skilfully presented so that the mildly deprecating language attributed to the nursing sister ('bugger's still fighting') only serves, by covertly praising him, to boost Ben's own heroic status. It is noteworthy too that the nurse's evaluation is presented as reported speech ('he says she ... said') thus fortifying the evaluative locus of the story. Labov emphasises that this technique (of attributing evaluations to others present) 'is used only by older, highly skilled narrators from traditional working-class backgrounds. Middle-class speakers are less likely to embed their evaluative comments so deeply in the narrative' (1972: 373).

The interviewer's subsequent question: 'so they'd given up on you?' is itself evaluative, and permits Ben to reformulate *his* evaluation.

24	RG	yeah so they'd given up on you?
25	BC	well (.) when you've got a hundred and seven point five
26		you you=
27	RG	=you should be dead
		[
28	BC	getting a bit close to it

Whereas the two previous evaluations are 'external' (reported speech and action), the speaker now provides what Labov terms a *comparator* (1972: 381). Comparators compare the events which did occur to those which might have, could have, but did not in fact occur. Often the effect is to 'spice up' the story. In this case the comparator is achieved through the speculation that had the nurse not pulled the sheet back and found him 'still fighting' he would have been buried alive:

29	BC	they bury you the same day out there you know (.)
30		no (.) they don't keep you very long

Toolan (1988: 161) writes that the *coda* 'signals the "sealing off" of a narrative, just as the abstract announces the "opening up"'. It renders the asking of 'and then what happened?' absurd. The coda also removes the narrative from another spatiotemporal context and returns us to the present. Ben Coates' *coda* happily fulfils both these conditions:

so that's my first *real* illness (ll. 31)

with which statement Ben 'pushes away' and 'seals off' (Labov 1972: 366) the preceding narrative events.

Apart from fulfilling the criteria of a mini-narrative, the opening of Ben Coates' interview provides the kind of background to his personal history that is often helpful in identifying an individual's explanatory model of illness. We have learned that Ben was a volunteer soldier (since he was in India before World War Two), that he perceives his recovery from this bout of fever as being somewhat exceptional (he had been given up for dead), and that he self-presents in an heroic – or mock-heroic – mould ('bugger's still fighting'), ostensibly (or ostentatiously) making light of the alternative outcome of his illness ('they bury you the same day out there you know'). He has told us how, despite contracting sand fly fever, he 'doped [him]self and carried on' which insinuates the kind of stoic individualism observable in many accounts by males of his generation and background (Williams 1990; Gwyn 1997).

'Personal stories', write Rosenwald and Ochberg, 'are not merely a way of telling someone (or oneself) about one's life; they are the means by which identities may be fashioned' (1992: 1). Most significantly, then, in the context of research interviewing, this extract illustrates how the first story that a respondent provides can do much more than simply prefix the interview with a neatly-structured narrative; it helps the speaker to establish *who* they are in relation to the *what* of illness. That the same degree of detailed analysis could be expected of health care workers in the consulting room is unrealistic, but such a method does provide a comprehensive and straightforward approach to narrative analysis which might serve as a useful and reflexive analytical tool for health care workers.

ACKNOWLEDGEMENT

This Chapter has been adapted from pages 139–150 of *Communicating Health and Illness*, Richard Gwyn (Sage Publications, 2002).

REFERENCES

Barthes, R. (1993) 'Introduction to the structural analysis of narratives', in Sontag, S. (ed.) *A Barthes Reader*, London: Vintage.

Blaxter, M. (1983) 'The causes of disease: women talking', *Social Science and Medicine* 17 (2): 56–69.

Cortazzi, M. (1993) *Narrative Analysis*, London: Falmer Press.

Gwyn, R. (1997) *The Voicing of Illness: Narrative and Metaphor in Accounts of Illness Experience*, Unpublished PhD thesis: Cardiff University.

Greenhalgh, P. and Hurwitz, B. (1999) *Narrative Based Medicine*, London: BMA.

Herzlich, C. (1973) *Health and Illness*, London: Academic Press.

Hillman, J. (1983) *Healing Fiction*, Woodstock, CT: Spring Publications.

Kierkegaard, S. (1987) *Either/Or Part II*, Princetown: Princetown University Press.

Labov, W. (1972) *Language in the Inner City*, Oxford: Blackwell.

Labov, W. and Waletsky, J. (1967) 'Narrative analysis: oral versions of personal experience', in Helms, J. (ed.) *Essays on the Verbal and Visual Arts*, Seattle: University of Washington Press.

Mishler, E. (1986) *Research Interviewing*, Cambridge, MA: Harvard University Press.

Riessman, C. (1993) *Narrative Analysis*, Newbury Park, CA: Sage.

Rosenwald, G.C. and Ochberg, R.L. (1992) 'Introduction: life stories, cultural politics, and self-understanding', in Rosenwald, G.C. and Ochberg, R.L. (eds) *Storied Lives: the Cultural Politics of Self-understanding*, New Haven, CT: Yale University Press.

Sackett, D., Scott Richardson, W., Rosenberg, W. and Haynes, R. (1997) *Evidence Based Medicine: How to Practice and Teach EBM*, New York: Churchill Livingstone.

Toolan, M.J. (1988) *Narrative: A Critical Linguistic Introduction*, New York: Routledge.

Williams, R. (1990) *A Protestant Legacy: Attitudes to Death and Illness Among Older Aberdonians*, Oxford: Oxford University Press.

Wolfson, N. (1976) 'Speech events and natural speech: some implications for sociolinguistic methodology', *Language in Society* 5: 189–209.

CHAPTER 16

PREPARING FOR LINGUISTICALLY SENSITIVE PRACTICE

Richard Pugh

INTRODUCTION

A linguistically sensitive practice is one informed by a sound understanding of the social, psychological, political and sociological significance of language and linguistic variation. It is based upon a developed awareness of the complex role that language plays in constructing and communicating culture, identity and power. Regrettably, language is a dimension of social difference that is frequently ignored or underplayed in the education of health and social care professions (Kornbeck 2001). This chapter provides an introduction to the subject, a more detailed exposition can be found in Pugh (1996, 2003a).

Language issues have tended to be subsumed under discussions of 'race', or alternatively, considered too narrowly in terms of communicative efficiency. The conflation of language with 'race' is mistaken because it assumes that language difference is only an issue when working with black and ethnic minorities who do not speak English as their first language. This erroneous assumption only prompts consideration of language as a relevant factor when other forms of difference such as skin colour are noted. Although there is obvious merit in considering the effectiveness of communication processes, an overly narrow focus upon this technical aspect, omits consideration of the broader social context in which language is used, and in particular, neglects the powerful role that it plays in constructing social life.

It can be difficult for those raised in monolingual environments to appreciate the extent to which their understandings of the world are constructed by this experience. They may not realise the subtle role that language has in establishing perceptions of what is considered to be 'normal' or 'traditional'. As Steiner observed:

> *We are so much the products of set feeling patterns, Western culture has so thoroughly stylized our perceptions, that we experience our 'traditionality' as natural. In particular we leave unquestioned the historical causes, [and] the roots of determinism which underlie the 'recursive' structure of our sensibility and expressive codes.*
>
> (Steiner, cited in Husband 1977: 213)

The 'naturalness' of English to monoglot English speakers fosters an ethnocentric perception towards other languages. At its most basic, this can be seen in the way in which English becomes the normal unmarked standard against which other languages are contrasted, usually less favourably. For example, the phrase 'promoting Welsh' is often used to describe Welsh language initiatives, whereas the everyday presumption of English as the norm goes unremarked. This echoes the assimilationist premise that immigrants should 'fit in', and embodies a static and homogeneous conception of culture. A conception which ignores the historical diversity of influences upon British culture, and presumes a monolithic culture which is supposedly shared by all who speak English.

This apparent 'naturalness' derives from the ways in which language both *conveys* and *embodies* particular cultural perspectives upon the world. Perspectives we remain largely unaware of. For example, Cameron in her account of the role that language plays in constructing gender points out the false dichotomy of sexual polarity in language. She cites a study by Rosenthal in which people were presented with pairs of words such as knife/fork, Ford/Chevrolet, salt/pepper, vanilla/chocolate, and asked which word in each pair was feminine and which was masculine (Cameron 1992: 82–83). Given that English is not gendered language in the same way that French and German are, this was an unusual task for them. What was remarkable, were the high levels of agreement in the answers (knife, Ford, pepper and chocolate were commonly picked as masculine). The powerful role of metaphorical gender is revealed. An organising construct so powerful that it can be mobilised reliably and predictably by different individuals even when presented with novel tasks.

LANGUAGE MYTHS

Preparation for linguistically sensitive practice requires that practitioners become aware of some of the common myths about language and its use.

ENGLISH IS A SUPERIOR LANGUAGE

The increasing popularity and prevalence of English is sometimes taken as evidence of its technical superiority over other languages, but there is little evidence to support this view. While English certainly has a larger vocabulary than many languages, much of this is due to the ease with which it has incorporated loan words from other languages. Sociolinguists generally agree that there is little basis for assuming that some languages are intrinsically better than others at performing the communicative functions required in particular societies (Crystal 1987).

Concerns are often expressed about the use of Creole, Patois, slang, and other language varieties, which are perceived as limited and inferior forms. However, such perceptions fail to appreciate two important features of language use. First, that many of those using such forms are also able to participate effectively using other 'standard forms', i.e. that their linguistic repertoire is not necessarily limited to one form. They may be using a linguistic device known as code switching, a crucial aspect of communicative competence and which involves switching from one register to another within a language, or from one language or dialect to another (Trudgill 2000). For example, professionals may use a particular speech form or jargon for their work in formal settings, one which signals competence and knowledge, and then switch to a more casual register for informal conversation, to signal friendliness or intimacy. Second, when conversationalists share a common context and have good knowledge of each other, then language need not be highly specific for it to be effective. In contrast, in situations where conversationalists lack a common context, high specificity may be needed to avoid misunderstanding.

MONOLINGUALISM IS THE NORM

The assumption that monolingualism is the norm throughout the world and that multilingualism is exceptional is mistaken. There are many countries where people routinely use more than one language, or where the state recognises a linguistic plurality. In some African countries, many people speak a tribal dialect, a broader language like Swahili, as well as a European language such as English or French (Trudgill 2000). Belgium has two official languages and two linguistically separated health and social care systems (Flemish and French), an arrangement that is also found in Quebec in Canada (English and French). While in Switzerland there are four recognised languages, French, German, Italian and Romansch, each of which is dominant in different cantons. Nonetheless, the idea that the nationality of a country and its people are constituted through the use of a common language remains influential and this can result in the marginalisation of minority languages and their speakers (May 2001).

MINORITY LANGUAGE USE IS RELATIVELY LIMITED

There is a surprising degree of linguistic variation within the British Isles (Alladina and Edwards 1991). For example, a survey of children in London schools found over 300 different home languages and English was the first language in just under 68 per cent of homes (Baker and Mohieldeen 2000). Although this diversity is exceptional, a conservative estimate of the numbers of people throughout the UK using a language other than English was at least two millions (Pugh and Jones 1999). These other languages include the older languages of the British Isles such as Gaelic, Irish and Welsh; sign languages such as BSL (British Sign Language); well established newer languages such as Cantonese, Gujerati and Urdu; and more recently an increase in the numbers using languages such as Arabic, Farsi and Pushtu.

MINORITY LANGUAGES WILL INEVITABLY DECLINE

This belief is understandable given the numbers of languages that have disappeared. The UNESCO Red Book on Endangered Languages suggests that in Europe there are 38 indigenous languages that are endangered and another 26 that are seriously endangered (Salminen 1999). Nonetheless, one should be wary of assuming that all minority languages will inevitably decline. For example, the 2001 census in the UK revealed that the numbers speaking Welsh in Wales had increased and constituted 28.4 per cent of all those aged over three years of age. This increase is also evident in the fact that a third of all school children are receiving their primary education in Welsh, obviously including many from non-Welsh speaking homes.

Generally, in regard to the 'newer languages', although many of the second and third generations born to immigrants do not learn to speak their parents' or grandparents' language, some do. The language may be needed for participation in community activities and maintaining links overseas, but for those subject to social marginalisation, it may be a crucial cultural resource in maintaining group identity and resisting discrimination.

BILINGUALISM IS PROBLEMATIC

Attitudes to bilingualism in Britain are inconsistent and imbued with racist assumptions about superior and inferior languages. In schools an elite form of bilingualism is promoted, where 'white' languages such as French and German receive support, while others, such as those originating in Africa and the Asian subcontinent, do not. Baker contends that in regard to bilingualism, many people assume a situation of competition and conflict, where 'positive consequences for one language imply negative consequences for another' (Baker 1992: 77). This leads to a deficiency model of bilingualism in which it is believed that two languages can rarely exist satisfactorily in the same person or society. For example, it is often assumed that bilingualism creates a cognitive struggle within the speaker's brain whereby one language is learned and becomes dominant at the expense of the other. Superficially, this appears to be borne out by language testing of bilingual people which shows that few have equal competence in all aspects of both languages, such as formal and informal speech, reading and writing. But this is a misconception about what bilingualism is. Few bilinguals have equal facility, instead they develop differing levels of skill according to the requirements of the domains of use. Thus, many speakers of minority languages who use them competently in informal situations, such as at home and among friends, might score relatively poorly when tested for formal written competence. Failure to recognise the situated or contextual nature of language use frequently leads to negative assumptions being made about the competence of bilingual speakers.

CULTURAL EQUIVALENCE

The presumption that there is a close or direct equivalence in the words and ideas embodied within different languages may result in an unwitting ethnocentrism. While there is evidence for this assumption in the terms used for familiar physical objects or natural phenomena, there is considerable variation in regard to social relationships and other abstract concepts.

For example, in English the terms 'brother-in-law' and 'sister-in-law' are used to identify the siblings of a person's partner but do not differentiate in any other way among them. Whereas, in some cultures these relationships are linguistically marked and differentiated because of the special obligations that an older brother has towards the partners of his younger brothers if they are widowed.

This assumption of cultural equivalence can have serious consequences when professionals are making assessments about bilingual people. In fact, many studies on psychiatric interventions have shown how differences in self-concept, linguistic expression, and cultural references, influence the assessment of the patient (Nazroo 1997; Rack 1982). For example, Ely and Denney noted the confusion that arose when a woman of Asian origin was asked by a psychiatrist 'How do you feel in yourself'? She seemed to have difficulty answering the question, and when she replied that her family were well, the doctor took this apparently indirect response as evidence of her mental confusion. However, its meaning lay in her conception of herself as a mother, wife and daughter. That is, in relation to the health and well-being of significant people in her life, and her social roles, relationships and responsibilities (Ely and Denney 1987: 176).

LANGUAGE AND IDENTITY

The general question of identity is a difficult and complex one (Woodward 1997). If one accepts that identity is potentially fluid (changing according to context as well as over time), that is created and recreated through social interaction, and that language both represents and shapes constructions of identity, then it follows that it has an important role in mediating relationships between people and groups. For most people, language is the predominant means by which they develop their ideas of themselves and of others, and there is a significant element of reflexivity in this:

> *Everyday life, is above all, life with and by means of the language I share with my fellow men [sic] ... What is more, I hear myself as I speak: my own subjective meanings are made objectively and continuously available to me and* ipso facto *become 'more real' to me ... I objectivate my own being by means of language.*
>
> (Berger and Luckman 1966: 52)

For those who are bilingual, the situation is even more complex. Baker in rebutting one common misconception has noted that a:

> *bilingual person is not two monolinguals in one frame, but a unity uniquely different from a monolingual ... to be bicultural is not to own two monocultures. The way two cultures are blended, harmonised and combined is unique and not simply the sum of two parts.*
> (Baker 1992: 78)

While this may be commonplace among children in the stable context that Baker is discussing, it is often the case that those who migrate and attempt to learn another language later in life, feel less comfortable in the new language. They experience a sense of dislocation as they attempt to straddle two cultures. They may also experience a loss of self confidence as they perceive themselves as less competent in their new context. Indeed, Gumperz (1982) has shown how monolinguals from the dominant language group in a society typically construe difficulties in communication with linguistic minorities as evidence of social and intellectual inadequacy.

The survival of minority languages is not simply a function of their utility for communication, they may be a 'continuing bond and a potential rallying point for ethnic identity if required' (Edwards 1977: 266) especially for those who experience discrimination. This is illustrated by the increased use of Patois by British-born black Afro-Caribbean youth during the 1970s and 1980s (Edwards 1986), where a previously unfashionable language form became remobilised as a form of resistance to racism.

CONCLUSION

Ahmed observed that 'the language barrier has been one of the most oppressive factors in denying many black and ethnic minority ethnic families their right to services, simply because the service agencies are not able to communicate with them in their own languages' (Ahmed 1991: 6). Despite some valuable initiatives such as Language Line (www.languageline.co.uk) and the availability of excellent guidance on interpretation and translation services (Sanders 2001), this still remains the case. Many providers of public services remain ill-prepared in terms of policies, practical arrangements and training (Pugh 2003b; Williams 2003).

The legal position in regard to minority language provision is not encouraging. International law such as the 1992 *United Nations Declaration on the Rights of Persons Belonging to National or Ethnic or Religious Minorities* and the 1996 *Draft Universal Declaration of Linguistic Rights* allow individual states considerable discretion as to which elements of the declaration they choose to apply (May 2001). This mirrors the situation in UK law, where with the exception of the Welsh Language Acts of 1967 and 1993, there are no formal language rights. Indeed, much of the legislation which underpins current service provision, such as the Mental Health Act and the Children Act encourages or permits workers to consider the cultural background of the service user, but leaves it to workers to decide whether language is a relevant issue.

In the widespread absence of education and training in linguistically sensitive practice, it is likely that this discretion is not exercised as well as it might be, and even when used positively, it may still result in poor or inappropriate provision (Pugh and Jones 1999). Although services may be made accessible in a minority language, problems can still arise because of the lack of understanding of how issues of power, identity and culture may impact upon the interaction between the professional and the service user. Even service providers who allow users some choice of language may not appreciate how this may be shaped by other factors, such as a fear of being thought ill-educated, or the desire to 'fit-in'. Thus, services may be delivered ineffectively and may also unintentionally reinforce some of the damaging and assimilationist assumptions made about minority languages. Finally, the use of interpreters raises a number of issues in regard to; their availability, their competence and suitability, the conditions under which they are used, and the adequacy of professional preparation for working skilfully through a third party.

To conclude, while the development of linguistically sensitive practice must be based upon improving professional awareness and knowledge, it also requires other steps. These should include efforts to:

- develop language policies which state the primacy of consumer choice;
- establish clear practice guidance in relation to the use of professional discretion and interpreting services;
- promote innovation in developing non-traditional means of access to services, such as community outreach through existing social institutions;
- recruit a work force that is representative of the communities served;
- develop the capacity of workers to use minority languages in a professional context through the publication of professional dictionaries and glossaries, support in developing confidence, and ensuring competence in both oral and written language;
- acquire accurate knowledge about minority language communities, i.e. the range of languages used, the extent to which speakers commonly read and write them, the existence of shared languages between ethnic groups, and the significance attached to the use of particular languages;
- improve agency collaboration in researching local needs and developing access to the services, i.e. joint registers of interpreters, common policies, sharing best practice.

REFERENCES

Alladina, S. and Edwards, V. (eds) (1991) *Multilingualism in the British Isles*, Volumes 1 and 2, Harlow: Longman.

Ahmed, B. (1991) 'Preface', in Baker, P., Hussain, Z. and Saunders, J. *Interpreters in Public Services*, Birmingham: Venture Press.

Baker, C. (1992) *Attitudes and Language*, Clevedon: Multilingual Matters.

Berger, P. and Luckman, T. (1967) *The Social Construction of Reality*, Harmondsworth: Penguin.

Baker, P. and Mohieldeen, Y. (2000) The languages of London's schoolchildren, in Baker, P., Eversley, P. and Eversley, J. (eds) *Multilingual Capital: London*, Battlebridge Publication.

Cameron, D. (1992) *Feminism and Linguistic Theory*, Basingstoke: Macmillan.

Crystal, D. (1987) *The Cambridge Encylopedia of Language*, Cambridge: Cambridge University Press.

Edwards, J.R. (1977) 'Ethnic identity and bilingual education', *European Monographs in Social Psychology* 13: 250–269

Edwards, V. (1986) *Language in a Black Community*, Clevedon: Multilingual Matters.

Ely, P. and Denney, D. (1987) *Social Work in a Multi-Racial Society*, Aldershot: Gower.

Gumperz, J.J. (1982) *Language and Social Identity*, Cambridge: Cambridge University Press.

Husband, C. (1977) 'A case study in identity maintenance', *European Monographs in Social Psychology* 13: 212–250.

Kornbeck, J. (2001) 'Language training for prospective and practising social workers: a neglected topic', *British Journal of Social Work* 31: 307–316.

May, S. (2001) *Language and Minority Rights: Ethnicity, Nationalism and the Politics of Language*, Harlow: Longman.

Nazroo, J. (1997) *Ethnicity and Mental Health: Findings from a National Community Survey*, London: Policy Studies Institute.

Pugh, R. (1996) *Effective Language in Health and Social Work*, London: Chapman and Hall.

Pugh, R. (2003a) 'Research into practice', *Community Care* 20–26 February: 45.

Pugh, R. (2003b) 'Understanding language practice, policy and provision in social work', in Kornbeck, J. (ed.) *Language Teaching in the Social Work Curriculum*, Mainz: Logophon Verlag.

Pugh, R. and Jones, E. (1999) 'Language and practice: minority language provision within the Guardian ad litem service', *British Journal of Social Work* 29: 529–546

Rack, P. (1982) *Race, Culture and Mental Disorder*, London: Tavistock.

Salminen, T. (1999) *UNESCO Red Book on Endangered Languages: Europe*, www.helsinki.fi/~talsalmin/europe_index.html.

Sanders, M. (2000) *As Good as Your Word: A Guide to Community Interpreting and Translation in Public Services*, London: The Maternity Alliance.

Trudgill, P. (2000) *Sociolinguistics*, Harmondsworth: Penguin.

Williams, D. (2003) 'Unpublished survey of UK social work departments', in preparation for PhD, Wrexham: NEWI.

Woodward, K. (ed.) (1997) *Identity and Difference*, London: Open University/ Sage.

CHAPTER 17

EMBARRASSMENT, SOCIAL RULES AND THE CONTEXT OF BODY CARE

Jocalyn Lawler

[...]

This chapter illustrates the extent to which body care is located in context, how that context is constructed and managed, what the taken-for-granted rules are which sustain the processes of care, and how important and fundamental the notion of embarrassment is to a somological understanding of the body in nursing practice.

During illness people are confronted with what Parker (1988: 10) called 'the boundedness of embodiment' such that their need for assistance with privatised body functions can be both embarrassing and unprecedented in adult life. It can also be a time when patients experience a loss of control over the body, and that loss of control can also become a source of embarrassment. In a society which has privatised the body and (some) bodily functions, embarrassment is a powerful means of social control. However, we know very little about the management of embarrassment in social situations generally, and almost nothing about its management in situations when people need assistance with body care. I will argue here that the concept of embarrassment is central to understanding how nurses manage the body – but embarrassment in a nursing sense is a much richer concept than that which is used in popular language in relation to 'normal' social life.

Source: *Behind the Screens: Nursing, Somology and the Problem of the Body* (1994): 135–154, Edinburgh: Churchill Livingstone.

THE NATURE AND MEANING OF EMBARRASSMENT

[...]

Many sources of embarrassment we experience in social life relate to the body, its attire, its functions, and our capacity to control bodily processes such as burping, crying and yawning. We are taught, through mechanisms which act to maintain social order, to control ourselves in public life and to control embarrassment, or the potential for embarrassment. The literature on embarrassment consists predominantly of works in which the ideas of Goffman (1955, 1956) and Gross and Stone (1964) have been influential. [...]

Edelmann defines embarrassment as 'a common and often dramatic experience' consisting of 'a highly uncomfortable psychological state, which can have a severely disruptive effect on social interaction' (Edelmann 1981: 125) because it 'can be attributed to the violation of social expectations which govern and define desirable behaviour' (Edelmann 1981: 126). He also argues that embarrassment must be differentiated from shame because the former is possible only in the presence of a real or imagined audience and that it is, therefore, an interpersonal process, while the latter is a personal and private experience. That is not to say that the two cannot co-exist. However, 'the crucial condition necessary for embarrassment to occur is that an individual behaves in a manner inconsistent with the way in which he or she would have wished to behave' (Edelmann 1981: 132).

There is a high level of consensus among those who have written on this topic that social rules are fundamental to embarrassment and that embarrassment occurs when rules are broken. However, embarrassment does not necessarily follow if the rule-breaker is unaware of the rules or deliberately chooses to break them (Edelmann 1981: 132).

There are several problems with the research on embarrassment. The first problem is that the literature is predominantly psychological and experimental to the extent that, with the exception of Weinberg's (1965, 1968) work, embarrassment has been studied under contrived conditions, usually, but not always, involving public places. As one would expect of psychology, it has focused on the effects of embarrassing situations on individuals. Second, little work has been done on establishing the rules which define some things as embarrassing and others as not embarrassing. Why, for example, did the researchers choose to use Tampax as an item which could induce embarrassment? Third, these studies have all been conducted on healthy 'normal' people, and not people who are ill and for whom, therefore, there may be little scope to initiate socially restorative mechanisms. [...]

THE CIVILISED BODY AND EMBARRASSMENT IN NURSING

In a 'civilised' society, people cover their bodies and there are rules which govern the circumstances in which it is socially acceptable to be naked, or to be relatively naked. For example, examination of the body by a medical practitioner is an occasion when it is acceptable to expose the body (see Emerson 1971), but there are strict taken-for-granted rules which apply. In the circumstances which often prevail during hospitalisation, however, both patient and nurse must negotiate the process of 'handing over' (on the part of the patient) and 'taking over' (on the part of the nurses) the body for its physical care. Consequently, there are rules which normally apply in society to be considered, such as the expectation that people will show some modesty about body exposure, there are rules which make it acceptable for nurses to take other people's clothes off, wash their bodies and help them with toileting, and there are rules which govern the timing of the 'handing over' 'taking over' process. However, Weinberg's (1968) two organising factors, the definition of the situation and the intended or unintended nature of the act, mean that managing embarrassment can be problematic for the patient and the nurse.

Defining the situation correctly requires knowledge of what is expected and acceptable. Experienced patients know these rules but nurses constantly encounter patients who are experiencing their first episode of hospitalisation. What is more, because nurses 'do for' patients in private and out of public view, there is a limit to what a patient *can* know unless the patient has had previous experience with hospitalisation. In addition, while patients may have been taught that some bodily functions ought to be done in private, when they are hospitalised they may not be able to do this, and so they must re-define situations. There is an added difficulty when patients lose control of bodily functions and as a consequence they are embarrassed about unintended acts on their part – acts which in normal circumstances they could control. [...]

It is only socially acceptable for nurses to have access to the body in keeping with the patient's condition.

NURSES' DEFINITION AND MANAGEMENT OF EMBARRASSMENT

Fundamental to helping patients with their bodies during illness, with their situated dependence, is help to manage embarrassment. When it is applied to what they perceive patients experience, nurses use the term embarrassment in a richer and more global sense than the definition provided by Edelmann (1981), and it means more than rule-breaking. Integral to nurses' construction of embarrassment are notions associated with the patient's vulnerability, dependence, and social discomfort and they regard embarrassment as a consequence of inadequate protection of the patient's 'privacy'. They also use embarrassment to describe how patients react when they are experiencing physical changes to their bodies. Before it is possible for nurses to help patients, they must first learn to manage their own embarrassment, but like so many other aspects of body care in nursing, this is not an explicit subject of instruction or education.

NURSES' MANAGEMENT OF THEIR OWN EMBARRASSMENT

[...]

Managing embarrassment has an element of teaching and coaching whereby the nurse leads the patient in defining situations that may be novel for the patient. If nurses are not embarrassed, it gives permission for the patient also to feel no embarrassment, but nurses must firstly learn to manage their own embarrassment and to convey the impression that they are not feeling uncomfortable. Managing one's own embarrassment gets easier with experience and with age, although age does not necessarily bring less embarrassment. One of the interviewees, who worked for many years teaching student nurses, had observed that mature age students cope no better with embarrassment than their younger colleagues. The crucial element would appear to be experience. Experience not only brings greater skill, which enables the nurse to feel more technically competent, but it also brings a greater sense of confidence and knowledge, which make the situation more manageable.

There is another crucial element in the management of embarrassment, and that is the sense of purpose associated with having to perform particular nursing acts. If there is a purpose which is explicit and accepted, potentially embarrassing situations become manageable. [...]

There are particular methods that nurses use to manage their own embarrassment. They use speed as a way of minimising the time they are exposed to certain situations, although this tends to be a technique which they use less and less as they become more experienced. They also talk among their colleagues and share their experiences so that the collegial sense of understanding makes it manageable – if others have had similar experiences it becomes something inherent in the nature of their work and not a personal failing if they feel embarrassment. In this sense shared reality is manageable reality. Nurses also adopt a sort of fatalistic approach to these things that is summarised in their notion, 'it has to be done', which means they can define a situation as unavoidable. This notion is extremely common and I heard it many times, not only with respect to embarrassment, but also with reference to many things in nursing which are aesthetically unpleasant. [...]

If the patient is not perceived by the nurse to be embarrassed, then it is very likely the nurse will also feel little embarrassment – there will be a reciprocity of perspective that makes the situation much easier to manage for both patient and nurse.

> *I think they [patients] can make you or break you ... You get a person who understands the situation and they make it very easy for you and then again you get someone ... [who gets embarrassed very easily] – they make it jolly hard.*

Nurses' perceptions of what indicates embarrassment are central to how they approach the patient, how they feel themselves, and how the encounter with the patient will be managed. Recognition of the potential for embarrassment is, however, fundamental to viewing the encounter in context and viewing it somologically. If the patient's embarrassment is an issue for the nurse when nursing care involves 'invading' the patient's body, there is a mutual recognition of the embodied experience of the patient. Non-recognition of potential embarrassment for the patient, on the other hand, reduces the patient to an object.

RECOGNISING PATIENTS' EMBARRASSMENT

The literature suggest that there are well recognised behaviours which indicate embarrassment, some of which are universal in humans, such as blushing, and some are culturally defined. Edelmann and Hampson (1979, 1981a, 1981b) have established that embarrassment is indicated by reduced eye contact, increased body movement, smiling, and changes in speech patterns, and Fink and Walker (1977) have noted that humour is often also used. [...] In their use of humour nurses take their cues from what they know about patients' personalities, and sometimes it is the patients who indicate that humour is a way of managing some things, in which case it is relatively easy for the nurse to share in that humour. There are other indicators nurses interpret as meaning that the patient is embarrassed.

> *They [patients] go red, they get sweaty or giggly, or they keep saying they're sorry ... or keep apologising.*

> *[Patients will] change the subject. Usually turn red, they look uncomfortable, fidget, pull the covers up, avoid the situation altogether.*

> *They might hedge around...*

> *Some people just tell you.*

> *They sort of wrap their arms up a bit, around themselves and hang on to the sheets or whatever, put it round themselves, firmly. Sitting up in chairs they will cover urine bags – things like that – hide them.*

> *They hide. They tend to cover themselves very quickly. Sometimes they will say things like 'I'll do it, I'll do it, it's alright'. Sometimes they can and sometimes they can't.*

As in most things related to nursing care, knowledge of the patient is important and the perception of embarrassment is based, in part, on that knowledge of how the patient behaves in other situations. The following account illustrates the importance of locating individual patient behaviour in the context of that patient's established way of responding.

> *Obviously there are clear things like blushing ... but I don't think blushing is as common as looking at the ceiling and excessive chatter, on the other hand extreme silence for some that may talk a lot anyway – to be suddenly very quiet, and turn away. I think they're the best indicators for me, but that comes from knowing the patient as well...*

[...]

Sometimes there are very subtle changes in the way patients respond which are interpreted as embarrassment. For example, one midwife, as well as illustrating the need to know the patient 'in the situation', contrasted how a patient's responses to two different nursing procedures indicates embarrassment. One situation requires access to the patients arm – a 'safe' area to touch (Jourard 1966, 1967, Jourard and Rubin 1968) and the other procedure is vaginal examination during labour.

> *It depends. And it is hard if you have never come across this particular patient before. But if you've worked with the patient doing non-*

embarrassing things then just the change in their tone, their attitude, their body language or – again it's how long you've known the person. It's little things other people mightn't notice because they all give signs that they're embarrassed. They don't all go red, or pull the sheet up over their head. They all give signs that they are embarrassed ... You will go in there [to the patient] and say 'I'm going to take your blood pressure' she'll stick our her arm, but if you go in there and say 'I've got to examine you' and instead of quickly getting themselves organised their movements are a little slower ... facial expression may not change all that much, but just enough to notice.

From the point of view of illness experience, many things which nurses do with and for patients, and many of the things which patients do when the nurse is present, break rules that would ordinarily apply in society. However, by the way they manage their own responses and by their lack of embarrassment (affect), nurses re-define situations for patients so that the patient need not feel embarrassed. It is a way of indicating to the patient that it is permissible to vomit in front of someone else, and to have someone help them with defaecation. It is a way of showing the patient that a situation is manageable. It is also a way of indicating to the patient that the body and body functions, irrespective of how privatised they are normally, can be integrated into experience.

BODY CARE FOR OTHERS AND BASIC SOMOLOGICAL RULES

In the context of hospitalisation, people will let nurses do things to them and with them that would be impossible and unthinkable for many in 'normal' social life. People in hospital are amazingly compliant with nurses' requests and give nurses permission to have the sort of intimate contact with their bodies that many have never experienced before, and which many will never again experience except during subsequent hospitalisations. [...]

Several important interrelated factors operate to form a system of basic rules which nurses learn from practice and which they expect the patient to respect, and there are also specific contextors which nurses need to use in order to create a nursing environment. Some of these rules appear self-evident and obvious, but they nevertheless need to be made explicit because they form part of the taken-for-granted social environment in which nursing is practised – a kind of social ecology to the extent that they form a system. [...]

THE GOOD PATIENT AND BASIC RULES IN THE CONTEXT OF NURSING

Central to a 'good' working relationship between the nurse and the patient is an understanding that patients are expected to comply with what the nurse wants them to do and that the patient does not resist or obstruct the nurse. [. . .]

The modesty rule means that the patient is expected to be neither too modest or embarrassed, nor too free to expose himself or herself, and that the nurse will protect the patient's privacy. The following two accounts illustrate, in particular, what this rule means and how it interrelates with the other three rules. In effect the patient is expected to let the nurse have control and to comply with the nurses' requests, to be appropriately modest, and for their part, nurses acknowledge a need for protection of patients – it is a reciprocal arrangement.

R. What makes a 'good' patient?

I. Ones that will let you do anything. (Laughter) No. I expect the patient to try and do things for themselves and you expect them to be a bit modest but they're in hospital and you've got to do these things for them so you expect them to let you do the things, whereas some patients won't let you near them, but you do expect – you just expect them to act like a patient! (Laughter) . . . Somebody sick in bed and you're caring for them so they should just let you do your duties.

R. They should let the nurse take control?

I. Yes. That's what you expect. I suppose we shouldn't really, because it's their own body and they should be in control of that.

I. A 'good' patient will make it easy for you by just chatting and not feeling embarrassed, they roll over when you tell them to roll over, they don't splash water all over the place. These are silly little things – interrupt the cycle by wanting to use a bedpan in the middle of a sponge, not questioning you a little too much.

R. So you expect the patient to be docile?

I. Oh yes! . . . That's a sad outlook, because I think that's when you get to know the people you're looking after the best, when you're invading their personal space like that, and that's when you need to be the most careful about what you say and almost not alarming them about anything.

The modesty rule is of particular relevance when nurses undress and expose patient's bodies, handle them and wash them – experiences which the patient may be having for the first time. Again there is an expectation that the patient is co-operative, and they are expected to show some modesty but not so much that they are 'too embarrassed' because they then become difficult for the nurse to manage. Patients who are very embarrassed at having their bodies exposed create their own particular kind of problems.

> *Some people are just so embarrassed, they've got their arms across their chest the whole time. You've got to prise them back and wash them ... Some people are just so shy and embarrassed – I think for the older [patients] that it was all taboo to be uncovered in front of anybody.*

[...]

In summary, nurses' work involves establishing social order when patients' everyday lives are disrupted. Nurses must deliberately construct a context which allows the body and the embarrassment associated with exposure, dependence, and illness to be managed in a particular occupational context – a context where the definition of the situation is not necessarily shared by patients. The definition of situations as nursing care rely on a set of rules that are learned through practice, and which may or may not be known (or adhered to) by patients. Those rules govern the management of the body and embarrassment during body care. They are social rules which are necessary in a society where the body and (some) body functions have been privatised and such rules are also used in order to make nursing practice socially permissible.

REFERENCES

Edelmann, R.J. (1981) 'Embarrassment: the state of research', *Current Psychological Review* 1: 125–138.

Edelmann, R.J. and Hampson, S.E. (1979) 'Changes in nonverbal behaviour during embarrassment', *British Journal of Social and Clinical Psychology* 18 (November): 385–390.

Edelmann, R.J. and Hampson, S.E. (1981a) 'The recognition of embarrassment', *Personality and Social Psychology Bulletin* 7 (1): 109–116.

Edelmann, R.J. and Hampson, S.E. (1981b) 'Embarrassment in dyadic interaction', *Social Behaviour and Personality* 9 (2): 171–177.

Emerson, J. (1971) 'Behaviour in private places: sustaining definitions of reality in gynaecological examinations', in Dreitzel, H (ed.) *Recent Sociology No. 2* London: Macmillan.

Fink, E.L. and Walker, B.A. (1977) 'Humorous responses to embarrassment', *Psychological Reports* 40 (2): 475–485.

Goffman, E. (1956) 'Embarrassment and social organisation', *American Journal of Sociology* 62 (November): 264–271.

Goffman, E. (1955) 'On facework', *Psychiatry* 18 (August): 213–231.

Gross, F. and Stone, G. (1964) 'Embarrassment and the analysis of role requirements', *American Journal of Sociology* 70 (1): 1–15.

Jourard, S.M. (1966) 'An exploratory study of body accessibility', *British Journal of Social and Clinical Psychology* 5: 221–231.

Jourard, S.M. (1967) 'Out of touch: the body taboo', *New Society* 10 (267): 660–662.

Jourard, S.M. and Rubin, J.E. (1968) 'Self-disclosure and touching: a study of two modes of interpersonal encounter and their interaction', *Journal of Humanistic Psychology* 8: 39–48.

Parker, J.M. (1988) 'Theoretical perspectives in nursing: from microphysics to hermeneutics', Paper presented at the Third Nursing Research Forum, Lincoln School of Health Science, Melbourne: La Trobe University, March.

Weinberg, M.S. (1965) 'Sexual modesty, social meanings and the nudist camp', *Social Problems* 12 (3): 311–318.

Weinberg, M.S. (1968) 'Embarrassment: its variable and invariable aspects', *Social Forces* 46 (3): 382–388.

CHAPTER 18

TECHNOLOGY, SELFHOOD AND PHYSICAL DISABILITY

Deborah Lupton and Wendy Seymour

INTRODUCTION

[...]

This chapter addresses the issue of the interface of technology and physical disability, drawing on a qualitative empirical study involving interviews with people with physical disabilities. The dominant research question was to explore the ways in which technologies contribute to the meanings and experiences of the lived body/self with disabilities. The study sought to investigate the understandings, beliefs and experiences of technology on the part of the interviewees, to identify their attitudes towards particular technological applications, to examine the relationship between type of disability and use of technology and to identify factors which may inhibit or enhance technological engagement on the part of people with disabilities.

The theoretical perspective adopted employs aspects of both social constructionist and materialist approaches to examining issues related to physical disability and technology. The constructionist approach includes examination of the ways in which the body with disabilities is socioculturally constructed via representation and the reproduction of meaning (e.g. Shakespeare 1994). The materialist argument addresses the ways in which disability is a form of social, political and material disadvantage, including restricted access to resources such as technologies (e.g. Oliver 1990). The two perspectives are interconnected, because material disadvantage is in

Source: *Social Science & Medicine* (2000) 50 (12): 1851–1862.

large part influenced by the tenor of sociocultural representations of and responses to impairment: [...]

The severely damaged body, the body that is culturally designated as 'disabled' compared with other bodies designated as 'normal', remains subject to a high level of stigmatisation and marginalisation (Oliver 1990; Hevey 1992; Davis 1995, and Thomson 1997). Unlike the typically 'absent' status of the 'normal' body (Leder 1990), the body of the physically disabled person is constantly 'present' to observers in its difference from other bodies. As Davis notes, 'The body of the disabled person is seen as marked by disability. The missing limb, blind gaze, use of sign language, wheelchair or prosthesis is seen by the "normal" observer. Disability is a specular moment' (Davis 1995: 12).[...]

In a society in which people with physical disabilities are still commonly represented and treated as lacking, as 'deviant' or 'grotesque' bodies expected to conform to social structures and expectations of mainstream society (Shakespeare 1994 and Stone 1995), for many the opportunity to use technologies in creative ways may be compelling. From a materialist perspective, therefore, technologies may be regarded as offering a tangible way of redressing sociocultural disadvantage and marginalisation.

People with disabilities have historically been excluded from full participation in society and active citizenship (Abberley 1987 and Oliver 1990). Williams argues that 'The reality of life for most disabled people is not the heroic overcoming of dramatic obstacles, but the daily struggle with the mundane activities through which identity is expressed and confirmed' (Williams 1993: 103). Technology offers the potential to greatly facilitate such mundane activities. In the process it has implications for the ways in which people with disabilities construct selfhood and interact with others. By augmenting or substituting particular bodily functions and transcending time and place, new technologies offer people with disabilities the possibility of facilitating entry and participation into previously inaccessible activities and domains. Computer technologies, for example, may lessen the importance placed on physical prowess and allow greater entree into the workplace for people with disabilities. As such, they may go some way towards redressing the disabling features of many work environments (Roulstone 1993; Roulstone and Roulstone 1998a and b).

However, technologies also bear with them negative meanings and implications. Among some members of the Deaf community, for example, there exists a trenchant resistance to using such technologies as cochlear implants (Davis 1995 and Yardley 1997). In this context, technology represents an 'artificial' invader of the body and a disruption of the subculture of the Deaf community, forced upon people who do not want it by advocates who continue to represent deafness as problematic and 'abnormal'. In such a context, technologies may be offensively represented as a 'correction' to or 'normalisation' of impairment, or as allowing people to 'overcome' their impairments, an approach which Roulstone (1998a) characterises as the 'deficit model' of technological aid.[...]

This research is extremely useful in providing some recent accounts of the lived experience of using technologies for people with disabilities. However, it is limited to the discussion of mainly computerised technologies specifically in the context of paid employment. It therefore does not provide insights into the other types of technologies that people with disabilities may use in other contexts. It is this lacuna that the present study sought to address.

THE STUDY

An in-depth interview study was undertaken with participants living in the city of Adelaide, the capital of the state of South Australia. The study was initially funded as exploratory and small-scale, the first phase in a series of related projects into technology and disability. [...] Those people who came forward and agreed to participate ranged in age from 19 to 46. Seven of the participants had suffered paralysis from a spinal injury, four had cerebral palsy, one had a lower limb amputation and three had a visual disability [...]

The questions in the interview schedule were arranged around four topic areas: the participants' broad attitudes towards and use of technologies; their ideas about the relationship between types of technology and bodily function or part; their negotiation of technologies; and their identification of barriers to the use of technology. Like Roulstone, we wished to avoid the 'deficit model' of technological aid, preferring to focus instead on the ways in which sociocultural contexts may be either enabling or disabling to the living and work practices of our participants. [...]

TYPES OF TECHNOLOGY USED

[...]

The participants all said that they used a broad range of technologies in their everyday lives. The technologies they used included both those that had been especially designed as an aid for a specific disability and those that were developed for the general community but were found useful by the participants in ways that were not necessarily planned by the manufacturers. The former type of technologies, for those with mobility problems and loss of limb function, included wheelchairs, modified household items such as doors that can be opened with a string by the teeth or by remote control and hydraulic lifts for getting in and out of bed or chairs. The participant with an amputated leg used a prosthesis. The people with visual disabilities said that they used such technologies as canes, closed-circuit television for enlarging print, ultrasound sensors, a water leveller, a 'talking' clock and 'talking' scales to weigh food. While they all also used guide dogs, they debated whether or not dogs should be considered a 'technology', given that they are living creatures rather than machines.

It was evident from this group of interviewees that computer technologies were extremely important in their lives. Some computer technologies were very commonly and regularly used across the group. These included voice-activated or talking personal computers, email and bulletin boards or discussion groups on the Internet, electronic organisers or memo machines, lap tops and scanners. Some of these computers had been specially adapted for the participants (for example, with voice-activated mechanisms) while others had not. Several people said that they used hands-free or mobile telephones. [...]

THE BENEFITS OF TECHNOLOGY

Regardless of their particular disability, several major attributes of the technologies to which they had access emerged as most important to the interviewees. These attributes were communication with others, mobility, physical safety, personal autonomy, control over one's body and life, independence, competence, confidence, the ability to engage in the workforce and participation in the wider community.

For example, Jo, a 35-year-old woman with quadriplegia, said that she highly values the technology she uses 'because it actually allows me to control my own life and without it I actually have less control'. Jo went on to emphasise that:

> *Control means being able to do things when I want to do them and make the decisions that I want to make as much as I can without having to involve another person.* [...]

Technologies also allow people to avoid the embarrassment associated with dependence on others for help with bodily functions. Sam talked about his discomfort about his urine catheter bag. He now has an electric device that allows him to empty it without another person's assistance. This meant that he was able to 'do that in a way that I don't have to rely on other people to do it. It's given me a whole larger range of independence and being able to do it in a way that is, can be reasonably discreet'. Jo also talked about her difficulties in relation to the elimination of bodily wastes. She commented how in an ideal world she would love to be able to access a technology that allowed her to toilet herself:

> *For me the nicest thing would be able to get on and off the toilet by myself, if I could do that. It actually doesn't bother me that I can't walk and I've often said. 'No, I think I am who I am and I'm okay with that'. My biggest frustration is that I can't get on and off the toilet by myself because my whole life revolves about people coming in and out to toilet me. So if I could do that, I mean, that would just be fabulous!*

TECHNOLOGY AND IDENTITY

The positive attributes of technology identified by the participants contributed to an integral aspect of selfhood and bodily experience: the opportunity to engage more easily in social relationships. For most of the participants, technologies were valued for allowing them to tame the disorderly aspects of their bodies and thus to facilitate social integration. They drew an important distinction, however, between the technologies they considered more 'normalising' and others which they saw as marginalising or stigmatising. All the participants felt strongly that their disability should not come to define their identities. As Tom argued:

> *I don't want to be particularly conspicuous on account of my particular way of dealing with my disability or because of my disability for that matter. I really want to be known as yes, a person that has a disability but has a lot of attributes too. So I'd like to be known in context rather than just one part of me being known. Often the visible technology that I use attracts attention to that.*

The notion of integration, thus, involved not only bodily functioning close to ideas of the norm, but also avoiding the use of technologies that overtly bespoke of a disability. The relative 'invisibility' or social acceptability of technologies was therefore important to people. For example, the people with visual disability discussed how they were treated when they used a guide dog compared with using a cane or an electronic sensor. They noted that when they used the dog, people tended to treat them in a more friendly and accepting manner. They suggested that the cane or ultrasound sensor may serve to make them look more alienating and 'different' to others. As Margie put it:

> *A dog is far more suitable than using something like a mote sensor and a sonic pathfinder, for example, which are electronic aids that are either hand-held, or one actually sits on your head, like a head band with ear plugs and a big thing across the forehead and stuff. I really believe that something like that is not – well, it's not that it's not socially acceptable, it's more from the point of view that it's socially frightening to a lot of people, because it doesn't look particularly attractive, it can cause a few reactions in some people. Whereas, for example, to walk around with a dog is completely and utterly socially acceptable. And I think with technologies, the more obtrusive it is, the more offensive it can become to some people.*

Several people noted that using technologies designed specifically for people with their disability may produce a response from others that was highly stigmatising. Tom commented, for example, that people often made offensive assumptions about his intelligence when he was using a cane, but did not do so when he used a technology that was in general use:

> *I think it's not so much the technology as what the technology refers back to the user of the technology. That is, as soon as you pull out a long white cane, then people start making assumptions, sometimes right, sometimes wrong, about your level of vision, about your level of intelligence or sorts of things like that, sort of indirect associations that are formed. And you know, I think the best example is something where that does not happen, like the little [electronic] business memo that I use. I have to explain to people, 'Look I'll just take a note of this, I'm going to speak into my business memo'. People think 'Gee, that's really cool', you know because anyone can use that, it's not specially related to people with disability.*

The wheelchair was often raised as a particular exemplar of how technologies may mark people out as 'different'. As Jenny, who is 30 and has paraplegia pointed out, 'a wheelchair is a signifier of disability'. She argued that the focus in general discourses on 'helping' people with disabilities with technologies is offensive. In her own case, as someone who uses a wheelchair for mobility, she was offended by:

all those soppy [women's magazine] articles that have these brave profiles – 'They told me I'd never walk again and I walked out of that hospital'. Yeah right! You could've been doing something useful, get yourself a decent wheelchair, go and learn how to use it and then go and do something useful!

Jenny criticised the idea put forward in such popular accounts that using a wheelchair is the worst thing that could happen to someone, the end of a useful and happy life. Such accounts, she observed, underline the position of people with disabilities as 'a lower human being'.

It was observed by other wheelchair-using participants that this technology tended to detract attention from the identity and individuality of the person using it. Jo was particularly vehement on this point, noting that:

The wheelchair is the topic of discussion whenever you get into a lift – how well it turns, can you reverse, do you have license, you know, all of those things. And sometimes you'd like to chuck it in the bin, I guess, just to say 'Excuse me, but it's about me!' You know, so it takes the focus from me.

Ian, however, could see both positive and negative aspects to using a wheelchair. He noted that his wheelchair both drew attention to his 'difference' but also enabled him to achieve a greater degree of mobility and interact with others:

I don't want people to feel sorry for me, that's one. And two, the chair just screams out ' Look at me!' and you get like crowds of people just staring at this chair ... [On the other hand], if I didn't use the wheelchair I'd be laid up in bed 24 hours, 7 days a week. So the advantage is yes, I can get around, it's a means of transport and yes, it's a little bit of quality of life.

Several people with cerebral palsy identified a particular technology that they found even more intrusive than a wheelchair – the communication board (involving using a pointer to point to letters consecutively to spell out words rather than speaking them) or its electronic version. Ron argued that a wheelchair was more socially acceptable than using an electronic communicator or computer to communicate with people face to face:

> *I can go into a party [in a wheelchair] and I'm Ron, but if I took a computer in there or a communicator I'd be viewed as Ron and the computer, or Ron and the communicator.*

[...]

The technologies Kate uses, she said, must address 'what I need them for but also they have to fit into my view of myself and the way that I want to present myself to the community'.

Several participants emphasised the point that where once using computers to communicate or perform work tasks might have singled out people with disabilities as 'different', this is no longer necessarily the case because these technologies are now used extensively in the workplace and at academic institutions. Tom commented, for example, that:

> *Certainly in terms of computerised technology, yes [it helps me fit in]. Although I'm obviously using it a different way, it makes me feel more like other people because everybody in my current workplace [a government department] uses PCs, it's a fairly major part of their work.*

Further, for a majority of the participants, computer technologies were seen to facilitate communication. People could have a choice whether or not they wished others to know about their disability and thus were able to avoid, to some extent, the discriminatory attitudes they otherwise encountered. As Ann, 35, who has cerebral palsy put it:

> *Because they can't see you, they don't know how disabled you are, they don't even know how you are accessing the keyboard. They're talking with you by your computer and disability doesn't even come into it because they speak to you like an able-bodied person. And especially when you have a speech disability, people on the outside think that because we speak slowly that we think slow and we get patronised all the time. But on the bulletin board I never get patronised, because they don't really know if you have a disability unless you tell them that you have got a disability.*

[...]

CONCLUSION

It was clear from this preliminary study that people with disabilities may attach great importance to some of the technologies they use. The participants identified and strongly affirmed a number of attributes offered by technology – communication with others, mobility, physical safety, personal autonomy, control, independence, competence, confidence, the ability to better engage in social relationships, the workforce and participation in wider community. These attributes are key components of their sense of self and wellbeing.

[...]

Technologies were conceptualised in two dominant ways by our participants: as tools assisting bodily function and as contributing to the body/self as it is experienced and presented to others. Some technologies allowed the participants to present themselves in ways which fitted with dominant values associated with functioning, capable individuals who need little help from others. The opportunity to construct and present this ideal self, contra to the meanings of passivity and helplessness that are commonly associated with disability, is clearly a choice that was of great importance to the people we interviewed. Such technologies, therefore, were incorporated unproblematically into their notions of self and body. In contrast, those technologies that served to underline the participants' status as 'disabled', to single them out as 'deviant bodies', tended to be greeted with greater ambivalence by the interviewees. Some people rejected these technologies outright, seeing them as barriers to presenting their preferred self even though they may have enhanced bodily capacities. These technologies were not incorporated, but rather were conceptually positioned as 'other' to oneself.[...]

REFERENCES

Abberley, P. (1987) 'The concept of oppression and the development of a social theory of disability', *Disability, Handicap & Society* 2 1: 5–19 *Abstract-PsycINFO.*

Davis, L. (1995) *Enforcing Normalcy: Disability, Deafness and the Body*, New York: Verso.

Hevey, D. (1992) *The Creatures Time Forgot: Photography and Disability Imagery*, London: Routledge.

Leder, D. (1990) *The Absent Body*, Chicago: University of Chicago Press.

Oliver, M. (1990) *The Politics of Disablement*, London: Macmillan.

Roulstone, A. (1998a) 'Researching a disabling society: the case of employment and new technology', in Shakespeare, T. (ed.), *The Disability Reader: Social Science Perspectives*, London: Cassell, 110–128.

Roulstone, A. (1998b) *Enabling Technology: Disabled People, Work and New Technology*, Buckingham: Open University Press.

Shakespeare, T. (1994) 'Cultural representation of disabled people: dustbins for disavowal?' *Disability and Society* 9 3: 283–299.

Stone, S. (1995) 'The myth of bodily perfection', *Disability and Society* 10 4: 413–424. *Abstract-PsycINFO*.

Thomson, R. (1997) *Extraordinary Bodies: Figuring Physical Disability in American Culture and Literature*, New York: Columbia University Press.

Williams, G. (1993) 'Chronic illness and the pursuit of virtue in everyday life', in Radley, A. (ed.) *Worlds of Illness: Biographical and Cultural Perspectives on Health and Disease*, London: Routledge, 92–108.

Yardley, L. (1997) 'The quest for natural communication: technology, language and deafness', *Health* 1 1: 37–56.

PART III

THE PERSON IN THE PROCESS

Anita Rogers

Part III focuses on the person in the communication process in health and social care. The chapters included here explore and expand on a number of related themes: attitudes, attributes and skills, the emotional impact of encounters for service users and practitioners, and the nature of difficult encounters.

The first group of readings in this section explore ways of thinking about the necessary attributes for interpersonal communication in care settings. In Chapter 19 (written in 1957) 'The necessary and sufficient conditions of therapeutic personality change', the American humanistic psychologist Carl Rogers describes the 'core conditions', a set of important attitudes and attributes that have become widely regarded as central to helping relationships. Chapter 20 'Compassion fatigue: how much can I give?' by Peter Huggard, a lecturer in primary health care, explores why practitioners in health care sometimes avoid interpersonal engagement in an attempt to protect themselves from burnout. In Chapter 21 'Do virtues have a role in the practice of counselling?', Anne Gallagher, a lecturer and mental health practitioner, suggests there is an ethical dimension to helping relationships. Taking a virtue ethics approach to core conditions or facilitative qualities, she suggests that they can be developed through practice.

The second group of chapters shifts the focus to the question of skills. In Chapter 22 'Are there universal human being skills?' Richard Nelson-Jones, a writer on the theory and practice of counselling, asks whether there are skills that all human beings possess that lead them toward cooperation and caring. Chapter 23 'To communicate and engage: relevant counselling skills' by Janet Seden, a social work educator, explores the kind of communication skills needed by social workers as they engage with service users. In Chapter 24 'Disability and communication: listening is not enough' Sally French and John Swain, who are both academics and writers on disability issues, take a critical stance towards attempts to develop effective communication in services for disabled people, emphasising the importance of issues of power and diversity.

The next three chapters explore the emotional impact of caring relationships. In Chapter 25 'Caring presence: a case study' Joan Engebretson, an American nurse educator, gives a powerful and moving account of what it means to be a 'caring presence' for both practitioner and service user in a tragic situation. Arlie Hochschild, an American sociologist who introduced the term 'emotional labour' to the language of health and social care, discusses how emotions are constructed and managed 'in context' in Chapter 26 'The sociology of emotion as a way of seeing'. In Chapter 27 'Divisions of emotional labour: disclosure and cancer', nurse educator Nicky James explores how responsibilities for the emotional agenda and the management of emotions are divided up among various medical practitioners and service users in the treatment of cancer.

The final two chapters focus in different ways on difficulties and challenges in communication and relationships in care work. In Chapter 28 'Rediscovering unpopular patients: the concept of social judgement', Martin Johnson and Christine Webb, both nurse educators, raise provocative issues about how service users are evaluated and judged, using research from the nursing context. Finally, in Chapter 29 'Steven' Valerie Sinason, a psychoanalytic psychotherapist, describes her six-year odyssey working with Steven, a boy with organic brain damage, offering glimpses into Steven's extraordinary world and her extraordinary work with him.

CHAPTER 19

THE NECESSARY AND SUFFICIENT CONDITIONS OF THERAPEUTIC PERSONALITY CHANGE

Carl R. Rogers

For many years I have been engaged in psychotherapy with individuals in distress. In recent years I have found myself increasingly concerned with the process of abstracting from that experience the general principles which appear to be involved in it. I have endeavoured to discover any orderliness, any unity which seems to inhere in the subtle, complex tissue of interpersonal relationship in which I have so constantly been immersed in therapeutic work. One of the current products of this concern is an attempt to state, in formal terms, a theory of psychotherapy, of personality, and of interpersonal relationships which will encompass and contain the phenomena of my experience.[1] What I wish to do in this chapter is to take one very small segment of that theory, spell it out more completely, and explore its meaning and usefulness.

THE PROBLEM

The question to which I wish to address myself is this: Is it possible to state, in terms which are clearly definable and measurable, the psychological conditions which are both necessary and sufficient to bring about

Source: *The Journal of Consulting Psychology* (1957) 21: 95–103.

constructive personality change? Do we, in other words, know with any precision those elements which are essential if psychotherapeutic change is to ensue?

Before proceeding to the major task let me dispose very briefly of the second portion of the question. What is meant by such phrases as 'psychotherapeutic change', 'constructive personality change'? This problem also deserves deep and serious consideration, but for the moment let me suggest a commonsense type of meaning upon which we can perhaps agree for purposes of this chapter. By these phrases is meant: change in the personality structure of the individual, at both surface and deeper levels, in a direction which clinicians would agree means greater integration, less internal conflict, more energy utilisable for effective living; change in behaviour away from behaviours generally regarded as immature and toward behaviours regarded as mature. This brief description may suffice to indicate the kind of change for which we are considering the preconditions. It may also suggest the ways in which this criterion of change may be determined.[2]

THE CONDITIONS

As I have considered my own clinical experience and that of my colleagues, together with the pertinent research which is available, I have drawn out several conditions which seem to me to be *necessary* to initiate constructive personality change, and which, taken together, appear to be *sufficient* to inaugurate that process. As I have worked on this problem I have found myself surprised at the simplicity of what has emerged. The statement which follows is not offered with any assurance as to its correctness, but with the expectation that it will have the value of any theory, namely that it states or implies a series of hypotheses which are open to proof or disproof, thereby clarifying and extending our knowledge of the field.

Since I am not, in this paper, trying to achieve suspense, I will state at once, in severely rigorous and summarised terms, the six conditions which I have come to feel are basic to the process of personality change. The meaning of a number of the terms is not immediately evident, but will be clarified in the explanatory sections which follow. It is hoped that this brief statement will have much more significance to the reader when he has completed the chapter. Without further introduction let me state the basic theoretical position.

For constructive personality change to occur, it is necessary that these conditions exist and continue over a period of time:

1 Two persons are in psychological contact.
2 The first, whom we shall term the client, is in a state of incongruence, being vulnerable or anxious.

3 The second person, whom we shall term the therapist, is congruent or integrated in the relationship.
4 The therapist experiences unconditional positive regard for the client.
5 The therapist experiences an empathic understanding of the client's internal frame of reference and endeavours to communicate this experience to the client.
6 The communication to the client of the therapist's empathic understanding and unconditional positive regard is to a minimal degree achieved.

No other conditions are necessary. If these six conditions exist, and continue over a period of time, this is sufficient. The process of constructive personality change will follow.

A RELATIONSHIP

The first condition specifies that a minimal relationship, a psychological contact, must exist. I am hypothesising that significant positive personality change does not occur except in a relationship. This is of course an hypothesis, and it may be disproved.

The remaining 5 conditions define the characteristics of the relationship which are regarded as essential by defining the necessary characteristics of each person in the relationship. All that is intended by this first condition is to specify that the two people are to some degree in contact, that each makes some perceived difference in the experiential field of the other. Probably it is sufficient if each makes some 'subceived' difference, even though the individual may not be consciously aware of this impact. Thus it might be difficult to know whether a catatonic patient perceives a therapist's presence as making a difference – a difference of any kind – but it is almost certain that at some organic level he does sense this difference.

Except in such a difficult borderline situation as that just mentioned, it would be relatively easy to define this condition in operational terms and thus determine, from a hard-boiled research point of view, whether the condition does, or does not, exist. The simplest method of determination involves simply the awareness of both client and therapist. If each is aware of being in personal or psychological contact with the other, then this condition is met.

This first condition of therapeutic change is such a simple one that perhaps it should be labelled an assumption or a precondition in order to set it apart from those that follow. Without it, however, the remaining items would have no meaning, and that is the reason for including it.

THE STATE OF THE CLIENT

It was specified that it is necessary that the client be 'in a state of incongruence, being vulnerable or anxious'. What is the meaning of these terms?

Incongruence is a basic construct in the theory we have been developing. It refers to a discrepancy between the actual experience of the organism and the self picture of the individual insofar as it represents that experience. Thus a student may experience, at a total or organismic level, a fear of the university and of examinations which are given on the third floor of a certain building, since these may demonstrate a fundamental inadequacy in him. Since such a fear of his inadequacy is decidedly at odds with his personal concept this experience is represented (distortedly) in his awareness as an unreasonable fear of climbing stairs in this building, or any building, and soon an unreasonable fear of crossing the open campus. Thus there is a fundamental discrepancy between the experienced meaning of the situation as it registers in his organism and the symbolic representation of that experience in awareness in such a way that it does not conflict with his own picture. In this case to admit a fear of inadequacy would contradict the picture he holds of himself: to admit incomprehensible fears does not contradict his self concept.

Another instance would be the mother who develops vague illnesses whenever her only son makes plans to leave home. The actual desire is to hold on to her only source of satisfaction. To perceive this in awareness would be inconsistent with the picture she holds of herself as a good mother. Illness, however, is consistent with her self concept, and the experience is symbolised in this distorted fashion. Thus again there is a basic incongruence between the self as perceived (in this case as an ill mother needing attention) and the actual experience (in this case the desire to hold on to her son).

When the individual has no awareness of such incongruence in himself, then he is merely vulnerable to the possibility of anxiety and disorganisation. Some experience might occur so suddenly or so obviously that the incongruence could not be denied. Therefore, the person is vulnerable to such a possibility.

If the individual dimly perceives such a personal incongruence, then a tension state occurs which is known as anxiety. The incongruence need not be sharply perceived. It is enough that it is subceived – that is, discriminated as threatening to the self without any awareness of the content of that threat. Such anxiety is often seen in therapy as the individual approaches awareness of some element of his experience which is in sharp contradiction to his self concept.

It is not easy to give precise operational definition to this second of the six conditions, yet to some degree this has been achieved. Several research workers have defined the self concept by means of a Q sort by the individual of a list of self-referent items. This gives us an operational picture of the self. The total experiencing of the individual is more difficult to capture. Chodorkoff (1954) has defined it as a Q sort made by a clinician who sorts the same self-referent items independently, basing his sorting on the picture he has obtained of the individual from projective tests. His sort thus includes unconscious as well as conscious elements of the individual's experience, thus representing (in an admittedly imperfect way) the totality of the client's experience. The correlation between these two sortings gives a crude operational measure of incongruence between self and experience, low or negative correlation representing of course a high degree of incongruence.

THE THERAPIST'S GENUINENESS IN THE RELATIONSHIP

The third condition is that the therapist should be, within the confines of this relationship, a congruent, genuine integrated person. It means that within the relationship he is freely and deeply himself, with his actual experience accurately represented by his awareness of himself. It is the opposite of presenting a façade, either knowingly or unknowingly.

It is not necessary (nor is it possible) that the therapist be a paragon who exhibits this degree of integration, of wholeness, in every aspect of his life. It is sufficient that he is accurately himself in this hour of this relationship, that in this basic sense he is what he actually is, in this moment of time.

It should be clear that this includes being himself even in ways which are not regarded as ideal for psychotherapy. His experience may be 'I am afraid of this client' or 'My attention is so focused on my own problems that I can scarcely listen to him'. If the therapist is not denying these feelings to awareness, but is able freely to be them (as well as being his other feelings), then the condition we have stated is met.

It would take us too far afield to consider the puzzling matter as to the degree to which the therapist overtly communicates this reality in himself to the client. Certainly the aim is not for the therapist to express or talk out his own feelings, but primarily that he should not be deceiving the client as to himself. At times he may need to talk out some of his own feelings (either to the client, or to a colleague or supervisor) if they are standing in the way of the two following conditions.

It is not too difficult to suggest an operational definition for this third condition. We resort again to Q technique. If the therapist sorts a series of items relevant to the relationship (using a list similar to the ones developed by Fiedler 1950, 1953 and Bown 1954), this will give his perception of his experience in the relationship. If several judges who have observed the interview or listened to a recording of it (or observed a sound movie of it) now sort the same items to represent *their* perception of the relationship, this second sorting should catch those elements of the therapist's behaviour and inferred attitudes of which he is unaware, as well as those of which he is aware. Thus a high correlation between the therapist's sort and the observer's sort would represent in crude form an operational definition of the therapist's congruence or integration in the relationship; and a low correlation, the opposite.

UNCONDITIONAL POSITIVE REGARD

To the extent that the therapist finds himself experiencing a warm acceptance of each aspect of the client's experience as being a part of that client, he is experiencing unconditional positive regard. This concept has been developed by Standal (1954). It means that there are no *conditions* of acceptance, no feeling of 'I like you only *if* you are thus and so'. It means a 'prizing' of the person, as Dewey has used that term. It is at the opposite pole from a selective evaluating attitude – 'You are bad in these ways, good in those'. It involves as much feeling of acceptance for the client's expression of negative, 'bad', painful, fearful, defensive, abnormal feelings as for his expression of 'good' positive, mature, confident, social feelings, as much acceptance of ways in which he is inconsistent as of ways in which he is consistent. It means a caring for the client, but not in a possessive way or in such a way as simply to satisfy the therapist's own needs. It means a caring for the client as a *separate* person, with permission to have his own feelings, his own experiences. One client describes the therapist as 'fostering my possession of my own experience ... that [this] is *my* experience and that I am actually having it: thinking what I think, feeling what I feel, wanting what I want, fearing what I fear: no "ifs," "buts," or "not reallys"'. This is the type of acceptance which is hypothesised as being necessary if personality change is to occur.

Like the two previous conditions, this fourth condition is a matter of degree,[3] as immediately becomes apparent if we attempt to define it in terms of specific research operations. One such method of giving it definition would be to consider the Q sort for the relationship as described under Condition 3. To the extent that items expressive of unconditional positive regard are sorted as characteristic of the relationship by both the therapist and the observers, unconditional positive regard might be said to exist. Such items might include statements of this order: 'I feel no revulsion at anything the client says': 'I feel neither approval nor disapproval of the client and his statements – simply acceptance'; 'I feel warmly toward the client – toward his weaknesses and problems as well as his potentialities'; 'I am not inclined to pass judgement on what the client tells me'; 'I like the client'. To the extent that both therapist and observers perceive these items as characteristic, or their opposites as uncharacteristic, Condition 4 might be said to be met.

EMPATHY

The fifth condition is that the therapist is experiencing an accurate, empathic understanding of the client's awareness of his own experience. To sense the client's private world as if it were your own, but without ever losing the 'as if' quality – this is empathy, and this seems essential to therapy. To sense the client's anger, fear, or confusion as if it were your own, yet without your own anger, fear, or confusion getting bound up in it, is the condition we are endeavouring to describe. When the client's world is this clear to the therapist, and he moves about in it freely, then he can both communicate his understanding of what is clearly known to the client and can also voice meanings in the client's experience of which the client is scarcely aware. As one client described this second aspect: 'Every now and again, with me in a tangle of thought and feeling, screwed up in a web of mutually divergent lines of movement, with impulses from different parts of me, and me feeling the feeling of its being all too much and suchlike – then whomp, just like a sunbeam thrusting its way through cloudbanks and tangles of foliage to spread a circle of light on a tangle of forest paths, came some comment from you. [It was] clarity, even disentanglement, an additional twist to the picture, a putting in place. Then the consequence – the sense of moving on, the relaxation. These were sunbeams'. That such penetrating empathy is important for therapy is indicated by Fiedler's research (1953) in which items such as the following placed high in the description of relationships created by experienced therapists:

> *The therapist is well able to understand the patient's feelings.*

> *The therapist is never in any doubt about what the patient means.*

> *The therapist's remarks fit in just right with the patient's mood and content.*

> *The therapist's tone of voice conveys the complete ability to share the patient's feelings.*

An operational definition of the therapist's empathy could be provided in different ways. Use might be made of the Q sort described under Condition 3. To the degree that items descriptive of accurate empathy were sorted as characteristic by both the therapist and the observers, this condition would be regarded as existing.

Another way of defining this condition would be for both client and therapist to sort a list of items descriptive of client feelings. Each would sort independently, the task being to represent the feelings which the client had experienced during a just completed interview. If the correlation between client and therapist sortings were high, accurate empathy would be said to exist, a low correlation indicating the opposite conclusion.

Still another way of measuring empathy would be for trained judges to rate the depth and accuracy of the therapist's empathy on the basis of listening to recorded interviews.

THE CLIENT'S PERCEPTION OF THE THERAPIST

The final condition as stated is that the client perceives, to a minimal degree, the acceptance and empathy which the therapist experiences for him. Unless some communication of these attitudes has been achieved, then such attitudes do not exist in the relationship as far as the client is concerned, and the therapeutic process could not, by our hypothesis, be initiated.

Since attitudes cannot be directly perceived, it might be somewhat more accurate to state that therapist behaviours and words are perceived by the client as meaning that to some degree the therapist accepts and understands him.

An operational definition of this condition would not be difficult. The client might, after an interview, sort a Q-sort list of items referring to qualities representing the relationship between himself and the therapist. (The same list could be used as for Condition 3.) If several items descriptive of acceptance and empathy are sorted by the client as characteristic of the relationship, then this condition could be regarded as met. In the present state of our knowledge the meaning of 'to a minimal degree' would have to be arbitrary.

SOME COMMENTS

Up to this point the effort has been made to present, briefly and factually, the conditions which I have come to regard as essential for psychotherapeutic change. I have not tried to give the theoretical context of these conditions nor to explain what seem to me to be the dynamics of their effectiveness.[. . .]

I have, however, given at least one means of defining, in operational terms, each of the conditions mentioned. I have done this in order to stress the fact that I am not speaking of vague qualities which ideally should be present if some other vague result is to occur. I am presenting conditions which are crudely measurable even in the present state of our technology, and have suggested specific operations in each instance even though I am sure that more adequate methods of measurement could be devised by a serious investigator.

My purpose has been to stress the notion that in my opinion we are dealing with an if-then phenomenon in which knowledge of the dynamics is not essential to testing the hypotheses. Thus, to illustrate from another field: if one substance, shown by a series of operations to be the substance known as hydrochloric acid, is mixed with another substance, shown by another series of operations to be sodium hydroxide, then salt and water will be products of this mixture. This is true whether one regards the results as due to magic, or whether one explains it in the most adequate terms of modern chemical theory. In the same way it is being postulated here that certain definable conditions precede certain definable changes and that this fact exists independently of our efforts to account for it.

THE RESULTING HYPOTHESES

The major value of stating any theory in unequivocal terms is that specific hypotheses may be drawn from it which are capable of proof or disproof. Thus, even if the conditions which have been postulated as necessary and sufficient conditions are more incorrect than correct (which I hope they are not), they could still advance science in this field by providing a base of operations from which fact could be winnowed out from error.

The hypotheses which would follow from the theory given would be of this order:

If these six conditions (as operationally defined) exist, then constructive personality change (as defined) will occur in the client.

If one or more of these conditions is not present, constructive personality change will not occur.

These hypotheses hold in any situation whether it is or is not labeled 'psychotherapy'.

Only Condition 1 is dichotomous (it either is present or is not), and the remaining five occur in varying degree, each on its continuum. Since this is true, another hypothesis follows, and it is likely that this would be the simplest to test:

> *If all six conditions are present, then the greater the degree to which Conditions 2 to 6 exist, the more marked will be the constructive personality change in the client.*

At the present time the above hypothesis can only be stated in this general form – which implies that all of the conditions have equal weight. Empirical studies will no doubt make possible much more refinement of this hypothesis. It may be, for example, that if anxiety is high in the client, then the other conditions are less important. Or if unconditional positive regard is high (as in a mother's love for her child), then perhaps a modest degree of empathy is sufficient. But at the moment we can only speculate on such possibilities.

SIGNIFICANT OMISSIONS

If there is any startling feature in the formulation which has been given as to the necessary conditions for therapy, it probably lies in the elements which are omitted. In present-day clinical practice, therapists operate as though there were many other conditions in addition to those described, which are essential for psychotherapy. To point this up it may be well to mention a few of the conditions which, after thoughtful consideration of our research and our experience, are not included.

For example, it is *not* stated that these conditions apply to one type of client, and that other conditions are necessary to bring about psychotherapeutic change with other types of client. Probably no idea is so prevalent in clinical work today as that one works with neurotics in one way, with psychotics in another, that certain therapeutic conditions must be provided for compulsives . . ., etc. Because of this heavy weight of clinical opinion to the contrary, it is with some 'fear and trembling' that I advance the concept that the essential conditions of psychotherapy exist in a single configuration, even though the client or patient may use them very differently.[4]

It is *not* stated that these six conditions are the essential conditions for client-centered therapy, and that other conditions are essential for other types of psychotherapy. I certainly am heavily influenced by my own experience, and that experience has led me to a viewpoint which is termed 'client centered'. Nevertheless my aim in stating this theory is to state the conditions which apply to *any* situation in which constructive personality change occurs, whether we are thinking of classical psychoanalysis, or any of its modern offshoots, or Adlerian psychotherapy, or any other. It will be obvious then that in my judgement much of what is considered to be essential would not be found, empirically, to be essential. Testing of some of the stated hypotheses would throw light on this perplexing issue. We may of course find that various therapies produce various types of personality change, and that for each psychotherapy a separate set of conditions is necessary. Until and unless this is demonstrated, I am hypothesising that effective psychotherapy of any sort produces similar changes in personality and behaviour, and that a single set of preconditions is necessary.

It is *not* stated that psychotherapy is a special kind of relationship, different in kind from all others which occur in everyday life. It will be evident instead that for brief moments, at least, many good friendships fulfil the six conditions. Usually this is only momentarily, however, and then empathy falters, the positive regard becomes conditional, or the congruence of the 'therapist' friend becomes overlaid by some degree of façade or defensiveness. Thus the therapeutic relationship is seen as a heightening of the constructive qualities which often exist in part in other relationships, and an extension through time of qualities which in other relationships tend at best to be momentary.

It is *not* stated that special intellectual professional knowledge – psychological, psychiatric, medical, or religious – is required of the therapist. Conditions 3, 4, and 5, which apply especially to the therapist, are qualities of experience, not intellectual information. If they are to be acquired, they must, in my opinion, be acquired through an experiential training – which may be, but usually is not, a part of professional training. It troubles me to hold such a radical point of view, but I can draw no other conclusion from my experience. Intellectual training and the acquiring of information has, I believe, many valuable results – but becoming a therapist is not one of those results.

It is *not* stated that it is necessary for psychotherapy that the therapist have an accurate psychological diagnosis of the client. Here too it troubles me to hold a viewpoint so at variance with my clinical colleagues. When one thinks of the vast proportion of time spent in any psychological, psychiatric, or mental hygiene center on the exhaustive psychological evaluation of the client or patient, it seems as though this *must* serve a useful purpose insofar as psychotherapy is concerned. Yet the more I have observed therapists, and the more closely I have studied research such as that done by Fiedler (1953) and others, the more I am forced to the conclusion that such diagnostic knowledge is not essential to psychotherapy.[5] It may even be that its defence as a necessary prelude to psychotherapy is simply a protective alternative to the admission that it is, for the most part, a colossal waste of time. There is only one useful purpose I have been able to observe which relates to psychotherapy. Some therapists cannot feel secure in the relationship with the client unless they possess such diagnostic knowledge. Without it they feel fearful of him, unable to be empathic, unable to experience unconditional regard, finding it necessary to put up a pretence in the relationship. If they know in *advance* of suicidal impulses they can somehow be more acceptant of them. Thus, for some therapists, the security they perceive in diagnostic information may be a basis for permitting themselves to be integrated in the relationship, and to experience empathy and full acceptance. In these instances a psychological diagnosis would certainly be justified as adding to the comfort and hence the effectiveness of the therapist. But even here it does not appear to be a basic precondition for psychotherapy.[6]

Perhaps I have given enough illustrations to indicate that the conditions I have hypothesised as necessary and sufficient for psychotherapy are striking and unusual primarily by virtue of what they omit. If we were to determine, by a survey of the behaviours of therapists, those hypotheses which they appear to regard as necessary to psychotherapy, the list would be a great deal longer and more complex.

IS THIS THEORETICAL FORMULATION USEFUL?

Aside from the personal satisfaction it gives as a venture in abstraction and generalisation, what is the value of a theoretical statement such as has been offered in this chapter? I should like to spell out more fully the usefulness which I believe it may have.

In the field of research it may give both direction and impetus to investigation. Since it sees the conditions of constructive personality change as general, it greatly broadens the opportunities for study. Psychotherapy is not the only situation aimed at constructive personality change. Programmes of training for leadership in industry and programmes of training for military leadership often aim at such change. Educational institutions or programmes frequently aim at development of character and personality as well as at intellectual skills. Community agencies aim at personality and behavioural change in delinquents and criminals. Such programmes would provide an opportunity for the broad testing of the hypotheses offered. If it is found that constructive personality change occurs in such programmes when the hypothesised conditions are not fulfilled, then the theory would have to be revised. If however the hypotheses are upheld, then the results, both for the planning of such programmes and for our knowledge of human dynamics, would be significant. In the field of psychotherapy itself, the application of consistent hypotheses to the work of various schools of therapists may prove highly profitable. Again the disproof of the hypotheses offered would be as important as their confirmation, either result adding significantly to our knowledge.

For the practice of psychotherapy the theory also offers significant problems for consideration. One of its implications is that the techniques of the various therapies are relatively unimportant except to the extent that they serve as channels for fulfilling one of the conditions. In client-centred therapy, for example, the technique of reflecting feelings has been described and commented on (Rogers 195: 26–36). In terms of the theory here being presented, this technique is by no means an essential condition of therapy. To the extent, however, that it provides a channel by which the therapist communicates a sensitive empathy and an unconditional positive regard, then it may serve as a technical channel by which the essential conditions of therapy are fulfilled. In the same way, the theory I have presented would see no essential value to therapy of such techniques as interpretation of personality dynamics, free association, analysis of dreams, analysis of the transference, hypnosis, interpretation of life style, suggestion, and the like. Each of these techniques may, however, become a channel for communicating the essential conditions which have been formulated. An interpretation may be given in a way which communicates the unconditional positive regard of the therapist. A stream of free association may be listened to in a way which communicates an empathy which the thereapist is experiencing. In the handling of the transference an effective therapist often communicates his own wholeness and congruence in the relationship. Similarly for the other techniques. But just as these techniques *may* communicate the elements which are essential for therapy, so any one of them may communicate attitudes and experiences sharply contradictory to the hypothesised conditions of therapy. Feeling may be 'reflected' in a way which communicates the therapist's lack of empathy. Interpretations may be rendered in a way which indicates the highly conditional regard of the therapist. Any of the techniques may communicate the fact that the therapist is expressing one attitude at a surface level, and another contradictory attitude which is denied to his own awareness. Thus one value of such a theoretical formulation as we have offered is that it may assist therapists to think more critically about those elements of their experience, attitudes, and behaviours which are essential to psychotherapy, and those which are nonessential or even deleterious to psychotherapy.

Finally, in those programmes – educational, correctional, military, or industrial – which aim toward constructive changes in the personality structure and behaviour of the individual, this formulation may serve as a very tentative criterion against which to measure the programme. Until it is much further tested by research, it cannot be thought of as a valid criterion, but, as in the field of psychotherapy, it may help to stimulate critical analysis and the formulation of alternative conditions and alternative hypotheses.

SUMMARY

Drawing from a larger theoretical context, six conditions are postulated as necessary and sufficient conditions for the initiation of a process of constructive personality change. A brief explanation is given of each condition, and suggestions are made as to how each may be operationally defined for research purposes. The implications of this theory for research for psychotherapy, and for educational and training programmes aimed at constructive personality change, are indicated. It is pointed out that many of the conditions which are commonly regarded as necessary to psychotherapy are, in terms of this theory, nonessential.

NOTES

1 This formal statement is entitled 'A theory of therapy, personality and interpersonal relationships, as developed in the client-centered framework', by Carl R. Rogers. The manuscript was prepared at the request of the Committee of the American Psychological Association for the Study of the Status and Development of Psychology in the United States. It will be published by McGraw-Hill in one of several volumes being prepared by this committee.

2 That this is a measurable and determinable criterion has been shown in research already completed.

3 The phrase 'unconditional positive regard' may be an unfortunate one, since it sounds like an absolute, an all or nothing dispositional concept. It is probably evident from the description that completely unconditional positive regard would never exist except in theory. From a clinical and experiential point of view I believe the most accurate statement is that the effective therapist experiences unconditional positive regard for the client during many moments of his contact with him, yet from time to time he experiences only a conditional positive regard – and perhaps at times a negative regard, though this is not likely in effective therapy. It is in this sense that unconditional positive regard exists as a matter of degree in any relationship.

4 I cling to this statement of my hypothesis even though it is challenged by a study by Kirtner (1955). Kirtner has found, in a group of 26 cases from the Counseling Center at the University of Chicago, that there are sharp differences in the client's mode of approach to the resolution of life difficulties, and that these differences are related to success in psychotherapy. Briefly, the client who sees his problem as involving his relationships, and who feels that he contributes to this problem and wants to change it, is likely to be successful. The client who externalises his problem, feeling little self-responsibility, is much more likely to be a failure. Thus the implication is that some other conditions need to be provided for psychotherapy with this group.[...]

5 There is no intent here to maintain that diagnostic evaluation is useless. We have ourselves made heavy use of such methods in our research studies of change in personality. It is its usefulness as a precondition to psychotherapy which is questioned.

6 In a facetious moment I have suggested that such therapists might be made equally comfortable by being given the diagnosis of some other individual, not of this patient or client. The fact that the diagnosis proved inaccurate as psychotherapy continued would not be particularly disturbing, because one always expects to find inaccuracies in the diagnosis as one works with the individual.

REFERENCES

Bown, O.H. (1954) 'An investigation of therapeutic relationship in client-centered therapy', Unpublished doctor's dissertation, University of Chicago.

Chodorkoff, B. (1954) 'Self-perception, perceptual defense, and adjustment', *J. Abnorm. Soc. Psychol.* 49: 508–512.

Fiedler, F.E. (1950) 'A comparison of therapeutic relationships in psychoanalytic, non-directive and Adlerian therapy', *J. Consult. Psychol.* 14: 436–445.

Fiedler, F.E. (1953) 'Quantitative studies on the role of therapists' feelings toward their patients', in Mowrer, O.H. (ed.) *Psychotherapy: Theory and Research*. New York: Ronald.

Kirtner, W.L. (1955) 'Success and failure in client-centered therapy as a function of personality variables', Unpublished master's thesis, University of Chicago.

Rogers, C.R. (1951) *Client-centered Therapy*, Boston: Houghton Mifflin.

Standal, S. (1954) 'The need for positive regard: a contribution to client-centered theory', Unpublished doctor's dissertation, University of Chicago.

CHAPTER 20

COMPASSION FATIGUE: HOW MUCH CAN I GIVE?

Peter Huggard

An increasing number of publications examine the disturbing effects on clinicians of witnessing or learning of trauma experienced by their patients. This vicarious traumatisation is described in various terms, including secondary victimisation, secondary survival, emotional contagion, counter-transference, burnout and compassion fatigue. It is generally accepted that, while they have significant similarities, there are also differences between these phenomena. Central to these processes is the use of empathy by clinicians. What is the role of empathy in the doctor–patient relationship?

> *Clues ... were ignored, with the doctor usually exploring the diagnostic aspects of symptoms.*

The nature of empathy and its role in a helping relationship has been debated from a variety of theoretical viewpoints over several decades. Reynolds' (2000) review of the role of empathy illustrates the development of the construct and presents a view that it is multidimensional and has emotive, moral, cognitive and behavioural components. Definitions of empathy vary. Gerald Egan, (1994) reviewing the work of Carl Rogers, (1980) describes empathy as 'a way of being', where the helper, without judgement, enters the private world of the client. Egan further describes a deeper level of empathy, where the helper gains an insight, beyond that of

Source: *Medical Education* (2003) 37: 163–164, Oxford: Blackwell Publishing.

the client, into the client's own story. A study by Suchman *et al.* (1997) of doctors working in a primary care setting showed this empathic understanding of the 'story behind the story' to be lacking. The study found that both clues and direct expression of affect were ignored, with the doctor usually exploring the diagnostic aspects of symptoms. Reynolds (2000) extends Rogers' definition by including the communication of this understanding of the 'story behind the story' to the client as a means of validating the client's world. Other research has indicated that there is a relationship between clinicians' empathy and compassion and the quality of the care they provide (Bellet and Maloney 1991). If this is the case, why is it that empathy and compassion often appear to be lacking in therapeutic relationships?

Central to these processes is the use of empathy by clinicians.

Halpern (2001) gives the following reasons why doctors might seek detachment from, rather than emotional engagement with, their patients: protection from burnout, improved concentration, rationing of time, maintenance of impartiality, and that the fact that 'emotions are inherently subjective influences that interfere with objectivity'. She also reports that detachment does not protect doctors from burnout; rather, burnout can be linked to time pressures and other organisational issues that prevent the development of doctor–patient relationships. Research on burnout has shown that it is a process that begins gradually and progressively worsens, and that a key element of it is emotional exhaustion (Figley 1995). Figley has researched the field of stress related to the use of empathy and compassion and has described a stress response that emerges suddenly and without warning and that includes characteristics such as a sense of helplessness and confusion, feelings of isolation from supporters and symptoms that are often disconnected from their real cause. However, there appears to be a faster recovery rate from this particular stress response than there is from burnout. Figley uses the term 'compassion fatigue' to describe this process, which he regards as secondary traumatic stress, or the stress resulting from the learning of, or witnessing of, a traumatising event involving some other significant person.

Detachment does not protect physicians from burnout.

While empathic engagement with patients may be independent of the development of burnout, Figley describes the use of empathy as one of the particular reasons why trauma workers are especially vulnerable to compassion fatigue. While only a portion of clinicians is exposed on a frequent basis to traumatic material, those who are may experience emotions similar to those of their patients. Elsewhere in Figley's book, the development of compassion fatigue is described as being possibly due to an over-intensive identification with the survival strategies adopted by patients, and inappropriate or lacking personal survival strategies.

> *'Compassion fatigue', or secondary traumatic stress, results from the learning of, or witnessing of, a traumatising event involving some other significant person.*

Pearlman and Saakvitne (1995) describe a process for managing and treating compassion fatigue. Their interventions are grouped into personal, professional and organisational categories. Personal strategies include identifying and making sense of disrupted schemas, striking an appropriate work-life balance, undertaking personal psychotherapy, identifying healing activities and attending to spiritual needs. Professional strategies include undertaking regular professional supervision with an experienced senior colleague where patients can be discussed and the clinician's own responses to them examined without embarrassment and fear of censure, engaging in appropriate self-care practices, developing and maintaining professional networks, having a realistic tolerance of failure, and being aware of work and personal goals. Organisational strategies include developing a workplace environment that is as comfortable as possible, and ensuring a culture of support and respect within the workplace that relates to employees as well as to patients.

> *Compassion fatigue is described as being possibly due to inappropriate or lacking personal survival strategies.*

What are the requirements of a medical education programme that will prepare doctors to manage the effects of processes such as compassion fatigue? Public opinion since ancient times has required that doctors be equipped with such characteristics as integrity, sacrifice and compassion. The quality of compassion is one of the key components in the development of the humanistic doctor (Novack *et al.* 1999). Although the 'fatigue of compassion' can be managed as described above, to do so requires the development of skills in self-awareness that enable medical students and doctors to more effectively engage empathetically with their patients and to gain insight into their own responses to their patients' stories. This path of personal growth will lead to greater well-being (Novack *et al.* 1999), to greater use, by doctors, of themselves as therapeutic agents (Novack *et al.*

1997) and to an increased capacity on the part of doctors to give of themselves in their therapeutic relationships with their patients. The humanistic educator-physician can have a major influence as a role model at one of the most important and impressionable times of a young doctor's life – namely, during their medical education.

In 'caring for the carers', the challenge for health care organisations lies in developing respect and care for their employees in the same way that they require their employees to care for patients. In doing this, health care organisations will support and assist their employees in sustaining and further developing their humanism. Health professionals will then be able to give of themselves in the therapeutic relationship in a manner that enhances the physician–patient relationship and the lives of both the caregiver and the patient.

REFERENCES

Bellet, P.S. and Maloney, M. (1991) 'The importance of empathy as an interviewing skill in medicine', *JAMA* 266: 1831–1832.

Egan, G. (1994) *The Skilled Helper*, California: Brooks/Cole Publishing Co.

Figley, C.R. (1995) *Compassion Fatigue*, New York: Brunner/Mazel.

Halpern, J. (2001) *From Detached Concern to Empathy: Humanising Medical Practice*, Oxford: Oxford University Press.

Novack, D.H., Epstein, R.M. and Paulsen, R.H. (1999) 'Towards creating physician-healers. Fostering medical students' self-awareness, personal growth and well-being', *Acad. Med.* 74: 516–520.

Novack, D.H., Kaplan, G., Epstein, R.M., Clark, W., Suchman, A.L., O'Brian, M. *et al.* (1997) 'Personal awareness and professional growth: a proposed curriculum', *Med. Encount.* 13: 2–8.

Pearlman, L.A. and Saakvitne, K.W. (1995) 'Treating therapists with vicarious traumatisation and secondary traumatic stress disorders', in Figley, C.R. (ed.) *Compassion Fatigue*, New York: Brunner/Mazel 150–177.

Reynolds, W.J. (2000) *The Measurement and Development of Empathy in Nursing*, Aldershot: Ashgate Publishing.

Rogers, C.R. (1980) *A Way of Being*, Boston: Houghton Mifflin.

Suchman, A.L., Markakis, K., Beckman, H.B. and Frankel, R. (1997) 'A model of empathic communication in the medical interview', *JAMA* 277: 678–682.

CHAPTER 21

DO VIRTUES HAVE A ROLE IN THE PRACTICE OF COUNSELLING?

Ann Gallagher

INTRODUCTION

Ethics and counselling are inextricably linked. Ethics is concerned with right conduct and good character – with the questions 'how should I act'? and 'how should I live'? Ethics regulates our relationships with others. Counselling involves persons and relationships and has the potential to help alleviate suffering and to enable the individual to make progress. There is also much potential for harm should counsellors lack the necessary competence to practice or exploit the vulnerability of clients. Counselling organisations, such as BACP (British Association for Counselling and Psychotherapy), acknowledge the importance of ethics and publish codes of ethics emphasising values, principles and personal moral qualities (See *http://www.bac.co.uk* (accessed 11/12/02)).

Debates about the most appropriate ethical theories continue and are as applicable to counselling as to other practices. One of the most significant debates asks whether the correct focus of ethics should be on action or on the character of the agent, in this case, the counsellor.

This chapter will explore the relationship between virtue ethics and person-centred counselling or therapy. MacIntyre's exposition of a 'practice' will be applied to counselling providing a backdrop to a discussion of specific virtues. Key features of virtue ethics – the role of character, eudaimonia and the doctrine of the mean – will be considered and specific virtues (empathy and respectfulness) discussed in relation to counselling.

PERSON-CENTRED CONDITIONS

The conditions for person-centred counselling include unconditional positive regard, empathy and congruence. Unconditional positive regard and empathy are particularly challenging in terms of definition and in application. The former has been related to 'unconditional valuing' and to 'absolute respect' (Purton in Thorne and Lambers 1998). Rogers (1951: 21) says of respect: 'by use of client-centred techniques, a person can implement his respect for others only so far as that respect is an integral part of his personality make-up ...' Respect (or respectfulness) is not just demonstrated in action but is, it can be argued, a personal quality or virtue. But what does this respect mean in practice? What is it respect for? Can a counsellor respect too much or too little?

Empathy in therapy has been described as 'an empathic identification where the counsellor is perceiving the hates and hopes and fears of the client through immersion in an empathic process, but without himself, as counsellor, experiencing those hopes and fears' (Rogers 1951: 29). In addition to the role of perception, communication is also acknowledged in definitions of empathy (see Reynolds *et al.* 1999, Gagan 1983). So how might empathy appear as a virtue? Is empathy always possible? Again, can it be too much or too little?

Before these questions can be explored further, something needs to be said about the key features of virtue ethics.

VIRTUE ETHICS

Until recently, perspectives on ethics focused almost exclusively on doing the right thing, on right action. The justification for right action was generally framed in terms of duty (it is right to do what it is our personal or professional duty to do); in terms of consequences (doing the right thing involves doing what brings about the most happiness for the most people); or in terms of principles (principles provide guidelines for action). These approaches to ethics are predominantly rationalist. There may be an assumption that there is a straightforward movement from thinking to doing – I know what it is my duty to do and I ought to and will do it; I have calculated the consequences and I will do what optimises happiness or utility; I will follow the dictates of principles. The moral life is, however, more complicated than these approaches imply. Counsellors, as other practitioners, are not rational automatons and an approach to ethics which implies this is inadequate. As Beauchamp and Childress state:

> *Often, what counts most in the moral life is not consistent adherence to principles and rules, but reliable character, good moral sense, and emotional responsiveness. Even specified principles and rules do not convey what occurs when parents lovingly play with and nurture their children or when physicians and nurses exhibit compassion, patience, and responsiveness in encounters with patients and families. Our feelings and concerns for others lead us to actions that cannot be reduced to instances of rule-following and we all recognise that morality would be a cold and uninspiring practice without various emotional responses and heart-felt ideals that reach beyond principles and rules.*
>
> (Beauchamp and Childress 2001: 26)

Whereas the approaches to ethics outlined above, focus on the rightness or wrongness of individuals' actions, virtue ethics prioritises judgements about the internal world of the individual – their motives, dispositions and about their character.

The virtues have a long, varied and distinguished history. They appear in the wide-ranging writings of Homor, Sophocles, Aristotle, the New Testament, Jane Austen and Benjamin Franklin (MacIntyre 1985: Ch: 14). There has, however, been a revival of virtue in the context of ethics over the last four decades. This revival is usually traced back to a paper, by Elizabeth Anscombe, published in 1958 which recommended a move from a duty-focus to virtue (Anscombe 1958). Since then, virtue ethics has made substantial theoretical inroads to mainstream moral philosophy through, for example, the work of MacIntyre (1985, 1999), Hursthouse (1987, 1999), Foot (1978), Geach (1977), Slote, Stocker and Driver (See Crisp 1996). In the United States, bioethicists such as Edmund Pelligrino and Beauchamp and Childress (2001) have considered the approach in relation to biomedicine. In the UK, in relation to professional ethics, writers such as Anne Scott (1995) and Derek Sellman (1997) have advocated virtue ethics for nursing practice. Peter Toon (1993: 18) stated that 'medical ethics needs to consider how to cultivate moral virtue in medical practitioners'. Contemporary writing on the virtues has, to a lesser or greater extent, been influenced by the Greek philosopher Aristotle (384 to 323 BC – for an accessible introduction to his work see Hughes 2001).

Virtue ethics has been defined as:

> *. . . a theoretical perspective within ethics which holds that judgements about the inner lives of individuals (their traits, motives, dispositions, and character), rather than judgements about the rightness or wrongness of external acts and/or consequences of acts, are of the greatest moral importance.*
>
> (Loudon in Chadwick 1998)

Virtue ethics accepts the place of the emotions in the moral life and this is significant in relation to the practice of counselling. The expression of the emotions is, according to Aristotle, regulated by the doctrine of the mean, which will be discussed below. Virtue ethics has also been described as an ethics of aspiration, where individuals aspire to a kind of flourishing, to 'eudaimonia'. Before discussing eudaimonia, something needs to be said about character.

Virtue ethics relates the rightness of actions to the character of the individual who acts. The good counsellor is then more than the counsellor who merely does the right thing, fulfils his or her duty, adheres to principles or calculates consequences. Rather, the good counsellor is the counsellor who acts from good internal motives and dispositions. The good counsellor is not only someone who acts well but is also a certain kind of person.

The good counsellor demonstrates virtues (morally desirable character traits) consistently and reliably. Hefty challenges may be launched against a character-based approach to ethics but these are not insurmountable. Surely, it might be asked, what is important is what the counsellor *does* not what he or she is inside? Isn't it unrealistic to expect counsellors to possess and demonstrate virtues on cue? Finally, it might be objected, as there is no consensus as to what virtues are necessary and sufficient for counselling, it seems preferable to focus on action.

It is, of course, important that counsellors act ethically, that they do the right thing, are competent and demonstrate appropriate behaviour. It is better if they are disposed to do so, enjoy and want to do it. Counsellors can, and do, follow action guidelines which support therapeutic relationships and forbid exploitation. However, there may be a gap between what counsellors know they should do and their having the wherewithal to do it. At times, for example, counsellors will need to be courageous. They, and the clients they work with, will also benefit from the possession of the virtue of prudence or practical wisdom. Counsellors can act 'as if' they possess virtues such as empathy and respectfulness but it is better if they truly possess these virtues. Regarding the question as to how realistic it is to expect counsellors to 'be' something on cue, to demonstrate the appropriate virtues, to feel in the appropriate way, it must be said that it is not so. It seems inevitable that, at times, counsellors will work with clients who challenge and in situations where virtues such as empathy and respectfulness do not emerge spontaneously. In such a situation, emotional labour may be necessary. There is a view within virtue ethics that if individuals act virtuously habitually, then they will become so.

The third objection concerns the identification of the virtues. A wide range of virtues are evident in the literature (courage, prudence, temperance, justice, faith, hope, compassion, integrity and so on) so which of these should the good counsellor demonstrate? The personal moral qualities outlined by the BACP (web-site accessed 11/12/02) are compatible with, and go beyond, the conditions mentioned above – empathy, sincerity, integrity, resilience, respect, humility, competence, fairness, wisdom and courage. The possibility that there may not be a consensus regarding virtues is not damning for virtue ethics. There is likely to be a good deal of agreement. It is also the case that there is unlikely to be a complete consensus in relation to action guidelines.

It has been said that one of the strengths of virtue ethics lies in its ability to accommodate the emotions. One relationship between virtues and the emotions is explained by Aristotle's doctrine of the mean. Unlike approaches to ethics where the suppression of the emotions is considered desirable, virtues are described as the right expression or moderation of the passions 'in the right place and at the right time' (Carr 1991: 50) or as Aristotle states:

> *virtue aims to hit the mean ... to have those feelings at the right times on the right grounds towards the right people for the right motive and in the right way ... is the mark of virtue.*
>
> (Aristotle 1976: 101)

Aristotle's view is that virtues are flanked on either side by a vice – on one side, a vice of excess and, on the other, of deficiency. The virtue of courage, for example, has foolhardiness (excess) on one side and cowardice (deficiency) on the other.

So how might this relate to the virtues of empathy and respect or respectfulness? In relation to courage, the emotion in question is generally taken to be fear (although some accounts consider also confidence); the situation is not so straightforward in relation to empathy and respectfulness. Definitions of empathy vary but identified components would seem to include: the ability to perceive, to reason and to communicate 'an understanding of the client's world' (See Reynolds *et al.* 1999, Wiseman 1996). It is not clear what the relevant emotion is in relation to empathy but it is arguable that some degree of care and concern is indicated. It seems possible that counsellors could fail in relation to empathy in ways other than by lacking the relevant emotions. They may lack the necessary perceptual skills to, for example, 'see' a client's needs or distress. It seems likely also that they may fail should they lack reasoning and communication skills.

The emotion(s) underpinning respectfulness is again not so straightforward. It seems generally to be the case that judgement plays a more important role in relation to respect than the emotions. Generally 'respect' is related to respectworthiness, to reasons why an individual deserves respect. It has been pointed out that Rogers' view of unconditional positive regard implies unconditional respect and this is described as 'puzzling'

(Purton in Thorne and Lambers 1998). It is asked 'how, with some clients, can one possibly embody the core conditions of congruence and unconditional respect at the same time'?(1998: 26). Purton's (1998: 27–29) suggestion is to distinguish between the empirical self (with all its blemishes) and the essential self (which contains the possibilities and potential of the person) – a focus on the latter is said to be compatible with unconditional respect. Another possibility is that we demonstrate respectfulness on the basis of concern or even love for our common humanity. If counsellors acknowledge their own human fallibility and vulnerability, it is likely they will feel more warmly toward those who are also less than virtuous.

In relation to the doctrine of the mean, it is at least plausible that empathy and respectfulness might appear as follows:

Excess	*Virtue*	*Deficiency*
Over-involvement Or over-identification	Empathy	Moral blindness or indifference
Unreflective or servile disrespectfulness Deference	Respectfulness	

David Carr states that:

> *the doctrine of the mean is the perfectly reasonable idea that the passions and appetites are not as some philosophers have suggested merely sources of temptation to be controlled by the virtues, but actually necessary conditions for the expression of them. By this I mean not only that courage would not be possible without fear but also that charity and compassion would not be possible in the absence of genuine human feelings of love and concern for other people.*
>
> (Carr 1991: 55–56)

Although the emotions which underpin empathy and respectfulness as virtues are not so obvious as fear in relation to courage, it seems possible that care, concern, love and perhaps warmth are close approximations. It might well be asked what virtues are for anyway?

In relation to counselling, it seems clear that both counsellor and client can benefit from the counsellor possessing virtues. It is not always the case, however, that those who possess and demonstrate the virtues are better off. Supposing, for example, a counsellor blows the whistle on bad practice, it may well be that job prospects and even health may suffer as a consequence. However, the counsellor may still feel that he or she did the right thing and managed to maintain his or her integrity. What the virtues contribute to then may not be happiness as we normally think of it, but rather a sense of individual flourishing or 'eudaimonia'.

The Greek word 'eudaimonia' is usually translated as happiness and it has been pointed out that this is misleading. Hughes states:

> *'Happiness' in English suggests a feeling of one kind or another, perhaps a feeling of contentment, or delight, or pleasure. Aristotle makes it clear that he does not have any such feeling in mind at all. (In book 10) he says that eudaimonia is achieving one's full potential ... It is more closely connected with what one has made of one's life.*
>
> (Hughes 2001: 22)

Similarly, Barnes points out that eudaimonia is not just a mental state but also relates to 'well-living' and 'well-acting'.

> *The* eudaimon *is the man who makes a success of his life and actions, who realises his aims and ambitions as a man, who fulfils himself.*
>
> (Barnes in Aristotle 1976: 33–34)

Here three aspects of virtue ethics have been introduced in relation to counselling: the significance of character and the virtues; the role of the doctrine of the mean; and the significance of eudaimonia. Demonstrating the virtues does not guarantee that the counsellor will be 'happy' in the everyday sense but it is likely that he or she will have a sense of flourishing and of living well.

COUNSELLING AS A MORAL PRACTICE

Counselling can be described as a moral practice. This is defined by MacIntyre as:

> *...any coherent and complex form of socially established cooperative human activity through which goods internal to that form of activity are realised in the course of trying to achieve those standards of excellence which are appropriate to, and partially definitive of, that form of activity, with the result that human powers to achieve excellence, and human conceptions of the ends and goods involved, are systematically extended...*
>
> (MacIntyre 1985)

To explain 'goods internal' to a practice and distinguish them from 'goods external' to a practice, MacIntyre gives the example of a child playing chess. Two kinds of goods are possible in playing chess – if the child plays purely to win sweets, then the goods are external to the practice. If the child plays for reasons specific to chess, for example, for the particular analytical and strategic skills and competitiveness, then the goods can be described as 'internal' to the practice. A further example is given of portrait painting. There are goods external to that practice, for example, money, fame, status and possibly, power. Goods internal to that practice concern the performance of the painter and the excellence of the portrait, both described as 'products'. External goods then can become an 'individual's property and possession' and are 'characteristically objects of competition'. Internal goods may also be the outcome of:

> *competition to excel, but it is characteristic of them that their achievement is a good for the whole community who participated in the practice.*
>
> (MacIntyre 1985)

The 'goods external' to the practice of counselling would include financial gain, status and perhaps power. Goods internal to the practice would include the performance of the counsellor and also benefits to the client and to the community. However, the 'product' of counselling is somewhat controversial. The BACP Code states that the 'overall aim of counselling is to provide an opportunity for the client to work towards living in a way that he or she experiences as more satisfying or resourceful'. It is possible that the way of living chosen by the client is immoral and also that counselling itself militates against morality. Phillips has, for example, written of the 'therapeutic sensibility':

> *... the contemporary age is therapeutic, not religious. People ... hunger not for personal salvation but 'for the feeling, the momentary illusion, of personal well-being, health and psychic security' ... Whatever problems he or she may have are defined as arising not from weakness of character or lack of inner-control, but increasingly as 'psychic' difficulties. For many today, evil and morally wrong actions are dissolved into sickness and social maladjustment...*
>
> (Phillips in Sterpa 1998)

It is not suggested here that counselling should be about instilling morality nor is it suggested that ethics/morality is reducible or equal to religion. Lessons from the past where women were incarcerated in asylums, for having children outside of marriage, and populations oppressed for not practicing the prevailing religion highlight the dangers of such positions. What is being questioned is the role of counselling as a moral practice. But is the 'therapeutic sensibility' necessarily immoral? Is it a practice with internal goods?

Phillips' view is that the 'therapeutic sensibility' is that people are:

> *guided almost entirely by considerations of self-interest and, so far as possible, act to choose the least costly means (for themselves) of achieving their own private ends or means, conflict seems inevitable ... Since such persons view social relationships as reducible to individual desires or to a calculation of means and ends, moral discourse is not even possible for them. Moral judgements, they believe, are reducible to questions of the most subjective personal taste. ('if it feels good, do it'.)*
>
> (Phillips in Sterpa 1998: 30)

The search for authenticity is aligned with the therapeutic sensibility. The 'moral' view, on the other hand, is concerned with what people 'ought to do' rather than what they 'want to do'. Authenticity, according to Phillips, involves a preoccupation with self whereas morality is mainly concerned with our involvement in interpersonal relationships.

A number of things can be said about Phillips' view. First, it seems that it misrepresents (perhaps caricatures) what it is many counsellors may think of as 'therapeutic' activity. It is, of course, possible that counselling could become exclusively self-indulgent pandering to egocentricity and colluding with clients' wishes to satisfy desires, whatever the cost. However, it seems more likely that engagement in any 'therapeutic' activity necessarily involves better equipping individuals to live in the world and that requires better understanding of, and engagement in, interpersonal relationships. It does not seem to be the case that this rules out morality but rather it implies it. Second, if we understand authenticity as better understanding ourselves and desiring to be ourselves, it does not seem to follow that this implies a disregard for others. A concern with authenticity does not rule out an aspiration to be something better. In this case the therapeutic sensibility is not necessarily immoral and counselling implies internal goods which warrants the label moral practice.

In addition to general challenges to the practice of counselling, a further challenge to counselling involves the use of counselling skills in other practices such as nursing, medicine and social work. The philosophies and activities of these practices may conflict with those of counselling, In mental health work, for example, nurses, doctors and social workers may simultaneously assume a therapeutic role as counsellor and also be involved in depriving that same client of his liberty by sectioning him under the Mental Health Act.

CONCLUSION

This chapter has discussed some aspects of virtue ethics in relation to counselling. It was suggested that while right action is crucially significant, good character is likely to be more reliable and fills gaps when individuals know what to do but feel unable to do it. Courage is relevant when fear is experienced and prudence (practical wisdom) when individuals have uncertain ends or means.

Some of the challenges to a character-based ethics were responded to. It is unrealistic to expect an individual to demonstrate the virtues on cue. There are likely to be situations when counsellors have to act 'as if' the appropriate virtue was possessed. It may be that with habitual practice, this acting 'as if' will become the virtue. It is unlikely that there will be complete agreement on the virtues which are necessary and sufficient for the practice of counselling. It may be helpful to consider rather what counselling would be like if or when counsellors lacked certain virtues – virtues such as empathy and respectfulness. It was further suggested that the charge that the 'therapeutic sensibility' was incompatible with morality was unfounded.

So 'do the virtues have a role in the practice of counselling'? It seems they do. They have a role in supporting the ethical reliability of the counsellor and in filling the gap between knowing what to do and in being able to do. It seems that counsellors and clients will benefit from the virtues. Counsellors will benefit in terms of eudaimonia or individual flourishing and clients from having respectful, empathic/empathetic, courageous and wise counsellors. There is no plea here to abandon other approaches to ethics. Virtue ethics is not incompatible with action-based ethics. However, an approach to ethics which focuses solely on external factors, on what people do, is an impoverished account.

REFERENCES

Anscombe, E. (1958) 'Modern moral philosophy', *Philosophy* 33: 1–19

Aristotle (1976) *The Ethics of Aristotle – The Nicomachean Ethics*, London: Penguin Books.

Beauchamp, T.L. and Childress, J.F. (2001) *Principles of Biomedical Ethics*, Oxford: Oxford University Press.

British Association for Counselling and Psychotherapy (accessed 11/12/02) *Code of Ethics and Practice for Counsellors http://www.bac.co.uk/members_visitors/public_information/public?code?counsellors.*

Carr, D. (1991) *Educating the Virtues – An Essay on the Philosophical Psychology of Moral Development and Education*, London: Routledge.

Crisp, R. (ed.) (1996) *How Should One Live? Essays on the Virtues*, Oxford: Oxford University Press.

Foot, P. (1978) *Virtues and Vices and Other Essays in Moral Philosophy*, Oxford: Basil Blackwell.

Geach, P. (1978) *The Virtues – The Stanton Lectures 1973–4*, London: Cambridge University Press.

Hughes, G.J. (2001) *Aristotle on Ethics*, London: Routledge.

Hursthouse, R. (1987) *Beginning Lives*, Oxford and Buckingham: Blackwell in Association with the Open University Press.

Hursthouse, R. (1999) *On Virtue Ethics*, Oxford: Oxford University Press.

Loudon, R.B. 'Virtue Ethics' in Chadwick, R. (Editor-in-Chief) (1998) *Encyclopedia of Applied Ethics*, 4 San Diego: Academic Press.

MacIntyre, A. (1985) *After Virtue – a Study in Moral Theory*, London: Duckworth.

MacIntyre, A. (1999) *Dependent Rational Animals: Why Human Beings Need the Virtues*, London: Gerald Duckworth & Co. Ltd.

Purton, C. (1998) 'Unconditional regard and its spiritual implications', in Thorne, B. and Lambers, E. (eds) *Person-Centred Therapy: A European Perspective*, London: Sage Publications.

Phillips, D.L. (1998) 'Authenticity or morality'? in Sterpa, J.P. (ed.) *Ethics: The Big Questions*, Oxford: Blackwell Publishers Inc.

Reynolds, W.J., Scott, B. and Jessiman, W. (1999) 'Empathy has not been measured in clients' terms or effectively taught: a review of the literature', *Journal of Advanced Nursing* 30 (5): 1177–1185.

Rogers, C.R. (1951) *Client-Centered Therapy*, London: Constable and Company Ltd.

Scott, A. (1995) 'Aristotle, nursing and health care ethics', *Nursing Ethics* 2 (4): 279–285.

Sellman, D. (1997) 'The virtues in the moral education of nurses: Florence Nightingale revisited', *Nursing Ethics* 4 (1): 3–10.

Toon, P. (1993) 'After bioethics and towards virtue?' *Journal of Medical Ethics* 19: 17–18.

Wiseman, T. (1996) 'A concept analysis of empathy', *Journal of Advanced Nursing* 23 (6): 1162–1167.

CHAPTER 22

ARE THERE UNIVERSAL HUMAN BEING SKILLS?

Richard Nelson-Jones

The issue of what constitutes a skilled human being is fundamental to counselling and psychotherapy. Furthermore, multicultural counselling and therapy is based on the two primary assumptions of common humanity and cultural diversity. However, nowhere have I seen in the psychotherapy theory and the multicultural literature the issue addressed of whether there are universal human being skills that underlie and transcend cultural diversity. By 'universal human being skills' I mean skills that characterise the good or effective person regardless of the culture or country in which they live. Arguably the widespread possession of such human skills throughout the world is fundamental to creating happiness and avoiding suffering on a daily basis. Furthermore, the survival of the species depends on the existence of sufficient good or skilled human beings to protect the interests of future generations.

THE ISSUE OF SKILLS

To date, curiously enough, the theory and practice of counselling and therapy has not placed a major emphasis on explicitly identifying and imparting skills to clients. Psychoanalysis, analytical therapy, person-centred therapy and gestalt therapy do not clearly advocate teaching skills to clients. Even the psycho-educational approaches to therapy, such as

Source: *Counselling Psychology Quarterly* (2002) 15 (2): 115–119.

Ellis' rational emotive behaviour therapy, Beck's cognitive therapy and Lazarus's multimodal therapy are not predominantly framed in the language of training clients in skills. However, in the cognitive-behavioural literature references are made to skills, such as assertion and friendship, but rarely to cognitive or mind skills. The multicultural counselling and therapy literature stresses therapist competencies or skills (for example, Sue *et al.* 1998) independently of training clients in skills. Furthermore, professional training in the West heavily emphasises teaching counselling and clinical skills to students without acknowledging that counsellors and therapists are only skilled to the extent that they can impart skills to their clients. If we can have skilled counsellors, therapists and helpers, why can't we have skilled clients too?

It is high time for counsellors and therapists to put client skills and human being skills at centre stage. Skills can be defined by area, for instance active listening skills, by level of competence, for instance good or poor listening skills, and by the sequences of choices involved in good or poor performance of a skill. This latter way of defining skills locates it clearly in people's minds and, as such, potentially under their influence. Though the areas overlap, a further distinction can be made between mind skills and communication/action skills. What distinguishes humans from other animals is their capacity for symbolic thought. Humans can not only think, but they can think about how they think, sometimes known as meta-cognition. Elsewhere, I have identified seven central mind skills: namely creating awareness, rules, perceptions, self-talk, visual images, explanations and expectations (Nelson-Jones 2001).

Communication/action skills are observable and consist of verbal, vocal, bodily, touch and action-taking messages and various mixtures of these messages. Communication/action skills contain mental components that can enhance or impede how well people enact them: for instance, mental processes influence communicating active listening to speakers. Feelings and physical reactions are not skills in themselves since they represent humans' animal nature, but can be influenced by how well or poorly people use their mind skills and communication/action skills.

Another way of thinking of human being skills is in terms of level of functioning or developing human potential. Here a distinction exists between possessing sub-normal, normal and supra-normal skills. For genetic, social learning and economic reasons, some humans function at below the norm for the human race. The vast majority of people possess a mixture of good and poor human being skills that place them within the range of normal functioning. However, some people develop their human being skills to the point where their level of functioning is clearly superior. Though not using the word skills, Maslow, in his study of self-actualising people, tried to identify some of the characteristics of supra-normalcy (Maslow 1970).

What are some advantages of using a skills framework or skills language? First, attempts can be made to identify and define the skills human beings and clients require if they are to function effectively. Second, the concept of skills provides a focus for training people in human being skills. Already much successful training takes place without using the concept of skills. For example, children reared in loving and nurturing environments are more likely to possess the skills of relating to other people warmly than those children who are emotionally abused or deprived. Nevertheless identifying and articulating what are desirable human being skills might lead to better child rearing practices. Third, in therapy, the use of skills language provides a framework for assessing clients and for identifying the mind skills and communication/action skills they need to improve. Furthermore, derived from such assessments, therapists and clients can select interventions designed to build clients' skills. Fourth, the concept of skills provides both clients and human beings with a self-help framework for monitoring, improving and, where necessary, self-correcting how well they use their mind skills and communication/action skills.

THE ISSUE OF UNIVERSALITY

A starting point for discussing the issue of universality is that of the biological basis of human nature. Over thousands of years, humans have evolved as a distinct species whose behaviour is influenced by their thoughts rather than solely determined by instinct. Nevertheless the role of instinct remains strong: for instance in regard to meeting biological needs, reproducing the species, nurturing the young and caring for the sick.

Every individual has a biologically based inner nature comprised of elements that are common to the species and those that are unique to that individual. Charles Darwin referred to humans possessing an 'instinct of sympathy' and this would appear to be an important survival instinct for the species (Dalai Lama and Cutler 1998). However, much of Western thinking sees human nature as egoistic, selfish and destructive, summed up in one of Freud's favourite quotes, which came from the Roman writer Plautus: 'Man is a wolf to man'. This 'bad animal' view of humans might be seen as based on humans who are not at a high level rather than on the healthiest human beings (Maslow 1971). Furthermore, it ignores the ample evidence that humans can be co-operative and caring as well as hostile and uncaring (Argyle 1991; Beck 1999). How people act appears to be largely a matter of training and of how much their animal nature is lovingly nourished or frustrated.

Much research points to the conclusion that humans across the world share many common or universal characteristics. For example, Ekman and Friesen (1971) have identified seven main facial expressions for emotion across cultures: happiness, interest, surprise, fear, sadness, anger and disgust or contempt. Another example is that of Schwartz (1992) who classified values into ten types: power, achievement, hedonism, stimulation, self-direction, universalism, benevolence, tradition, conformity and security. Based on information from 20 countries in six continents, he confirmed that each of the ten values was found in at least 90 per cent of the countries he surveyed, suggesting that his value types were near universal.

THE ISSUE OF CULTURAL DIVERSITY

Alongside universality, there is also diversity. Humans across the world have had to face the tasks involved in human existence within the contexts of different physical environmental circumstances, such as climate, topography and natural resources. Throughout history, people in different locations have been in a constant process of evolving their cultures. Though some of the distinctiveness of individual cultures increasingly risks being eroded by globalisation resulting from technological advances (Hermans and Kempen 1998), a huge range of cultural diversity still exists.

Despite the overly rosy view sometimes presented in the multicultural literature, cultural diversity can be a two-edged sword. Taking the world as a whole, a clear advantage of diversity is the range of options for dealing with the human condition that different cultures offer. Such variety may add spice and depth to life and, where it is life-affirming, should be celebrated and cherished. Members of different cultures can learn from one another and each be enriched in the process. However, culture can divide as well as unite as external wars and civil wars show. Societies require a minimum level of cultural cohesion if they are to function well in the interest of all their members. Furthermore, cultures differ in the extent to which they restrict or enhance the full humanness of their members.

Maslow (1971) was cautiously optimistic about the biological nature of human beings. However, he thought that positive instinctual aspects of human nature, such as altruistic concern for others, were frequently weak, needed a benign culture for their appearance, and could be inhibited or shattered by bad cultural conditions. The noted anthropologist Ruth Benedict used the notion of *synergy* to describe the healthy interaction between individual and society (Benedict 1942). Probably there is a reciprocal interaction between the development or lack of development of individuals and the cultures or societies to which they belong.

TOWARDS UNIVERSAL HUMAN BEING SKILLS

Perhaps I can draw together this chapter by making a number of points.

- Viewing human functioning in skills terms is important. At present there are many different psychological theories about how human beings and clients function, but they tend not to be couched in skills terms. The world has a long history of human misery as well as of the overcoming of suffering and of happiness. Currently humans in their dealings with one another are not nearly as skilled as they should be to make the world a happier and safer place. Not to apply the concept of skills to human functioning leaves a huge gap in thinking about how to improve the human condition.
- Yes, almost certainly there are universal human being skills. Furthermore, humans have the potential to develop such skills to a high level. Though family and social environments differ across cultures, certain characteristics or skills of the good person almost certainly transcend culture. One possible reason for this is that such skills are ultimately grounded in human biology and evolutionary requirement of survival of the species.
- Probably it is more important to define universal mind skills than universal communication/action skills. Coming from the framework of Western psychotherapy, two of the central mind skills are the ability to reality-test and alter unrealistic perceptions, the main characteristic or skill of Beck's cognitive therapy, and the ability to dispute and restate irrational beliefs or rules, the main skill of Ellis's rational-emotive behaviour therapy. Such mind skills are important whatever continent and culture people come from. One of the Buddha's sayings is 'As the shadow follows the body, as we think, so we become'. Put another way, skilful communication and action follows from skilful thinking. For instance, compassionate actions are likely to follow from compassion-enhancing perceptions and beliefs. When identifying what are universally desirable mind skills, the wisdom and traditions of Eastern and other cultures as well as those of the West must be drawn upon.
- Diversity within universality is desirable. Partly because they are observable, human beings may have more latitude for cultural diversity in communication and action skills than in mind skills. Positive cultural diversity, reflecting life-affirming variations of universal human being skills, requires nurturing and encouraging.
- Much more effort needs to be put into identifying what are universal human being skills before it is too late. The human race's technological ability to destroy itself far outreaches its capacity for skilful and harmonious living. What is needed may be a large-scale international research project, similar to the Human Genome Project, to crack the biologically influenced code of what are universally desirable human

being skills. All counsellors, therapists and people in general make a series of assumptions about what are desirable ways of thinking and communicating/acting. The practice of counselling and psychotherapy, whether it be with clients from the same or different cultures, would be much more soundly based than presently the case if much more large scale research on desirable human being skills were to be conducted. The findings of any such research would merit wide dissemination in a practitioner-friendly fashion.

- Once desirable universal human being skills are more validly and clearly identified, further research work needs to be performed on how best to disseminate them. As well as focusing on how to improve counselling and therapy, such broad-spectrum research should focus on what sort of kinship and societal frameworks are synergistic rather than antagonistic to helping people to develop and maintain their full humanness.

REFERENCES

Argyle, M. (1991) *Cooperation: The Basis of Sociability*, London: Routledge.

Beck, A.T. (1999) *Prisoners of Hate: The Cognitive Basis of Anger, Hostility, and Violence*, New York: Harper Collins.

Benedict, R. (1942) Unpublished lectures on 'Synergy in Society', Bryn Mawr, PA.

Dalai Lama and Cutler, H.C. (1998) *The Art of Happiness: A Handbook for Living*, Sydney: Hodder.

Ekman, P. and Frisen, W. (1971) 'Constants across cultures in the face and emotion', *Journal of Personality and Social Psychology* 17: 124–129.

Hermans, H.J.M. and Kempen, H.J.G. (1998) 'Moving cultures: the perilous problems of cultural dichotomies in a globalizing society', *American Psychologist* 53: 1111–1120.

Maslow, A.H. (1970) *Motivation and Personality*, New York: Harper & Row.

Maslow, A.H. (1971) *The Farther Reaches of Human Nature*, Harmondsworth: Penguin Books.

Nelson-Jones, R. (2001) *The Theory and Practice of Counselling and Therapy*, London: Continuum.

Schwartz, S.H. (1992) 'Universals in the content and structure of values: theoretical advances and empirical tests in 20 countries', in Zanna, M. (ed.) *Advances in Experimental Social Psychology*, 1: 1–65 New York: Academic Press.

Sue, D.W., Carter, R.T., Casas, J.M., Fouad, N.A., Ivey, A.E., Jensen, M., Lafromboise, T., Manese, J.E., Ponterotto, J.G. and Vazquez-Nuttal, E. (1998) *Multicultural Counselling Competencies: Individual and Organizational Development*, London: Sage.

CHAPTER 23

TO COMMUNICATE AND ENGAGE: RELEVANT COUNSELLING SKILLS

Janet Seden

[...]
Communication in social work practice involves more than imparting information. It is a process where thoughts, feelings, ideas and hopes are not only exchanged between people, but also need to be understood together. Verbal and non-verbal communications are used to:

- transmit and share information;
- establish relationship;
- exchange ideas and perceptions;
- create change;
- exchange attitudes, values and beliefs;
- achieve worker and user goals.

It is important that in this exchange workers respect the values and beliefs of others as far as is consistent with their professional authority and function. Meanings must be carefully checked, and in each exchange, care needs to be taken to be aware of, and reduce, the blocks to communication that can come from the many differences between individuals, such as authority and power, language, ability and disability, personality, background, gender, health, age, race, class. Other barriers may impede communication, such as environment, the pressure of limited available

Source: *Counselling Skills in Social Work Practice* (1995) Maidenhead: Open University Press/McGraw-Hill.

time, the involvement of other people, the physical environment or interruptions. Genuine communication is only achieved if the barriers are considered and worked through or removed.

Lago and Thompson (1996: 40), writing about cultural barriers to communication in counselling, suggest a similar range of possible dimensions:

> *language, time, context, purpose of meeting, views and attitudes towards each other, location of meeting, customs/ rituals, smell, age, touch, disability, decoration, adornment, jewellry, personal institutional power, expectations, perceptions of previous personal history, context of meeting, why they are meeting, conventions of greeting and meeting behaviour, gender, notions of acceptable/unacceptable behaviour, system of ethics/morals, interpersonal projections, political differences, personal theories of communication, physical appearance, height, weight, non verbal behaviour.*

Each meeting between two human beings, carrying their own cultural conditionings, can be seen to have several dimensions of difference and assumptions as well as similarities. Lago and Thompson (1996: 41) suggest that the 'counsellor may have considerable difficulty in fully offering one of the core therapeutic conditions as defined by Rogers (1961) for successful therapy to occur, that of acceptance or non-judgementalism'. They also usefully remind the reader that awareness of cultural dimensions of counselling should not be used to conceal prejudice or racism within the counsellor.

These dimensions of difference can also be barriers in social work [and other care] practice. [. . .]

Communication can be viewed as an interactive process involving the giving, receiving and checking out of meaning. Communication occurs on many levels and may not always be congruent. Role relationships are an important dimension and barriers to communication should be considered. It is crucial that interviewers tune into the potential barriers created by differences such as age, class or ethnicity. Communication is a process of which the outcome is engagement, the beginning of a further process where the parties are able to work together, to be involved, to achieve mutual understanding, to hold attention and to contract to a purpose.

Communication skills have been the bedrock of social work practice, and other professions need abilities in communicating. For example, medicine is finding that the failure of doctors to communicate well is at the root of many complaints (Moore 1997; Smith and Norton 1999). Consequently, more attention has been paid to communication skills in doctor and nurse training. Social workers in hospitals frequently find themselves using their own counselling skills in communication to clarify miscommunication and the subsequent lack of engagement. Social workers aim for the active involvement of people, so that they can be empowered to change their own situations or have more control and knowledge within them.

PRACTICE EXAMPLE

The following narrative shows how a block in communication, which was producing conflict between a patient and his doctor, was resolved through the use of counselling skills by a hospital social worker.

Mr Mistry was a hospital patient being cared for on a medical ward. He was a black man born in India, and his first language was Gujerati. The social worker was a white woman, born in Britain, whose first language was English. The doctor was a white man, born in Britain, but of Eastern European ancestry. His first language was English.

The service user was in hospital after experiencing a stroke. He had completed his drug therapy and was described as medically stable by the doctor. He was referred to the social work team, because he was reluctant to comply with further treatment, which included physiotherapy and occupational therapy. He had refused to go to the gym for exercise. The doctor described the patient as having become 'lazy' and adopting the 'classic sick role'. Exploration of this with the doctor brought out that he thought that the patient enjoyed the sick role and liked the idea of people doing everything for him, including dressing and feeding him. The conclusion from this was that the service user would be best placed in a nursing home, where he could remain dependent and be looked after by other people.

The social worker's first step was to visit the service user, but with an interpreter to check that the communication between the user and worker was accurate. The service user clearly stated that he did not want to go into a nursing home, and that he wanted to go home. He knew that as he lived alone he would need to be able to wash, dress and feed himself in order to be safe. In this interview he did not appear to be enjoying the sick role and seemed to want to return home as soon as possible (skills used here: *active listening, attending, listening to body language, use of interpreting service, checking, so enabling worker and patient to communicate, empathy*).

At the end of this first interview there was a contradiction between what the service user was saying and the original referral information. At the next meeting, the worker shared with the service user her puzzlement over what was happening (*immediacy*). She asked why, if he was wanting to get better, he didn't comply with the treatment (*exploratory open-ended question*). He replied that he had complied, as he had taken all of his tablets. The worker then understood from Mr Mistry that he saw medicine as treatment. He thought that the doctor no longer believed that he had been ill and was sending him to the gym for exercise to prove that he was no longer ill. Since then there had been a block in communication and understanding between Mr Mistry and the ward and he had not been enabled to participate in the follow-up treatment.

The social worker had established that there was miscommunication and now decided to observe the interaction between the doctor and the patient. She reflected on the use of language between the two people. Her conclusion was that both the medical stance and the language used were moralistic, judgemental and authoritarian. The client was judged as lazy, a decision about him that had been made quickly, without checking, and in an authoritarian mode of knowing best. The worker considered that the medical model of communication was often from a controlling parent ego-state (*ego psychology/transactional analysis theoretical model*). This was possibly arousing resistance (*a defence*) in the service user. As she reflected upon Mr Mistry's language, he was using phrases like 'I will not. He cannot make me', reflecting the kind of responses which can come from the dependency of childhood, and which may be aroused in adults through illness and helplessness. The anger and resistance that can accompany such feelings where there is a parental attitude in the helper reinforce the difficulties of dependency (*child ego-state*).

The worker recognised that neither of the two parties was being helpful to the other, and that they were instead reinforcing polarised attitudes. The more the doctor acted as a controlling parent, the more the service user refused to work as he was prescribed. This analysis enabled the worker to focus clearly on the way in which the doctor and patient were reinforcing their miscommunication.

The worker suggested a meeting between the doctor and Mr Mistry, with herself present. She invited the doctor to explain to the service user the treatment benefits being suggested, in that it would build up his muscles, improve his ability to walk and enable him to gain strength before being at home alone. She asked Mr Mistry to explain that he had refused the treatment because he had thought that he needed to be really fit to use a gym, and that rest was the best cure. He had thought that the doctor regarded him as fit. (Here the worker used her empathy for the views of both people to set up a meeting to clarify and summarise the actual intentions of both people, using counselling skills in mediation as she challenged the authority model constructively.) At this meeting, the two 'sides' were able to exchange information and perceptions as one adult to another. The service user was able to hear and understand that physiotherapy was offered to increase his possible rehabilitation. The doctor began to understand that the service user was reluctant to use the gym for other reasons, not from laziness or unexplained reluctance (*challenge to perspectives, the enabling of the lowering of defences on the patient's part*).

The worker, by her early involvement of the interpreter, had checked that two-way communication could happen. She reduced the power imbalance between the hospital and the service user, who was able to have his voice heard. By valuing both people equally and by *attentive listening*, she established where the misunderstanding was, and examined the frames of reference of both people carefully. She used her skills (*listening, summarising, use of questions, empathy*) to facilitate a meeting to work out a solution. She did this by her *immediacy* and understanding to facilitate a three-way conversation that unblocked the impasse and enabled Mr Mistry to receive the services to which he was entitled in dignified and adult mode.

The worker's analysis of her actions demonstrated her knowledge, values and skills. She explored the cultural context in which she was working and considered how far her theoretical model was applicable. There was a clear cultural difference between the doctor's belief that the patient would improve with active rehabilitation and the patient's belief that he should rest and pass the time quietly to improve. There were power differentials created by role and status. Her role was to remain non-judgemental and objective, while acknowledging boundaries that both supported the client and provided a service for the hospital. The worker discussed the boundaries of her role with the client and doctor, so as to be explicit about their transactions. [...]

REFERENCES

Lago, C. and Thompson, J. (1996) *Race, Culture and Counselling*, Buckingham, Open University Press.

Moore, W. (1997) 'Speak to me before it's too late', *Health Service Journal* 2 January 20–22.

Norton, S. and Smith, K. (1999) *Counselling Skills for Doctors*, Buckingham, Open University Press.

Rogers, C.R. (1961) *On Becoming a Person*, Boston, Houghton Mifflin.

CHAPTER 24

DISABILITY AND COMMUNICATION: LISTENING IS NOT ENOUGH

Sally French and John Swain

The usual starting point for professionals in considering 'disability and communication' is the development of effective communication. The improvement of health and social care services is equated with better conveyance of information and, quintessentially, better listening – improved skills and their use. The imperative of effective communication has had clear mandates for many years and it would be difficult to find a text within the professional literature that did not emphasise the need to listen to clients.

Taking a more critical stance is not an easy position as it seems to fly in the face of common sense. There are, however, a number of related foundations for taking such a stance which we would like to explore in this chapter.

- The dominant, common sense notions of what it means to be disabled have been challenged by disabled people themselves. Disabled people and their allies have developed a social as opposed to an individual, or medical, model of disability.
- The barriers to effective two-way communication are ingrained in institutional discrimination, for example in the ways in which meetings are conducted. 'Listening' could, in a broader sense, involve a collaborative approach to remove such barriers between professionals and clients.
- The barriers to effective two-way communication are also ingrained in the power relations between professionals and clients. For example

professionals have control of the timing of consultations and how much of the budget is spent in making communication accessible.

- Active listening is responsive – it can transform health and social care into a working alliance between disabled clients and professionals and create a communication environment in which disabled clients have control.

UNDERSTANDING DISABILITY

Disabled people and their allies have generated a social model of disability over the past 30 years. We shall characterise this model here by comparing it with the individual, and particularly the medical, model of disability, that has been increasingly challenged but still remains the dominant view of disability. So, looking from the two viewpoints what is 'the problem'? From the point of view of the medical model it is the individual, the impairment or the medical condition. Problems of communication emanate from the fact that the individual is deaf, or 'has aphasia' or is a 'stroke victim'. From the viewpoint of the social model, the problem is the disabling society that is geared by and for non-disabled people – for 'normal' communication. What of individual change? The medical model is orientated towards normality – to walk, to hear, to see. The social model, however, is directed towards transforming consciousness, that is towards the affirmation that disability is a political issue. What of changing services? From the medical model, what is needed is more of the same, for example more speech therapy provided by trained speech therapists. From a social model viewpoint, it is control by disabled clients of their own services that is of paramount importance, for example direct payments has been a significant development for many disabled people. And political change? From the medical viewpoint it is empowerment of powerless people by those who possess the power. Looking from the social model, the politics of change are in the struggles by those who lack power. Finally what of the future? From the viewpoint of the medical model it is the maintenance of a normal society with more effective services to cure or care for those rendered or deemed to be abnormal. For the social model the vision of the future is full participatory citizenship and equal rights for all disabled people.

There has been considerable discussion about the social model over the years (Swain *et al.* 2003). Mairian Corker (1998) has argued that social model accounts have tended to exclude those people for whom language and communication are the foundations of oppression and exclusion. She argues that this exclusion is perpetuated by the disabled people's movement which has failed to analyse culture and discourse in the construction of disability. She writes:

> *Without the full integration of cultural processes into the model, reference to the cultural construction of disability and deafness seem somewhat hollow...*
>
> (Corker 1998: 38)

It is important to recognise, however, that Corker and others, who have an interest in language and discourse, are not attempting to abandon the social model but rather are 'encouraging its reflexive use' (Corker 1999: 209). This involves the recognition and liberation of silent 'voices' and a greater range of positions from which disabled people can subvert forces of oppression and discrimination.

In terms of the analysis in this chapter, the unfair and unequal treatment of disabled people is not just built into institutional organisations, and their policies and practices, at a structural level, it is built into the language, communication and client-professional discourse. Simply to improve professionals' communication skills, for instance listening skills, may only strengthen unequal client-professional relations. There are many ways that this can be manifest, as we shall see below, but it is underpinned by control by the professional. Norell (1987) believes that the desire to say the 'right' thing and respond in the 'correct' manner has become something of a preoccupation. He believes that a spontaneous response can be superior to the 'painfully laboured, contrived, self-conscious effort of the "trained" doctor' (1987:14) and that one measure of a good relationship is that it can survive disagreement and conflict. He states:

> *The doctor who decides for instance not to conceal his disappointment or disapproval may be helping to develop a more productive relationship than if he were to assume the outward appearance of tolerance while fuming inwardly.*
>
> (Norell 1987: 14)

Harry (interviewed by French, forthcoming) speaks of an incident where a physiotherapist spoke to him in an unorthodox manner which, nonetheless, led to a good result:

> *I was in the physiotherapy department, they all knew me well, I was part of the furniture, and I remember saying to one of the physios, 'Why isn't there any counselling'? I said, 'There really should be counselling offered to people who've had strokes and who have communication problems'. ... and this physio said, 'Harry, I'm fed up with you moaning about this, I agree with you entirely but why don't you do*

> *something about it? Why don't you do a counselling course because I think you'd be really good at it? ... so stop moaning and do something about it'. I wandered around for weeks afterwards thinking 'I wonder' and 'maybe'. The thing that helped me so much was her belief that I could do it.*
>
> (French, forthcoming in 2004)

Harry subsequently became a fully qualified counsellor and now works with people with aphasia.

EXPERIENCING DISABLING COMMUNICATION BARRIERS

This takes us into disabled people's experiences of services, concentrating on barriers to communication, recognising that any analysis of barriers to communication needs to identify the complexities of the communication process itself and the diversity of disability. Such an analysis also needs to recognise the inequality of the professional-disabled client relationship.

Attitudinal barriers are commonly referred to by disabled clients. Boazman had mixed responses from health professionals when she became aphasic following a brain hemorrhage:

> *Their responses towards me varied greatly, some showed great compassion, while others showed complete indifference. I had no way of communicating the fact that I was a bright, intelligent, whole human being. That is what hurt the most.*
>
> (Boazman 1999: 18–19)

Similar mixed experiences were reported by people with aphasia interviewed by Parr and Byng. One person, talking of doctors, said:

> *...when you can't communicate they treat you like a kid and that is just so frustrating – A handful of doctors were just awful. You just wanted to say, 'Do you know what this is like'?*
>
> (Parr and Byng 1997: 74)

In another small-scale study involving people with speech disabilities, it was found that most difficulties were encountered within medical services and doctors' and dentists' receptionists were singled out for particular criticism. One participant recalled:

> *My most embarrassing incidents have been with my doctor's and dentist's receptionists. I have had more trouble with them than with any other group. They were impatient and rude when I tried to make appointments, and would talk to my carer when I was trying to ask questions.*
>
> (Knight *et al.* 2002: 19)

Another participant described his encounters with hospital consultants:

> *They have excluded my carer from any discussion despite me indicating that I preferred to have my carer lip-read to avoid having to use my oesophageal voice.*
>
> (Knight *et al.* 2002: 19)

Another common complaint of the research participants in this study was the means of access to services which generally depended on the telephone.

People with speech impairments are often compelled to wait long periods of time for the communication equipment they need. A survey conducted by *Scope* (Ford 2000) found that nearly a fifth of people waited for more than a year. Professionals may also have control of when the equipment can be used. One of the research participants said:

> *Physiotherapists at school have recommended the Delta Talker be removed from situ during travelling because of possible safety problems. They also used to request removal of the talker at meal times.*
>
> (Ford 2000: 29)

Deaf people have complained about the insistence of professionals that they use speech rather than sign language. A deaf person interviewed by Corker states:

> *I hated learning speech – hated it – I felt so stupid having to repeat the s,s,s ... I was asking myself 'Why do I have to keep going over and over it, I don't understand what it all means' ... It was just so stupid, a waste of time when I could have been learning more important things.*
>
> (Corker 1996: 92)

In interviews conducted by Sally French (French, forthcoming), Sue spoke of her experience of occupational therapy:

> *It was a case of being treated like a patient. I felt like my feelings were being ignored, that they were just going through a routine and they would give me exercises to do which I couldn't understand the purpose of because they didn't explain. I had enough speech to ask, but I didn't ask, because I didn't have the confidence to ask.*
>
> (French, forthcoming)

Information can also be given in an insensitive way as Joan (interviewed by French *et al.*) explained:

> *When I came back for the negatives, oh it was terrible. He lifted them up to the light and he said to the nurse 'Macula degeneration in both eyes, sign a BDS form' or whatever it is. Then he turned to me and he said 'There's nothing we can do about it'. He said 'You'll always be able to see sideways but you've got no central vision' ... So I came home feeling very upset about it.*
>
> (French 1997: 37)

Being unable to access information is a problem faced in all areas of life by visually impaired people, with potentially hazardous consequences of unreadable notices and loss of privacy when documents are unreadable by the intended recipient. Vale (2001) reports that appointment letters continue to be sent out in standard-size print even by many hospital eye clinics, and only one third of NHS hospitals offer general patient information in large print.

It is important to recognise that disability is intersected by social divisions – for example gender, age and ethnicity – which also produce communication barriers in some instances. In their study of young black disabled people's experiences and views, Bignall and Butt (2000) conclude that:

> *...most of these young people did not have the relevant information to help them achieve independence. Hardly any knew of new provisions, such as Direct Payments, which would help with independent living. Most people did not know where to get help or information they wanted, for example, to move into their own place or go to university.*
>
> (Bignall and Butt 2000: 49)

Problems included language barriers: language is often seen as the main barrier to effective service provision. It is, therefore, assumed that an adequate supply of leaflets in appropriate languages and interpreters would solve the problem. However, communication consists of more than language skills and literacy. Research by Banton and Hirsch (2000) bear out the findings of previous research. They state:

> *Communication problems are identified in all work in this area. Such problems are partly to do with language differences, but also arise from the separate lives led by different ethnic groups in our society and the consequent unlikely coincidence of communications about services arising through informal contacts.*
>
> (Banton and Hirsch 2000: 32)

Morris interviewed women with spinal cord injuries. Their most common compliant about health professionals was their lack of concern with emotional issues. One woman said, 'There is no space allowed for us to express our grief ... There is often pressure put on us to "cope" and if we fail to live up to the standard demanded of us we are categorised as a problem' (Morris 1989: 24). They reported receiving little or no help in coming to terms with paralysis, and often felt compelled to be jolly and play a particular role: as one woman put it, '... the staff expected you to have a smile on your face all the time' (Morris 1989: 24). Some women experienced a need for counselling, and said that the only thing that made life bearable for them in hospital was their relationships with other patients. Morris states that the majority of women:

> *...found that communication of the vital information about paralysis was poor, that their emotional experience was ignored, that their needs as women were not addressed, and finally they were given little help in planning for the future.*
>
> (Morris 1989: 33)

Begum (1996) explored physical, communication and attitudinal barriers between disabled people and GPs. She found that such barriers deny opportunities to disabled women and can impede access to the services they require. Disabled women, for instance, often find that information is withheld from them. One of her respondents explained that she had not been told that multiple sclerosis had been diagnosed, yet her husband had been told two years before she was informed. It seems too that the flow of information from disabled women to GPs is liable to distortion and failures. This is, at least in part, due to GPs' responses to impairment. One respondent in the research said: 'Sometimes I find that a GP – particularly one who is only here for a short time and fairly new – is more interested in my sight problem, or my child's sight problem, than in what I've come to ask about' (Begum 1996: 183–184).

Age can also be a factor that distorts communication. Olwen (interviewed by French *et al.*) talking about the attitude of professionals to her loss of sight said, 'Even though I'm older they were "at your age what can you expect?" You know they talk to you like that'. (1997: 35) Davis (1998) found that, although 90 per cent of visually impaired people are over 60, only one per cent of the targets relating to visual impairment set by Social Service Departments pertained to older people.

Disabled professionals stand in an interesting position in an analysis of communication between professionals and disabled people. It can be argued both that the barriers to communication have discriminated against disabled people wishing to be service providers and also that the acceptance of more disabled people into the professions would be a significant factor in developing inclusive communication. A visually impaired physiotherapist interviewed by French spoke of poor communication with her colleagues:

> *I'm a registered blind person but they haven't got a clue ... If I stay in one building I'm fine, it's only when I go over to G ... that I get really lost ... and one of the physios says, 'So you're not talking today'! because I've walked right passed them ... and I've worked with them for years; oh dear ... I just say 'I didn't see you' but they don't seem to learn.*
>
> (French 2001: 140)

Other health professionals have spoken of the advantages they have when communicating with ill and disabled clients: A disabled doctor explains:

> *Very many people have told me they can talk to me because I know what it feels like to have an illness. Once you get over that hump of being accepted for training then you can use your disability.*
>
> (French 1988: 178)

TOWARDS INCLUSIVE COMMUNICATION

'Inclusion' has been seen by many as a process of social change, rather than a particular state (Oliver 1996) and this can be seen to apply equally to communication and relationships. Oliver and Barnes state that:

> *. . . without a vision of how things should and ought to be, it is easy to lose your way and give up in the face of adversity and opposition . . . we all need a world where impairment is valued and celebrated and all disabling barriers are eradicated. Such a world would be inclusionary for all.*
>
> (Oliver and Barnes 1998: 102)

To develop this conceptualisation, this vision of an inclusive communication environment, we shall conclude this chapter by tentatively offering some general principles based on our discussion.

PARTICIPATION

Priority needs to be given to the participation of disabled people in the planning and evaluation of changing policy, provision and practice in developing inclusive communication. The onus is on service providers to face the challenges of enabling true participation of disabled people in decision-making processes, recognising that disabled people wish to participate in different ways. These include the democratic representation of the views of organisations of disabled people. Participation also includes as wide a consultation process as possible. Disabled people often continue to be treated as passively dependent on the expertise of others yet control seems to have become increasingly central to social change for disabled people.

ACCESSIBLE COMMUNICATION

Much is known about the accessibility of information based on the views expressed by disabled people. Clark (2002) offers wide ranging recommendations which cover such areas as alternative formats, for example, large print, large print with pictures and symbols, Braille, video and audiotape. Suggestions are also made for plain written language; typeface and font size; signage; layout; and websites.

For some people, particularly those with communication disabilities, the issue of time can be crucial to an inclusive communication environment. For people with communication disabilities a slower tempo can be the only accessible pace to ensure understanding. A research participant of McKnight *et al.* explains:

> *I prefer to speak for myself and I would rather repeat myself several times than have someone say they understood me when they did not.*
>
> (Knight *et al.* 2002: 17)

Along similar lines, Pound and Hewitt (forthcoming) emphasise that access in meetings will require attention to their length and timing.

Ford emphasises the need for people with speech impairments to have the communication equipment they require and hopes that Article 10 of the Human Rights Act (1998) (freedom of expression) will cover this requirement. He states:

> *Speech-impaired people have a right to communicate in the same way as non-disabled people. If we want a society in which disabled people are as valued as non-disabled people, society must ensure that disabled people have the appropriate equipment to be able to communicate.*
>
> (Ford 2000)

Ensuring accessibility of information to disabled people is complex and must fully involve disabled people at every stage of the process. This philosophy was central to the research by Parr *et al.* where an accessible book *The Aphasia Handbook* (undated) was produced.

DIVERSITY AND FLEXIBILITY

A disabled client (in French, forthcoming) provides the foundation for this by questioning the focus on 'normality', rather than being flexible and taking the client's perspective into account.

> *What concerns me most of all is this focus on trying to make me 'normal' … I get a lot of referrals of 'this may help' and 'that may help'. They had a massive case conference before the adaptations – it was a case of 'how normal can we make her first? Are the adaptations necessary'?*
>
> (French)

The lists of recommendations for communication access, as produced by Clark (2002) and others, clearly challenge the imperatives of normality and emphasise the diversity of communication styles and formats. Nevertheless, there are diverse needs even within specific groups of people with impairments, which again puts the emphasis on listening to disabled people and allowing them to take control. People with visual impairments, for example, are frequently presented with large print even though the depth, font and colour contrast may be more important. There is also the danger of assuming a disabled person prefers the use of technical adaptations rather than human assistance. As a visually impaired physiotherapist explains:

> *I'm lucky that the helpers, and all the staff generally, help with all the extra bits of paper that are around. The truth of the matter is, that as a blind person, you could get involved in form filling by putting it on the computer, but what the hell's the point because it's going to take an awful lot of time.*
>
> (French 2001: 128)

There are, of course, many broad social factors to consider in any discussion of the diverse needs of disabled people. As Dominelli argues, for instance, 'translation services should be publicly funded and provide interpreters matched to clients' ethnic grouping, language, religion, class and gender' (Dominelli 1997: 107). Issues concerning funding are also emphasised by Ford:

> *Speech impaired people are being denied their fundamental human right to communicate for want of an efficient and properly resourced service. Despite having been professionally assessed as needing equipment, disabled people are not getting the devices they need from statutory organisations. Education says, 'It is a health responsibility', health says, 'Ask a charity' ... New investment for equipment and training is required as a matter of urgency.*
>
> (Ford 2000: 6)

This begs the questions, however, of the need for professional involvement in the allocation of such equipment and whether professionals need disabled people more than disabled people need them. As Davis states:

> *...those of us who are familiar with some of the history of the disabled people's movement will recognise that today's 'disability*

professionals' are on a career path that has been carefully and painstakingly carved out by generations of their predecessors. Our movement's long campaign to redefine disability has left little room for doubt that society has been constructed by able-bodied people in ways which serve and perpetuate their own interests. Yet these people have used our consequential marginalisation and dependence not as a starting-point for developing with us a struggle for social change and equal opportunities, but as a handy and convenient way to justify the development of all the inappropriate disability services with which we are now so familiar.

(Davis 1993: 198–199)

HUMAN RELATIONS

Communication is constructed and embedded in relationships between people. The notion of personal relationships can be seen as irrevocably intertwined with communication. Communication is a means of expressing a relationship; it is the medium and substance through which the relationship is defined and given meaning. A disabled client offered advice to therapists on the basis of her experience. She said:

Forget you're a therapist – just be yourself. I don't mean forget all your training – but be yourself. Don't be afraid of showing the real you because that's what makes people respond, when they're ill they respond more easily if the therapist is being real.

(French, forthcoming)

USE OF INCLUSIVE LANGUAGE

In part inclusion reflects the idea that language controls or constructs thinking. Sexism, ageism, homophobia, racism and disablism are framed within the very language we use. This has been characterised and degraded by some people as 'political correctness' (PC), often with reference to examples seen as trivial or fatuous (e.g. being criticised for offering black or white coffee). Use of language, however, is not simply about the legitimacy of words or phrases. As Thompson (1998) explains, language is a powerful vehicle within interactions between health and social care professionals and clients. He identifies a number of key issues:

- Jargon – the use of specialised language, creating barriers and mystification and reinforcing power differences.
- Stereotypes – terms used to categorise people that reinforce erroneous presumptions, e.g. disabled people as 'sufferers' or as having 'special' needs.
- Stigma – terms that are derogatory and insulting, e.g. 'mentally handicapped' and 'short sighted' (meaning lack of insight).
- Exclusion – terms that exclude, overlook or marginalise certain groups, e.g. the term 'Christian name'.
- Depersonalisation – terms that are reductionist and dehumanising, e.g. 'the elderly', 'the disabled' and even 'CPs' (to denote people with cerebral palsy).

In this light, questions of the use of language go well beyond listing acceptable and unacceptable words to examining ways of thinking that rationalise, legitimise and underline unequal therapist-client power relations.

CONCLUSION

It is clear from this chapter that disabled people have had much to say about the ways in which health and professional care workers communicate with them. We will conclude this chapter with two quotations (French, forthcoming) from Sue and Harry, disabled people who have valued their contact with health care workers:

> *She said 'Come in when you like and use all the equipment'. I was particularly lucky with my physio because she had the foresight that that was what I needed for my recovery – to be in control ... She treated me like a person, she spoke to me like a person and not a patient. I felt in control and that gave me more confidence in myself ... and she understood that.*
>
> (Sue)

> *I liked my speech therapist ... and I remember thinking, 'What a fantastic woman, what a fantastic job' ... she showed kindness, kindness is something that is not acknowledged enough. She was gentle and empathetic, I felt as if she was joining in with my struggle.*
>
> (Harry)

The development of inclusive communication is a complex process that includes, though goes well beyond, active listening. However, as Pound and Hewitt (forthcoming) state:

> *It will support people with and without language impairment to enrich communication practice, share power and celebrate the creativity and challenge of communication difference.*
>
> (Pound and Hewitt, forthcoming)

REFERENCES

Banton, M. and Hirsch, M.M. (2000) *Double Invisibility: Report on Research into the Needs of Black Disabled People in Coventry*, Warwickshire County Council.

Begum, N. (1996) 'Doctor, doctor ...: Disabled women's experience of general practitioners', in Morris, J. (ed.) *Encounters with Strangers: Feminism and Disability*, London: The Women's Press.

Bignall, T. and Butt, J. (2000) *Between Ambition and Achievement: Young Black Disabled People's Views and Experiences of Independence and Independent Living*, Bristol: Policy Press.

Boazman, S. (1999) 'Inside aphasia', in Corker, M. and French, S. (eds) *Disability Discourse*, Buckingham: Open University Press.

Clarke, L. (2002) *Liverpool Central Primary Care Trust Accessible Health Information: Project Report*, www.leeds.ac.uk/disability-studies.

Corker, M. (1996) *Deaf Transitions: Images and Origins of Deaf Families, Deaf Communities and Deaf Identities*, London: Jessica Kingsley.

Corker, M. (1998) *Deaf and Disabled, or Deafness Disabled?* Buckingham: Open University Press.

Corker, M. (1999) 'New disability discourse, the principle of optimization and social change', in Corker, M. and French, S. (eds) *Disability Discourse*, Buckingham: Open University Press.

Davis, K. (1993) 'The crafting of good clients', in Swain, J., Finkelstein, V., French, S. and Oliver, M. (eds) *Disabling Barriers – Enabling Environments*, London: Sage.

Davis, M. (1998) *Putting Vision Into Community Care*, London: Royal National Institute for the Blind.

Dominelli, L. (1997) *Anti-Racist Social Work*, Houndmills: Macmillan.

Ford, J. (2000) *Speak For Yourself*, Scope: London.

French, S. (1988) 'Experiences of disabled health and caring professionals', *Sociology of Health and Illness* 10, 2: 170–188.

French, S. (2001) *Disabled People and Employment: A Study of the Working Lives of Visually Impaired Physiotherapists*, Aldershot: Sage.

French, S. (forthcoming in 2004) 'Enabling relationships in therapy practice', in Swain, J., Clark, J., French, S., Reynolds, F. and Parry, K. (eds) *Enabling Relationships in Health and Social Care: A Guide for Therapists*, Oxford: Butterworth-Heinemann.

French, S., Gillman, M. and Swain, J. (1997) *Working with Visually Disabled People: Bridging Theory and Practice*, Birmingham: Venture Press.

Knight, B., Sked, A. and Garrill, J. (2002) *Breaking the Silence: Identification of the Communication and Support Needs of Adults with Speech Disabilities in Newcastle*, Newcastle: CENTRIS.

Morris, J. (1989) *Able Lives. Women's Experience of Paralysis*, London: The Women's Press.

Norell, J. (1987) 'Uses and abuses of the consultation', in Elder, A. and Samuel, O. (eds) *While I'm Here Doctor: A Study of the Doctor–Patient Relationship*, London, Tavistock Publications.

Oliver, M. (1996) *Understanding Disability: From Theory to Practice*, Houndmills: Macmillan Press.

Oliver, M. and Barnes, C. (1998) *Disabled People and Social Policy: From Exclusion to Inclusion*, London: Longman.

Parr, S. and Byng, S. (1997) *Talking about Aphasia*. Buckingham: Open University Press

Parr, S., Pound, C., Byng, S. and Long, (undated) *The Aphasia Handbook* (available from Ecodistribution, 117 Main Street, Woodhouse Eaves, Leicestershire, LE12 8RY. Also available on www.ah-ha.org).

Pound, C. and Hewitt, A. (forthcoming) 'Communication barriers: building access and identity', in Swain, J., Barnes, C., French, S. and Thomas, C. (eds) *Disabling Barriers – Enabling Environments*, London: Sage.

Swain, J., French, S. and Cameron, C. (2003) *Controversial Issues in a Disabling Society*, Buckingham: Open University Press.

Thompson, N. (1998) *Promoting Equality: Challenging discrimination and oppression in the human services*, Houndmills: Macmillan.

Vale, D. (2001) *Improving Lives: Priorities in Health Social Care for Blind and Partially Sighted People*, On behalf of the Improving Lives Coalition by the Royal National Institute for the Blind, London.

CHAPTER 25

CARING PRESENCE: A CASE STUDY

Joan Engebretson

INTRODUCTION

Caring presence, especially the use of silence, is a difficult concept to teach. The use of case study or story is an excellent method to teach this aspect of nursing care. This case, describing an event in a clinical rotation of an undergraduate student, has served as an exemplar for other students. A pedagogical discussion of caring presence as a nursing dynamic and the impact on the patient, nurse, and the environment of care is presented. This story also serves to illuminate the values of the culture of the health care system and the impact that the action of one nurse can have on the care environment.

Being present is a primary principle in healing and one of four universal powers described in Arrien's (1993) cross-cultural perspectives on healing. Patterson and Zderad (1976) defined presence as the quality of being open, receptive, ready, and available to the experience of another person through a reciprocal interpersonal encounter. Presence or more specifically, caring presence, is often cited as an important concept for nursing practice. (Dossey, Keegan, Guzzetta and Kolkmeier 1995: Dossey 1997: Gaut 1992: Snyder and Lindquist 1998). Nursing theorists such as Leininger (1981): Parse (1981), Rogers (1970), Watson (1985), and others have identified presence as an important aspect of nursing. Presence has also been recognised as a principal component of human caring (Gaut 1992). Presence is listed as a nursing intervention in the Nursing Interventions Classifications (NIC) (McCloskey and Bulechek 1996) with silence and touch included as specific actions.

Source: *International Journal for Human Caring* (2000) 4 (2).

Caring presence refers largely to non-instrumental aspects of the patient-provider relationship. Thus, it is an aspect of nursing that often does not translate well to the contemporary environment of health care delivery that emphasises technology and efficiency. Although many experienced nurses practice caring presence and can relate to the theoretical writings on the subject, a problem exists in conveying these concepts to the novice nurse who is accustomed to following step by step procedures or using direct and measurable applications of theory to a practice. The dynamic of presence often does not rely on the words or specific tasks that the nurse performs. Nursing presence and creating a space for healing are subtle and often difficult to describe and therefore hard for students to understand.

The following experience with an undergraduate student illustrates caring presence without words and exemplifies for me what that caring presence can be. Students have found this example useful in understanding such subtle aspects of the nursing role. It enables them to experience some of their personal feelings associated with caring presence as a precursor for being with patients. The story is followed with an analysis of the potential impact of caring presence on this particular patient and the environment of patient care. Names and non-essential facts have been changed to maintain confidentiality.

THE STORY

It was Brenda's third day of her Parent-Infant Care clinical rotation and her first day on the post-partum unit. She had previously completed course-work and clinical experience in Fundamentals and Medical Surgical Nursing. We had just covered labour and delivery in the didactic portion of the course. She arrived on the post-partum unit just prior to the 6:45 AM report. Her assignment was Mrs Q, an African-American woman recently married to an African-born husband who was not present at the delivery and was reportedly out of town. Mrs Q delivered a son at 23 weeks gestation at 4AM by emergency C-section. She had a history of six pregnancy losses and had never carried a pregnancy past 20 weeks. This newly delivered infant was the only live birth. The infant had been taken immediately to the Neonatal Intensive Care Unit (NICU). After report, Brenda checked Mrs Q's vital signs and assisted her with early morning care. Shortly after, Brenda received a call from the NICU that Mrs Q's son was unstable and she was invited to come to the nursery.

Brenda prepared to bring her patient to the nursery. She assisted her in getting ready and took her by wheelchair to the NICU. Brenda asked me what her nursing role should be. I must say the question caught me off guard. I thought immediately what type of things she could say to the woman and a number of communication strategies that would encourage the woman to express her feelings. Somehow, none of those techniques felt quite right for the situation. All I could muster up was that she needed to be there for Mrs Q and stay with her. Brenda immediately looked at me and asked, 'How do you do that'? I was at a loss for words and all I could tell her was 'You need to be with her'. I added that this was a time when 'being with' might be in silence and that it was OK not to talk. I finally replied 'Just be with her throughout the shift and I will check on you frequently. Stay with her and focus on her experience'. I began to think how poorly we prepared students for the reality of such experiences. Is it any surprise that nurses and other health care providers busy themselves with tasks to avoid this powerful and painful human interaction?

Brenda and Mrs Q entered the unit, a large open area with the isolettes in a semicircle around the nurse's station. Each isolette was attached to a wall unit with the usual maze of tubes, monitoring lines, and intensive care equipment. Monitors were beeping and throngs of men and women were rushing around all dressed in blue-green scrub suits, the ubiquitous uniforms of ICUs. Being more attuned to both the student and the new mother, I was reminded how overwhelming and alienating the atmosphere of intensive care units can be. It was difficult to see the tiny newborn amidst all the wires and tubes. Moreover, it must have been confusing for this mother to determine easily which one of this circle of infants was hers. The uniform appearance of the caregivers also created an apparent obstacle, as not only did they all appear too busy to interrupt, but also the uniformity of their dress and manner made all of us, patient, student and even faculty, feel very much like outsiders. I found myself wondering 'Oh where to start, who do we approach, where to start to enter this alien world'. The student, asking how she could find this woman's baby, reiterated this sense of overwhelming confusion. Since I knew several of the nurses in the unit this problem was somewhat abated as I explained the student's assignment and asked a couple of the nurses to be available for my student.

The student moved Mrs Q's wheelchair to a spot near her infant's isolette. Mrs Q was a woman of few words, but her expression on seeing her newborn was filled with feelings. For a period she sat and watched her infant and Brenda watched the two of them. Brenda moved to the nurses' station, conveniently located in the open area in the center of the circle of isolettes. Shortly after, I moved a chair next to Mrs Q's wheelchair. This was an unmistakable message to Brenda that she was to sit with Mrs Q. The two sat side by side in relative silence against a backdrop of the continual cacophony of human and mechanical noises. In addition to multiple conversations of doctors, nurses, and other providers, there was the ceaseless hum of machinery punctuated by the beeps of monitors going off. Adding to the feeling of instability of these fragile neonates who could and did often code with little warning, the majority of the fixtures in the unit were on wheels of some sort. Isolettes were movable, x-ray machines were wheeled in and out, and providers rode their chairs from one task to another: for example taking a phone call and rolling to the records at the other end of the desk.

As the morning advanced, the baby's condition became less stable and increasingly critical. The nurses invited Mrs Q to touch her infant very gently. Brenda sat with her occasionally touching her shoulder. Nurses and doctors moving to the infant's isolette, checking various monitors, and performing seemingly complicated tasks, frequently broke the continual buzz of activity in the background. I would often make rounds to this unit but needed to attend to other students on adjacent units. As I observed this situation from the other side of the unit, it began to become apparent that as the doctors, nurses, and various other providers approached Mrs Q and Brenda, there was a noticeable change in their manner. They moved a bit slower and spoke more softly. Their touch seemed to be kinder and gentler.

After some time, one of the nurses placed the infant in Mrs Q's arms. She gently cradled her newborn, softly caressing his head and stroking his back. Brenda lightly placed her hand on Mrs Q's shoulder, arm, or back. Brenda seemed to sense that appropriate touch in this case needed to be very gentle, stable, and unobtrusive, almost mirroring the touch Mrs Q used with her infant. As Brenda moved closer to Mrs Q and her infant a tableau was created. The staff in the NICU appeared to sense a special space in the unit extending about 3–5 feet around them. Staff walked around that area, not intruding unless they had a specific need to do so. The mood in the entire unit also changed: there was a dramatically less hectic atmosphere in the unit. Staff seemed to move with more care, equipment was moved with less banging and bumping, voices were softer, and people behaved differently. An aura of dignity was created throughout the unit. Several residents and other providers coming into the unit on rounds stopped and paused in silence watching Brenda and Mrs Q sitting vigil with the infant.

I would occasionally check with Brenda to see if she needed anything. I was amazed at how intrusive it felt to ask Brenda, even quietly, if she or Mrs Q might need anything. I could see that Brenda was very engrossed in the interaction between Mrs Q and the infant. She appeared completely engaged with them and quite oblivious to the rest of the unit.

As the morning wore on, more and more equipment was removed from the infant leaving only one EKG lead that recorded the infant's heart rate on the monitor. Watching from across the room, it felt like time was suspended. Mrs Q was totally absorbed with her infant. She typified what has been described in the maternal-infant attachment literature as 'engrossment', holding the infant in the 'en face' position and gently stroking and touching the infant.

By mid-morning, the unit became considerably quieter and staff had gathered in a semi-circle 4–6 feet away from the trio. Nurses and doctors would move to attend to other infants and other tasks and return to stand in this circle. In the center, Mrs Q seemed totally absorbed with her infant and Brenda with the other two. It felt like the staff had formed a human boundary to protect a space for what was about to happen. As Mrs Q comforted and cared for her infant, his heart rate dropped below 100. Mrs Q cradled her son and stroked his back, gently rocking back and forth. The circle of staff in the NICU sent a message to anyone entering the unit to slow down and be quiet, and their presence created a protected space for this mother and son. This was more profoundly and effectively communicated than any sign on the door to the nursery. Over the course of the next 1–2 hours, the infant's heart rate decelerated to 80 … 60 … 40 … and gradually stopped. As the infant's condition deteriorated, around the circle of health care workers there were few dry eyes. Brenda had silent tears rolling down her cheeks, as did Mrs Q. After the baby died, Mrs Q sat holding the infant for another 20–30 minutes. She paused and looked to Brenda who turned her head toward the nurses' station. With no more communication necessary, one of the nurses took the EKG lead off then and invited Mrs Q to go into a private room to spend time alone with the infant. Brenda asked her if she would like her to go with her and she replied nodding, 'for a little while'. Brenda wheeled Mrs Q into this room, while the nurse carried the infant, placing him in his mother's arms. After some time Mrs Q stated she was ready to return to her room.

Brenda transferred Mrs Q back to her room, gave her pain medication, as she was less than twelve hours post C-section, and assuring that she was comfortable, told her that she would be there if she needed anything and left her to sleep and rest. Brenda and I went into the nurses' lounge where we both cried and talked about the experience. Much to my surprise this did not take long. The tears came freely and Brenda expressed that although it was sad, it was a wonderful experience, and she felt fulfilled.

PEDAGOGICAL ANALYSIS

This experience was the topic for the post clinical group discussion and I have continued to use this story as an illustration of therapeutic use of personal presence. This clinical exemplar of caring presence has been used to make a connection with the literature on presence as a nursing dynamic. The discussions have focused on the impact that presence has on the patient, the nurses, and the environment in which care is given. This case can also be used to expand cultural awareness of the contemporary health care system. This subtle, silent, and immaterial intervention illuminates the contrasting cultural values of an orientation to future time, action, materiality, and direct effects or outcomes that pervade health care delivery.

As this story took place several years ago, one of the issues of discussion is the changing technology and philosophy of neonatal care. At the time of the incident, extreme measures were often not used with an infant less than 24 hours old and under 24 weeks gestation whose condition was deteriorating. This contrasts with the advancing technology today wherein all interventions are used to prolong the life of the infant. The following are some of the ideas and nursing issues from these discussions.

PRESENCE AS A NURSING DYNAMIC

Actions of the student nurse can be analysed from the three categories of presence described by McKivergin and Daubenmire (1994) as physical presence, psychological presence, and therapeutic presence. Actions of the student nurse included all three types of presence. Physical presence is body to body contact and includes skills of seeing, examining, touching, doing, hearing, and hugging. Physical presence was apparent in Brenda's sitting with the patient and touching her gently. This action may have encouraged Mrs Q to touch her infant gently as well. In this case, touch may have both material and symbolic effects.

Psychological presence is mind to mind and incorporates communication, active listening, reflecting, attending to, caring, empathy, being nonjudgemental, and accepting. Although there was little verbal exchange, the student was clearly accepting, in a nonjudgemental manner, of the new mother's vigil with her son. This provided some stability for the new mother in a very unstable environment and situation. Brenda also attended to the mother and infant's needs, which was conveyed to the staff who cared for the new mother by placing the infant in the mother's arms and attending to needs of the infant beyond the technological life support.

Therapeutic presence is described as spirit to spirit or centred self to centred self with the associated skills of centreing, intentionality, intuitive knowing, commenting, and loving. In discussions with the student after the mother had returned to her room, Brenda related being really scared at first, but she knew she had to be there for this patient. In order to make this connection to her patient she had to first make a connection with something within herself. The only way she could do that was to sit quietly with Mrs Q with intent to help and heal. She discovered that she could reach an 'internal knowing of what to do'. She described to her fellow students that going through that experience with a patient was one of the most profound experiences of her life and although it was sad, it was extraordinarily rewarding.

In a concept analysis of presence, Hines (1992) proposed the following attributes:

1 time with another;
2 unconditional positive regard;
3 transactional being with another including nonverbal communication;
4 valued encounter and action beyond the ordinary;
5 connectedness and sharing; and
6 sustaining memory.

Brenda spent time using silence and touch, both non-verbal communication actions. She approached Mrs Q with unconditional positive regard and the encounter was one of connection. The reactions of the staff attest to the fact that Brenda's actions were out of the ordinary and were valued. Thus, in this example, attributes 1–5 were clearly exhibited, and it is likely that both Brenda and Mrs Q had a sustained memory of the experience and that Brenda's actions were valued. These actions affected the student nurse, the patient (mother and infant), other health care providers, and the health care environment.

IMPACT ON THE PATIENT

The ultimate evaluation of any nursing dynamic is concerned with the effect on the patient. In this case example the impact needs to be assessed from the perspective of the new mother, the infant, and the relationship between the two. Birth and death are pivotal life experiences for the mother, the infant, and the family.

Comfort in dying. The infant is generally the focus of care in the NICU: in this case, the infant was dying. He was allowed to spend a significant portion of his less than 24-hour life cradled in his mother's arms rather than in an isolette with mechanical devices attached to his body and surrounded by the amplified sounds of monitors and other equipment. The closeness of being held and cradled against his mother's breast and being softly caressed allowed him to experience touch that was comforting in contrast to the primarily instrumental touch of the providers in the NICU. Permitting him to die with the comforting touch of his mother was surely the most compassionate way to provide a 'good death' for this infant. The inattention that is often paid to the comfort and dignity of infants who cannot express themselves in words is a sign of an over-reliance on words and the meanings of words as symbols of communication.

Positive experience as a mother. This mother had six previous pregnancy losses. This was the only child that had been born alive. Although his life was short, less than 24 hours, she was able to enact a quintessential mothering role, that of comforting her son at a time of great need. The attainment of the maternal role starts in pregnancy but it is foundational to the parenting role that a mother 'protect and care for' her infant after birth. In cases where the infant is premature or in fragile health, this becomes difficult and the process is disrupted if the mother is not permitted to 'tend to' her child. The comfort and love this mother gave to her infant through his dying was unique. No caretaker could provide that intangible 'caring presence' provided by his mother. Many mothers have a lifetime to 'care for' their children. This mother, although her child lived less than a day, cared for him in 'being with' him as he died. It would seem unconscionable to deny either of them that opportunity. After six previous pregnancy losses, this was the only time she was able to tend and care for her child.

Attachment and grieving. The family's or mother's bereavement after neonatal death is a complex process that defies normal grief as there are few memories of the neonate. It is also a reverse of the natural expectation of parents to care for and protect their children and to precede them in death. Only recently has much attention been paid to the needs of parents after a neonate expires. In the process of grief resolution, it is necessary for the mother (and father) to attach to the infant as part of an optimal grief process. Attachment is the tie between the mother and infant that reflects a reciprocal process. The mother begins an orientation to the infant during pregnancy that continues through the birth process where her focus concentrates on the neonate. This process is abbreviated and more difficult with preterm deliveries, as the infant often cannot respond to or give cues to the mother's actions. It is a nursing responsibility to facilitate this process of helping the pair to overcome the impediments of preterm delivery and the hospital environment. The caring presence of Brenda appears to have affected the physical and human environment that allowed the mother and infant to use their own abilities to make this attachment.

The cardinal indicators of maternal-infant attachment relate to positioning, attitude, and engaging in a spontaneous reciprocal interaction with the neonate. Positioning includes cradling the infant in her left arm, assuming an en face position, eye contact, stroking and caressing. The mother, supported by caring presence of the student nurse, exhibited all these behaviours. The mother's interest in and sensitivity to nurturing the infant was clearly demonstrated in her actions. She and her newborn infant developed a mutual synchronous, albeit subtle, rhythm of cues and responses. It appeared that the mother and neonate were engaged in an intimate dance of subtle cues and responses indicative of early attachment.

IMPACT ON THE NURSE

Although it was difficult for Brenda to express the extent of her experience, she often mentioned that this day had a profound effect on her and reaffirmed her decision to go into nursing. This type of experience was what made her choice of work meaningful.

IMPACT ON THE ENVIRONMENT IN WHICH CARE IS GIVEN

Brenda's very overt physical presence of sitting with Mrs Q established a private sacred space that staff seemed to respond to as they hesitated to intrude and in turn, created a human circle solidifying a special quiet space around the student and patient. Noise level has been a nursing concern since Nightingale (1969) and has recently become an active concern related to the environment of NICUs. Recent research-based nursing interventions for developmental care for pre-term neonates have focused on the environment, in particular noise and light levels. Reducing sound levels is a component in developmental care for very low birth weight infants (Lotas and Walden 1996).

BUILDING CULTURAL AWARENESS

Bishop and Scudder (1985) and Noddings (1984) discussed the importance of caring as important in the ethics of the patient-provider relationship. Being present and engaged is identified as an essential aspect of the patient-provider relationship which is, unfortunately, often not practiced (Reiser and Rosen 1984: Stewart *et al.* 1995). An understanding of some of the cultural orientations of contemporary health care delivery may be helpful to explain this disparity.

Biomedicine has been described as reflecting the core American values of individuality, efficiency, technology, and scientific expertise (Lock and Gorden 1988). Davis-Floyd (1992) also described the contemporary hospital birth as a 'technocratic model of birth', reflecting the core American values of technology and science over the human experience. This case illuminates through contrast of the student's caring approach to the family some of the cultural issues that mitigate against a caring presence that are reflected in contemporary health care systems.

Orientation to time. Most providers have, and the health care system promotes, a future orientation toward time. This is exemplified by a high concern with schedules and planning for the future. Providers are often thinking and making plans for the future while engaging in tasks. Caring presence requires the nurse to be fully present in the moment, totally engaged in 'being with' the client. According to the literature, a characteristic of African-American culture is a present-orientation to time (Giger and Davidhizar 1995). In this case, Brenda in addition to illuminating the future orientation of the hospital culture may have also related to the present time value of her African-American clients.

Use of silence. Very few words were exchanged between Brenda and Mrs Q. The culture of the hospital, reflecting American culture, was a word-oriented culture. We value the printed word and focus on the meanings of the actual words. We have transferred this to verbal communication and tend to pay more attention to the words people speak than other aspects of an exchange. Many cultures tend to rely on a total picture of communication that includes body language, sincerity, and respect of the person rather than focusing primarily on the meaning of the spoken words (Giger and Davidhizar 1995). Most nursing textbooks and beginning curricula stress the importance of non-verbal communication, however, students often feel very insecure it they do not know what words to say. Words are a comfortable tool as the non-verbal communication often relates to an inner state of being that is not easily taught. Many professionals are often terrified of being with someone in silence.

Being and doing. Americans have been described as a 'doing' rather than a 'being' or 'becoming' culture (Kluckholm 1976). This is exemplified in ICU units where tasks of 'doing something to' patients is highly valued. Often a nurse's competence is determined by skills at doing complicated procedures effectively and efficiently. This is in sharp contrast to 'being with' someone, which is devoid of technology, and instead uses the caring presence of oneself. Gilje (1992) describes presence as a state of being which can be in relationship to others and starts with being physically located in space and time. She also differentiated between 'being there' (physical presence and attending to tasks) and 'being with' (psychological presence and including an authentic connection of self). This story exemplifies the nursing act of being with a patient.

Material vs. immaterial. Material things that can be seen and measured have come to be the markers of reality in many health care settings. Philosophically, positivism that couples materiality (reality is that which can be measured and perceived by the five senses) with scientific reductionism has pervaded the health care setting (Lincoln and Guba 1985). Caring presence is neither material nor measurable, and it cannot often be reduced to a specific effect on a person. It is thus difficult to collect reimbursement for 'being with' someone. This vital component of health care has often been trivialised or completely ignored.

Subtle vs. direct effects. This case example illustrates the large impact of so-called small interventions.

Immaterial actions have been labelled the small (not vital or important) nursing actions. Such trivialisation of less intrusive actions stems from a materialistic philosophy that is focused on large effects from large interventions that are contiguous in time. This thinking has pervaded the health care system's orientation to outcomes and effectiveness appraisal of interventions. The subtle effects of caregiver actions may have very profound and long-term effects that are often overlooked.

Taylor (1992) related nursing presence as enacting an 'ordinariness'. She described nurses who 'were just themselves' implying an authenticity in relating to others. This paradox of powerful authenticity and the humble term ordinariness deserves more attention. It is through authentic human ordinariness that humans are bonded together. As Brenda discussed her experience of 'being with' Mrs Q she found a common humanness from which authentic nursing care emerged. She was able to move through her initial impulse to hide in the professional role, which would have diminished the authentic fulfillment of her professional role.

IMPLICATIONS FOR NURSING

As health care develops a business approach, less tangible nursing activities can be easily dismissed as unquantifiable and inefficient. Nursing interventions that have no instrumental tasks or words are particularly likely to be ignored. Nurses can link their caring actions to patient satisfaction and other outcomes, which are vitally important to a business model.

Additionally, more research using a variety of methods is needed to explore the long term and more subtle effects of these non-material interventions.

It is also important for nurses to discuss their stories as a way of transmitting these aspects of nursing both to the public as well as to other members of the profession. The personal sense of meaning and fulfilment related to the mission of nursing should be emphasised. Nurses have a theoretical and literature base that validates caring presence as a professional and autonomous nursing activity. This autonomous nursing action need not wait for administrator's or physician's orders. This is part of the professional contract between the nurse and patient.

This story illustrates how one student, silently being with a patient, created a space for an infant to die with comfort and dignity in his mother's arms. The steadfast presence of this student impacted the entire ICU in the reduction of noise and the changes in human behaviour throughout the unit. It illustrated how easily a unit can become focused on the tasks and complex technology and equally how quickly one person's caring presence can remind all of the essential human dignity of patients. On reflection, it is understandable how the dignity and sacredness of human life (especially a neonate who cannot speak and communicate in the terms of rational words) can be disregarded in the emphasis on saving lives and the press for efficiency. The impact of this student's actions on the entire unit speaks to the awareness of most providers and their ability to link to the common 'extraordinary ordinariness' of the essential human experience.

One provider exhibiting caring presence can affect the entire system. We, as nurses, often feel that as individuals we cannot impact or change the care environment. This case illustrates how one nurse, a beginning student, provided the space for an entire unit to be transformed. This raises questions regarding how our presence or absence of caring presence impacts individual patients, the nursing profession, and the health care environment.

REFERENCES

Arrien, A. (1993) *The Four-Fold Way*, San Francisco, CA: Harper.

Bishop, A.H. and Scudder, J.R. (1985) *Caring Nurse, Curing Physician, Coping Patient Relationships*, Tuscaloosa, AL: University of Alabama Press.

Davis-Floyd, Robbie E. (1992) *Birth as an American Rite of Passage*, University of California Press.

Dossey, B.M. (ed.) (1997) *Core Curriculum for Holistic Nursing*, Gaithersburg, TN: Aspen.

Dossey, B.M., Keegan, L., Guzzetta, C.E. and Kolkmeier, L.G. (1995) *Holistic Nursing: A Handbook for Practice*, Gaithersburg, TN: Aspen.

Gaut, D.A. (ed.) (1992) *The Presence of Caring in Nursing*, New York: National League of Nursing Press.

Giger, J.M. and Davidhizar, R.E. (1995) *Transcultural Nursing: Assessment and Intervention*, St. Louis: Mosby.

Gilje, F. (1992) 'Being there: An analysis of the concept of presence', in Gaut, D. (ed.) *The Presence of Caring*, New York: NLN Press, 53–67.

Hines, D.R. (1992) 'Presence: Discovering the artistry in relating', *Journal of Holistic Nursing* 10 (4): 294–305.

Kluckholm, F.R. (1976) 'Dominant and variant value orientations', in Brink, P.J. (ed.) *Transcultual Nursing: A Book of Readings*, Englewood Cliffs: Prentice-Hall, 63–81.

Leininger, M. (1981) 'The phenomenon of caring: importance, research questions and theoretical considerations', in Leininger, M. (ed.) *Caring: An Essential Human Need*, Detroit: Wayne State University Press, 3–16.

Lincoln, Y. and Guba, E. (1985) *Naturalistic Inquiry*, Newbury Park: Sage.

Lock, M. and Gordon, D. (eds) (1988) *Biomedical Examined*, Dordrecht, Netherlands: Kluwer Academic Publisher.

Lotas, M.J. and Walden, M. (1996) 'Individualized developmental care for very low-birth-weight infants: A critical review', *Journal of Obstetric, Gynecologic, and Neonatal Nursing* 25 (8): 381–391.

McCloskey, J.C. and Bulechek, G.M. (1996) *Nursing Interventions Classification* (2nd Edn) St Louis: Mosby.

McKivergin, M. and Daubenmire, J. (1994) 'The essence of therapeutic presence', *Journal of Holistic Nursing* 12 (1): 65–81.

Nightingale, F. (1969) *Notes on Nursing: What It Is, and What It Is Not*, New York: Dover.

Noddings, N. (1984) *Caring: A Feminine Approach to Ethics and Moral Education*, Berkeley: University of California.

Parse, R. (1981) *Man-Living-Health: A Theory of Nursing*, New York: John Wiley & Sons.

Patterson, J. and Zderad, L. (1976) *Humanistic Nursing*, New York: John Wiley & Sons.

Reiser, D.E. and Rosen, D.R. (1984) *Medicine as Human Experience*, Baltimore, MD: University Park.

Rogers, M. (1970) *An Introduction to the Theoretical Basis of Nursing*, Philadelphia: F.A. Davis Co.

Snyder, M. and Lindquist, R. (1998) *Complementary/Alternative Therapies in Nursing*, New York: Springer.

Stewart, M., Brown, J.B., Weston, W.W., McWhinney, I.R., McWilliam, C.L. and Freeman, T.R. (1995) *Patient-Centered Medicine: Transforming the Clinical Method*, Thousand Oaks: Sage.

Taylor, B.J. (1992) 'Caring: Being manifested as ordinariness in nursing', in Gaut, D. (ed.) *The Presence of Caring in Nursing*, New York: National League of Nursing Press.

Watson, J. (1985) *Nursing: Human Science and Human Care*, New York: National League of Nursing Press.

CHAPTER 26

THE SOCIOLOGY OF EMOTION AS A WAY OF SEEING

Arlie Russell Hochschild

[...]

What is it like to see the world from the point of view of the sociologist of emotion?[1] Perhaps the best way to convey this point of view is to look very closely at one small episode, and to compare different ways of seeing it. As my episode, my 'grain of sand', I have chosen one young woman's description of her wedding day in 1981, drawn from my book *The Managed Heart*. The young woman says this:

> *My marriage ceremony was chaotic and completely different than I imagined it would be. Unfortunately, we rehearsed at 8 o'clock the morning of the wedding. I had imagined that everyone would know what to do, but they didn't. That made me nervous. My sister didn't help me get dressed or flatter me and no one in the dressing room helped until I asked. I was depressed. I wanted to be so happy on our wedding day ... This is supposed to be the happiest day of one's life. I couldn't believe that some of my best friends couldn't make it to my wedding. So as I started out to the church thinking about all these things, that I always thought would not happen at my wedding, going through my mind, I broke down and cried. But I thought to myself, 'Be happy for the friends, the relatives, the presents'. Finally, I said to myself, 'Hey, other people aren't getting married,* you *are'. From down the long aisle I saw my husband. We looked at each other's*

Source: Bendelow, G. and Williams, S.J. (eds) (1998) *Emotions in Social Life*, London: Routledge.

eyes. His love for me changed my whole being from that point on. When we joined arms, I was relieved. The tension was gone. From then on, it was beautiful. It was indescribable.[2]

(Hochschild 1983: 59)

[...]

THE SOCIOLOGY OF EMOTIONS VIEW

How would a sociologist of emotion approach the same bride? Like the psychoanalyst, the sociologist of emotion notes that the bride is anxious, and links her anxiety with the meanings she attaches to the wedding. But the sociologist of emotion does not usually focus on a person's childhood development *per se*, or on injury and repair, but instead on the sociocultural *determinants* of feeling, and the sociocultural bases for defining, appraising and managing human emotion and feeling.

Three questions arise. Why did the bride feel 'nervous', and 'depressed', as she put it, and break down and cry? How did she define her feelings? And how did she appraise the degree to which they corresponded with what she thought she 'should' feel?

To answer the first question, we would need to discover far more about the bride's prior expectations and her current apprehension of the self-relevance of her situation. I would personally argue that emotion emerges as a result of a newly grasped reality (as it bears on the self) as it clashes against the template of prior expectations (as they bear on the self). Emotion is a biologically given sense, and our most important one. Like other senses, hearing, touch and smell, emotion is a means by which we continually learn and relearn about a just-now-changed, back-and-forth relation between self and world, the world as it means something just now to the self.

Most of us maintain a prior expectation of a continuous self, but the character of the self we expect to maintain is subject to profoundly social influence. To understand the bride's distress, we would need to understand the template of prior expectations she had about herself, as a daughter, a girlfriend, a woman, a member of her community, and her social class. We would need to know how close she felt she 'really was' to the friends who didn't appear at her wedding, to the sister who didn't reassure her. We would need to know just what she picked out to see and absorb as she saw her sister from the dressing-table, and what gestures caught her eye among participants at the rehearsal. From these details we might reconstruct the social aspects of the moment of disappointment and tears. To be sure, the social aspect isn't everything. Emotion always involves some biological component: trembling, weeping, breathing hard. But it takes a social element, a new juxtaposition of an up-until-just-now expectation and a just-now apprehension of reality to induce emotion. That is one aspect of emotion the sociologist of emotion studies.

Second, how does the bride define her feelings? She draws from *a prior set of ideas about what feelings are feel-able*. She has to rely on a prior notion of what feelings are 'on the cultural shelf', pre-acknowledged, pre-named, pre-articulated, culturally available to be felt. We can say that our bride intuitively matches her feeling to a nearest feeling in a collectively shared emotional dictionary. Let us picture this dictionary not as a small object outside herself, but as a giant cultural entity and she a small being upon its pages.

Matching her feelings to the emotional dictionary, she discovers that some feelings are feel-able and others not. Were she to feel sexual and romantic homosexual attraction in China, for example, she would discover that to most people, homosexual love is not simply considered 'bad'; it is considered not to exist.

Like other dictionaries, the emotional dictionary reflects agreement among the authorities of a given time and place. It expresses the idea that within an emotional 'language group' there are given emotional experiences, each with its own ontology. So, to begin with, the sociologist of emotion asks, first, to what array of acknowledged feelings, in the context of her time and place, is our bride *matching* her inner experience, and, second, is her feeling of happiness on her wedding day a perfect match, a near match, a complete mismatch? This powerful process of matching inner experience to a cultural dictionary becomes, for the sociologist of emotion, a mysterious, important part of the drama of this bride's inner life. For culture is an active, constituent part of emotion, not a passive medium within which biologically pre-formulated, 'natural' emotions emerge.

Third, we ask: what does the bride believe she *should* or shouldn't feel? If, on one hand, the bride is matching her emotion to a cultural dictionary, she is also matching it to a bible, a set of prescriptions embedded in the received wisdom of her culture. The bride lives in a *culture of emotion*. What did the bride expect or hope to feel on this day? She tells us a wedding 'is supposed to be the happiest day of one's life'. In so far as she shares this wish with most other young heterosexual women in America, she has internalised a shared feeling rule: on this day feel the most happy you have ever felt. Specifically, the bride may have ideals about *when* to feel excited, central, enhanced, and when not to (around age 25, not 15). She has ideas about *whom* she should love and whom not (a kind, responsible man, not a fierce one) and *how strongly* she should love (with a moderate degree of abandon; not complete abandon, but not too cool and collected either).

Her feeling rules are buttressed by her beliefs concerning *how important* love should be. The poet Lord Byron wrote, 'Man's love is of man's life a thing apart, 'tis woman's whole existence'.

Does love loom larger for our bride than it does for her groom? Or does she now try to make love a smaller part of her life, as men in her culture have tried to do in the past? What are the new feeling rules about the place of love in a modern woman's life? How desirable or valued is the emotion of love or the state of deep attachment?

According to the western 'romantic love ethic', one is supposed to fall 'head over heels' in love, to lose control or come close to doing so. Within western cultures, there are subcultural variations. In Germany, *romantische Liebe* has a slightly derogatory connotation that it lacks in the USA. In many parts of non-western societies, such as India, romantic love is considered dangerous. On the basis of interviews with Hindu men on the subject of love, Steve Derne found that the Hindu men felt that 'head over heels' romantic love was dangerous and undesirable. Such love occurred, but it inspired a sense of dread and guilt, for it was thought to compete with a man's loyalty to his mother and other kinspeople in the extended family. This dread, of course, mixes with and to some extent alters the feeling of love itself.[3]

So we do not assume that people in different eras and places feel 'the same old emotion' and just express it differently. Love in, say, a New England farming village of the 1790s is not the 'same old' love as in upper-class Beverly Hills, California in 1995 or among the working-class Catholic miners in Saarbrucken, Germany. Each culture has its unique emotional dictionary, which defines what is and isn't, and its emotional bible, which defines what one should and should not feel in a given context. As aspects of 'civilising' culture they determine the predisposition with which we greet an emotional experience. They shape the predispositions with which we *interact* with ourselves over time. Some feelings in the ongoing stream of emotional life we acknowledge, welcome, foster. Others we grudgingly acknowledge and still others the culture invites us to deny completely.

Finally, like any sociologist, the sociologist of emotion looks at the *social context* of a feeling. Is the bride's mother divorced? Is her estranged father at the wedding? And the groom's family? How unusual is it for friends not to attend weddings? How serious were the invitations? Mothers, fathers, siblings, step-parents and siblings, friends: what are the histories of their 'happiest days'? This context also lends meaning to the bride's feelings on her wedding day.

THE MODERN PARADOX OF LOVE

Given the current emotional culture (with its particular dictionary and bible) on the one hand, and the social context on the other, a society often presents its members with a paradox – an apparent contradiction that underneath is not a contradiction but a cross-pressure.

The present-day western paradox of love is this. As never before, the modern culture invites a couple to aspire to a richly communicative, intimate, playful, sexually fulfilling love. We are invited not to hedge our bets, not to settle for less, not to succumb to pragmatism, but, emotionally speaking, to 'aim high'.

At the same time, however, a context of high divorce silently warns us against trusting such a love too much.[4] Thus, the culture increasingly invites us to 'really let go' and trust our feelings. But it also cautions: 'You're not really safe if you do. Your loved one could leave. So don't trust your feelings'. Just as the advertisements saturating American television evoke '*la belle vie*' in a declining economy that denies such a life to many, so the new cultural permission for a rich, full, satisfying love-life has risen just as new uncertainties subvert it.

Let me elaborate. On one hand, the culture invites us to feel that love is more important than before. As the historian John Gillis argues, the sacredness once attached to the Church and expressed through a wider community has been narrowed to the family. The family has become fetishised, and love, as that which leads to families, elevated in importance. Economic reasons for a man and a woman to join their lives together have grown less important, and emotional reasons have grown more important.[5] In addition, modern love has also become more pluralistic.[6] What the Protestant Reformation did to the hegemony of the Catholic Church, the sexual and emotional revolution of the last thirty years has done to romantic love. The ideal of heterosexual romantic love is now a slightly smaller model of love within an expanding pantheon of valued loves, each with its supporting subculture. Gay and lesbian loves can, in some subcultures, enjoy full acceptance; single career women now have a rich cultural world in which a series of controlled affairs mixed with warm friendships with other women is defended as an exciting life. Some of this diversification of love expands the social categories of people 'eligible' to experience romantic love, whereas some of it provides alternatives. But on the whole, the ideal of romantic love has increased its powerful grip by extending and adapting itself to more populations.

Paradoxically, while people feel freer to love more fully as they wish, and to trust love as a basis of action, they also feel more afraid to do so because love often fades, dies, is replaced by a 'new love'. The American divorce rate has risen from about 20 per cent at the turn of the century and stands now at 50 per cent, the highest in the world. Norms that used to apply to American adolescent teenagers in the 1950s, 'going steady', breaking up, going steady again with another, now apply to the adult parents of children. The breakup rate for cohabiting couples is higher still. In addition, more women raise children on their own, and more women have no children.[7]

These combined trends present our young bride with a tease. She is inspired by the image of a greater love, but sobered by its 'incredible lightness of being'.[8] The promise of expressive openness is undercut by the fear of loss. For in order to dare to share our innermost fears, we need to feel safe that the individual we love, the person dearest to us, perhaps a symbol of 'mother' in the last instance, is not going to leave.

NEW DEMANDS FOR EMOTION MANAGEMENT

Faced with this paradox, the bride may resort to one of several strategies for managing emotion. An act of emotion management, as I use this term, is an effort by any means, conscious or not, to change one's feeling or emotion. We can try to induce feelings that we don't at first feel, or to suppress feelings that we do. We can – and continually do – try to shape and reshape our feelings to fit our inner cultural guidelines. These acts of emotion management sometimes succeed; often they are hopeless. But however hopeless they are, such acts provide a clue to who we are trying, inside, to be; an emotional 'strategy' as a larger plan guiding acts of emotion management.[9] What strategies might the young bride pursue? She might try to make love last by unconscious, 'magical' means. In one study of emotional responses to the 'divorce culture', the sociologist Karla Hackstaff discovered that some young lovers who grew up in divorced homes unconsciously warded off the 'evil eye' of divorce in their own love-life by creating a First-Love-That-Fails and a Second-Love-That-Works (Hackstaff 1991). Our bride could have met a perfectly nice boyfriend before she met her husband. But because she feels she is destined to suffer a divorce and is eager to avoid that, she projects on to a first lover 'everything bad'. She tries to fall out of love. She leaves. Then she meets a second young man, just like the first, on whom she projects 'everything good'. With him, she tries to stay in love. Through this unconscious magic, our bride makes her first marriage into a symbolic second one, and magically clears away the danger of divorce.

Alternatively, the bride might try to adapt to the disquieting uncertainties of love by protecting herself with emotional armour. She defends herself against 'dangerous' needs – her own and those of others. She becomes a 'cool modern' person who avoids problems by avoiding needs.[10] She tries to expect less. She tries to care less. She tries to feel that no one can hurt her. Ironically, in an era of sexual and emotional liberation, our bride 'trains' herself to be an emotional Spartan. Her emotional armour can be donned in a great many ways. In one recent study of single women, Kim De Costa found that women tried to limit their trust of men; to dampen their fantasies of rich, emotional bonds with men, and to expand their fantasies of great love for children.[11] With children, one could dare to 'fall in love', and could, perhaps, displace on to children the dependency needs one feels one cannot afford to feel with men. [. . .]

What forces are driving the modern paradox of love? The strongest force, I believe, is the runaway horse of capitalism. Capitalism is a culture as well as an economic system. As Anthony Giddens has argued in *Modernity and Self-Identity*, the economy, the state, the mass media have become vast, farflung empires, 'abstract systems' he calls them, which dwarf, undermine and 'disembed' local cultures.

Giddens (1991) is unclear about precisely how they do this. One mechanism is substitution. We watch television more and talk to each other less. We turn on the radio more, play musical instruments less. Listen to call-in television more, vote less. In these ways, an abstract system, the mass media, comes to 'substitute for' local customs and domestic folkways. But underneath such substitutions, a more pervasive and deep-seated mechanism may be at work: the adaptation of the metaphors of abstract institutions to the local, intimate, more 'traditional' sphere of private life.

Replacing the idea of love, devotion, sacrifice, in our collective unconscious, is the metaphor of emotional capital. This metaphor poses a new set of questions. Do people think of emotion as that which they invest or divest so that the self is ever more lightly connected to feeling? Does emotion itself take on the properties of 'capital'?[12] Can we speak of new emotional investment strategies so that people more easily invest and divest their emotional capital? Is this emotional capital now more 'mobile' across social territory than in previous eras? Can we speak of a deregulation of emotional life, so that it flows across new boundaries according to private notions of emotional profit? If so, how does this affect the emotion management of a young bride? Given that in one American study, half of the divorced fathers of children five years after divorce had not seen their child during the last year, we can also ask: How does it affect children?

I am not arguing that people automatically enter relationships 'more lightly' nowadays than they did thirty years ago, or that they think shallow connections are better than deep ones. I am suggesting, rather, that one strategy of emotion management may be to try to become capable of limiting emotional connection. That emotional strategy fits the uncertain, destabilised intimate life shaken by the flight plan of capitalism. For the uncertain, destabilised intimate life is a life of potential profit and loss. The task of emotion management is to rise to the opportunity, and prepare for the loss. But the stance of emotional entrepreneur is in no way a natural one. We need to feel attached to others, and we dread the loss of attachment in a very pre-modern way. In such late modern times, it requires an extreme degree of emotion work to feel 'normal'. For as we begin each relationship, we are forever practising the end 'just in case'. This is the emotional insurance policy, the emotional hardening required of the post-modern hunter and gatherer of love. Fleeting as they are, magnified moments of emotion management tell a great deal about the brief steps through which we embrace or resist a capitalist culture of intimate life. In the case of mild feelings, acts of self-control also actually help shape the emotion. We may try to alter the expression of our feeling and in doing so actually alter the inward feeling (surface acting). Alternatively, we can verbally prompt ourselves to feel one emotion and not another (one kind of deep acting). Or we can try to enter into a different way of seeing the world (this is the deep acting in which professional actors often engage, the so-called 'method acting'). Whatever the method of emotion management, the emotions managed are not independent of our management of them.

Emotions always involve the body; but they are not sealed biological events. Both the act of 'getting in touch with feeling' and the act of 'trying to feel' become part of the process that makes the feeling we get in touch with what it is. In managing feeling, we partly create it.

We can see the very act of managing emotion as part of what the emotion becomes. This idea gets lost if we assume, as do more organismic theorists such as Charles Darwin and Sigmund Freud, that how we manage or express feeling is extrinsic to the emotion itself. It gets lost if we see emotion as simply 'motored by instinct'. In fact, I believe that culture impinges at many points: at the point of recognising a feeling, at labelling a feeling, at appraising a feeling, at managing a feeling and expressing a feeling. Thus, an emotional strategy useful in defending oneself against the paradox of modern love, provides not simply an emotional armour, but, to some degree, the feelings that are armoured.[12]

Thus, through how it makes us see relations, define experience and manage feeling, the culture of capitalism insinuates its way into the very core of our being. Weaving together the tatters of a waning tradition, the bride seeks to enter a private emotional bubble, her happiest day. In this light, her wedding is both a holdover and an act of resistance. She wants this day to be the happiest day of her life, but the day is lodged in this wider context, and her wish forms part of a larger paradox of modern love. Ultimately, this may be the source of the bride's unease. This paradox itself is a product of a misfit between old feeling rules (a former emotional dictionary-cum-bible) and a newly emergent social context. But feeling rules change, and so do social contexts. History provides a moving series of paradoxes.

I therefore believe that the important questions for the sociologist of emotion to ask are these. What emotional paradox are we apparently trying to resolve in order to live the life we want to live? By what dialectical interaction between feeling rules and context is this emotional paradox produced? To the historian, we pass the question of what forces have produced shifts between one paradox and the next. In light of these paradoxes, what emotional strategies come to 'make sense'? What kind of emotion work does it demand? And we have not finished the job until we dare to ask the question that begs so many more: what social contexts produce the 'best' ways of feeling?

NOTES

1 Within American sociology, the sociology of emotions is one of over twenty subfields. It was established in the mid-1980s, and publishes a quarterly newsletter with notes about new articles and books in the field. The British Sociological Association has a 'study group', as does the International Sociological Association. Also in the mid-1980s, the International Association for Research on Emotion was established to bring together sociologists with psychologists and other social scientists interested in emotions. For exposure to a fuller range of perspectives and topics within the sociology of emotions, see Franks and McCarthy (1989) and Kemper (1989).

2 Hochschild (1983: 59). The wording is slightly modified for the sake of coherence.

3 Steve Derne, 'Hindu men's langues of social pressure and individualism: the diversity of South Asian ethnopsychology', *International Journal of Indian Studies* 2 (2) (1992): 40–71.

4 This paradox is parallel to but slightly different from that described by Beck and Beck-Gernsheim. In *The Normal Chaos of Love*, Ulrich Beck and Elisabeth Beck-Gernsheim note a contradiction between individual desires (e.g. for higher education and career) and love and family. I am drawing attention to the emotional dilemma created by cultural support for a strong desire for love (which evokes trust in feeling), and the modern chanciness of love (knowledge of which evokes a distrust of feeling).

5 Changes in intimate life are part of a long-term decline in the functions of the family as the economy, the state, and the professions and various services have taken over activities and purposes that the family used to fulfil. In addition, the social ecology around the family has become weakened too. Local communities, the Church, the world of volunteers that provided support and control for family life, all have declined. Meanwhile, national and global organisations that in new ways connect human beings together, through time and space, have increased in power and importance. The non-market sector has declined, the market sector risen. Some commentators, such as the English sociologist Anthony Giddens, see in these shifts bracing new opportunities, while others, such as the German sociologist Sigmund Bauman, see new dangers. See Anthony Giddens's *Modernity and Self-Identity* (1991; English edition, Cambridge: Cambridge University Press). Also see Zygmunt Bauman, *Legislators*

and Interpreters (1989). As Gillis notes: 'The Victorians were the first to make room for a spiritualised home, and create within their homes a series of special family times and places where an ideal family could experience itself free from the distractions of everyday life. Families have become fetishised'. See Gillis (1994).

6 I am indebted to Cas Wouters for this insight. Cultural norms have not, of course, remained untouched by history. Romantic love has a long social history. As the historian Denise de Rougemont notes, during the middle to end of the feudal period in Languedoc, France, unemployed knights who had lost their feudal lords came to worship unavailable noblewomen. Towards these women, the romantic lover had an unconsummated, sometimes unrequited love, in which he transferred to the unavailable woman of higher station a worshipful pose he might otherwise have expressed towards his missing employer. The objects of this archetypal romantic love, upper-class married women, were themselves locked into loveless matches which cemented economically useful alliances between families. Today, we seem to be in the midst of a move away from this model of love, as the paper argues.

From this moment in history, one can trace over time the transmutation of this ideal of love – its growing association with sexual expression, with marriage, with procreation and, indeed, with the institution of the bourgeois family. In the United States, this new cultural synthesis of romantic love, with marriage and procreation, came to fullest development in the 1950s when a full 95 per cent of the population married at some point in their lives.

7 The divorce rate has greatly affected the relations between fathers and children; one study found that half of American children, ages 11 to 16, living with their divorced mothers, had not seen their fathers during the entire previous year. An in-depth study of divorcing families in California found that half of the men and two-thirds of the women felt more content with the quality of their lives after divorce, though only one in ten children did. Half of the women and a third of the men were still intensely angry at their ex-spouses ten years after the divorce. Wallerstein and Blakeslee (1989). Arlie Hochschild, 'The fractured family', *American Prospect* (Summer 1991): 106–115.

8 I believe other sociologists miss this point. Niklas Luhmann in *Love as Passion* (1986) suggests that sexuality has become a 'communicative code', a language rather than an experience integrated with a full range of implied social ties and controls. Also see Alberoni (1983).

9 See Hochschild (1983) *The Managed Heart: The Commercialization of Human Feeling*.

10 See Hochschild (1994). Ann Swidler (1986) and Francesca Cancian (1987) argue that commitment plays a diminishing part in people's idea of love, while the idea of growth and communication plays a more important part. Data from national opinion polls also document a twenty-year decline in commitment to long-term love.

11 See Kim De Costa 'Rationalizing love with men, essentializing love of children' (MA paper in progress, University of California, Berkeley). The idea that people have become more guarded in the wake of greater freedoms runs counter to popular notions of the 1970s and 1980s as a period of the 'culture of narcissism', as the historian Christopher Lasch calls it.

12 Larrie Lauren, 'Emotional capital', unpublished paper; Laurie Schaffner,

'Deviance, emotion and rebellion: the sociology of runaway teenagers' (honors thesis, Sociology Department, Smith College, 1994). See Loic Wacquant's use of the term 'bodily capital' in 'The pugilistic point of view: how boxers think and feel about their trade' (*Theory and Society* 24 (1995): 489–535).

13 Hochschild (1983: 18).

REFERENCES

Alberoni, F. (1983) *Falling in Love*, New York: Random House.

Bauman, Z. (1989) *Legislators and Interpreters*, Cambridge, MA: Polity Press.

Beck, U. and Beck-Gernsheim, E. (1995) *The Normal Chaos of Love*, Oxford: Polity Press.

Cancian, F. (1987) *Love in America: Gender and Self-Development*, Cambridge, MA: Cambridge University Press.

Derne, S. (1995) *Culture in Action: Family Life, Emotion and Male Dominance in Banaras India*, New York: State University of New York Press.

Franks, D. and Doyle McCarthy, E. (eds) (1989) *The Sociology of Emotions: Original Essays and Research Papers*, New York: JAI Press.

Giddens, A. (1991) *Modernity and Self-Identity*, Stanford, CA: Stanford University Press.

Gillis, J. (1994) 'What's behind the debate on family values', plenary session, section on Sociology of the Family, American Sociological Association.

Hackstaff, K. (1991) 'Divorce culture: a breach of gender relations', unpublished PhD dissertation, Sociology Department, University of California, Berkeley.

Hochschild, A.R. (1983) *The Managed Heart: The Commercialization of Human Feeling*, Berkeley, CA: University of California Press.

Hochschild, A.R. (1994) 'The commercial spirit of intimate life and the abduction of feminism: signs from women's advice books', *Theory, Culture and Society*, 112 (2 May): 1–23.

Kemper, T. (ed.) (1989) *Recent Advances in the Sociology of Emotion*, New York: State University of New York Press.

Luhmann, N. (1986) *Love as Passion: the Codification of Intimacy*, Cambridge: Polity Press.

Swidler, A. (1986) 'Culture in action: symbols and strategies', *American Sociological Review* 51: 273–286.

Wallerstein, J. and Blakeslee, S. (1989) *Second Chances: Men, Women and Children a Decade After Divorce*, New York: Ticknor & Fields.

CHAPTER 27

DIVISIONS OF EMOTIONAL LABOUR: DISCLOSURE AND CANCER

Nicky James

... the nurses told me the night before not to get worried. Bill would be in intensive care and I'd see all these machines and everything, but not to worry that was normal. They warned Bill as well. Well when I went in in the afternoon ... he was sitting in a chair. And I thought that's odd. And I said to him, 'Have you had the operation?' 'Yes' he said. ... He said, 'Well I can tell you they found something, but didn't say anything'. ... Well me and my son went in [to see Sister] later on. And she said that she was very sorry to tell us there was nothing they could do for Bill. They had operated, they had put this thing in and he'd think he was getting better for a while. She said, 'I'm afraid we found a growth at an advanced stage'. She wasn't supposed to have told me ... Anyway it didn't sink in what she was saying. I'd been told by all the doctors, no, no, no [i.e. it's not cancer]. And my son was cringing because he knew that she wasn't supposed to tell me.

I think he'd gone and had a word with one of the doctors without me and Bill knowing. And this particular doctor had said to my son, Robert ... 'Don't tell your mother. The surgeon has to see her himself. And my son and I came out, and I didn't say anything to Bill naturally, and he was all right.

When Sister finished with me a doctor walked in. And one of the staff nurses said, 'Did you do Bill Jenkins' operation? This is his wife and son'. And the doctor said, 'I can't tell you much about it but

Source: Fineman, S. (ed.) (1993) *Emotions in Organisations*, London: Sage.

the surgeon will have a word with you, he'll explain better than me. But I don't want you to think things are worse than they are'. You see, they're still telling me now that everything is all right, but I knew what the Sister had already said ... but I didn't say anything.

So I went back up but my son followed the doctor ... and went into his room. And my son said, 'You're holding something back and I want to know what it is'. 'Well, you see, I'm not supposed tell you in front of your mother', the doctor said ... I just don't know why, I was his wife, I should have been told. Perhaps, they thought I wouldn't take it, I don't know ... We came out of the hospital and my son said 'Now look Mum, don't go thinking the worst, don't go thinking now there's cancer there'. He said, 'Dad's going to be all right'. I know he is saying this because of what the doctor had told him. 'Well, anyway', I said, 'whatever it is, the surgeon will tell us tomorrow'. We went in the following day. Fortunately Bill didn't see me. We went round to a little place to see the surgeon. He said he'd operated and fixed this tube in and that there was a huge growth by the side of it. And he said, 'I'm glad I've proved myself right, but I'm sorry that he's got cancer'. He said, 'I felt it all the time, but it wasn't showing up on the X-rays'. So of course when they operated they discovered it was more than there, it had risen right up, the cancer, gone right up. And never a pain but terrible discomfort ... I still couldn't believe it. My mind was blank. And yet, looking back, I had a feeling there was something...

(Mrs Jenkins, aged 67, widow. Report 1 – edited interview transcript)[1]

MANAGING EMOTION

Mrs Jenkins was one of 31 people I interviewed as part of a project on care of the terminally ill. The interviews, with unwaged carers, took place five to nine months after the death from cancer of the carer's close relative. The focus of this chapter is on one aspect of the project; that is the management of emotions during the disclosure of a diagnosis of cancer. Particular attention is paid to the divisions of emotional labour, where differences between lay and professional people are indicative of different roles, power and levels of personal involvement. I use interview data to identify *differential* divisions of emotional labour based on equal status work, and *deferential* divisions of emotional labour which are characterised by submissions to authority. I argue that these divisions shape the context of emotional labour in health (and other) organizations – but they are being challenged.

EMOTION LABOUR AND CANCER

The phrase 'emotional labour' is intended to highlight similarities as well as differences between emotional and physical labour, with both being hard, skilled, work requiring experience, affected by immediate conditions, external controls and subject to divisions of labour. Emotions can be regulated with varying sophistication and with various outcomes and, like other skills, emotional labour requires flexibility and adjustment. It involves anticipation, planning, pacing, timetabling and trouble-shooting. Emotions that are not acknowledged – whether our own or those of others – may be denied or suppressed, but full emotional labour involves working with feelings rather than denying them. At its most skilled emotional labour includes managing negative feelings in a way that results in a neutral or positive outcome.

Emotional labour is an integral yet often unrecognised part of employment that involves contact with people. It has been argued, and counter-argued, that emotional labour demands an individualised but trained response which exercises a degree of control over the emotional activities of the labourer, and thereby commodifies their feelings (Hochschild 1983; James 1989; Wouters 1989). Hearn and Parkin (1987) have noted that although male-dominated professions, such as medicine, may define the limits and action of emotion for other workers and clients, the problems of dealing with emotional control are primarily located through others. However, emotional labour also underpins domestic care work. The skills of emotional regulation are learned at home, predominantly from women, and transferred to workplace carework where they have to fit in with workplace priorities (Hochschild 1990; James 1992).

Cancer is a particularly apt disease to review in order to analyse the management, control and 'labour' of emotions in health organizations. In *Illness as Metaphor* Sontag showed how the word cancer is used as a figure of speech to suggest a 'profound disequilibrium between individual and society' (1979: 73). Phrases such as 'it is like a cancer spreading among us' convey a sense of slow but relentless invasion, of a battle to be fought and won before the disease annihilates us. Sontag also observes how the use of cancer as a malign adjective for social ills has ramifications for those who have cancer. *Illness as Metaphor* was written as a tool of liberation from the social overtones of the disease, for 'conventions of treating cancer as no mere disease but a demonic enemy make cancer not just a lethal disease but a shameful one' (Sontag 1979: 57).

Emotions are bound within a diagnosis of cancer in two ways. First, cancer was and still is explained as a disease resulting from certain emotions and experiences such as depression, lack of confidence, repression and past trauma. Second, there are the emotions evoked by a diagnosis of cancer – because of its physical implications and because of its social consequences. As Sontag notes:

> *Since getting cancer can be a scandal that jeopardises one's love life, one's chance of promotion, even one's job, patients who know what they have tend to be extremely prudish, if not outright secretive, about their disease.*
>
> (Sontag 1979: 8)

In a 1988 survey in Britain, carried out on behalf of the Cancer Relief Macmillan Fund, 40 per cent of respondents agreed with the statement that 'the fear of cancer is worse than the fear of death' (1988: 5). This sense of the intensity of emotions surrounding cancer is reflected in doctors' own attitudes to disclosure of cancer diagnosis. As an American doctor noted, of both the USA and Britain:

> *doctors believed, and many still do, that for patients to have to face a cancer diagnosis is terrible, and by giving them the diagnosis, you can do nothing other than be destructive ... the medical profession were representing the feeling of society in general about cancer, in keeping the secret from patients.*
>
> (Kfir and Slevin 1991: 5)

Yet cancer is hard to hide and, whether formally told or not, relatives, the person with cancer and professionals have to regulate their feelings. Even the diagnosis (or potential diagnosis) of cancer is surrounded by its own language – 'disclosure', 'communication' and 'insight' in health staff's terms; 'telling' and 'knowing' in lay terms. At a personal level cancer generates disbelief, fear, lies and chaos which are controlled through information, optimism, routine living and social expectation. One in three of us will get cancer at some time in our life and despite excellent survival rates for some cancers, one in four of us will, eventually die of it.

Those of us who are diagnosed as having cancer are likely to have sentiments ranging from informed pragmatism, fatalism and numbness, to total anguish and the feeling that an active death sentence has been imposed. Further, the social impact of a diagnosis of cancer is rapid with a powerful ripple effect, so it will always be people with cancer and their relatives and friends who have to manage the strongest emotions. They have to live with the disease and its consequences. Yet health staff have a role in shaping the division of emotional labour because they are involved in setting the context within which feelings are managed. Thus the symbolic nature of a diagnosis of cancer, and the physical and social consequences, mean that debates about 'disclosure' and 'telling' are not just a matter of passing on information, but are a surrogate means of talking about managing the emotions surrounding cancer. Whoever has knowledge of the cancer has some power to control, to fight and to protect.

Disclosure of cancer is governed by myriad formal and informal rules. In Britain those involved in this process meet through the network of the biggest formal organisation in Europe, the National Health Service, while also relying on a network of informal health care systems. Yet lay and professional groups are heterogeneous, and people with cancer, staff, relatives and friends work to regulate their own and others' emotions – and express them in forms which are personally, privately, publicly and professionally acceptable.

DIVISIONS OF EMOTIONAL LABOUR AND DISCLOSURE

The division of emotional labour is particularly important when considering the wide range of people brought together by the formal and informal health system through which cancer is managed: the person with cancer, their family, friends and neighbours, nurses, porters, domestics, doctors, radiotherapists, the taxi driver that takes someone to the 'cancer hospital'. These systems also divide through a series of hierarchies, roles, negotiations and conflicting personal and professional needs. The interviewees' reports in this chapter indicate ways in which the process of diagnosing and disclosing cancer cut across the divide of lay and professional while also showing the significance of those roles. Similarly, other dichotomies become mixed in the process of disclosure, those of organisation and individual, waged and unwaged, public and private, male and female, active and passive, with techno-scientific knowledge being challenged by 'personal' knowledge. The reports illustrate how people with cancer, the unwaged carers, the doctors and nurses are all active and reflective as the process of disclosure unfolds. All are more or less logical and skilled in the management of their own and others' emotions, though some manage by denying emotions rather than engaging them.

While rejecting the adequacy of any single dichotomy in explaining the division of emotional labour in disclosure, I suggest that the division of emotional labour can be understood by recognising *different levels of involvement with the feelings* associated with cancer, but explained as resulting from *competing forms of status and knowledge*.

Divisions of emotional labour will be affected, first, by the depth of the feelings generated. In this respect, lay and professionals are likely to be differentially involved. A second element is the public context within which feelings are expressed and regulated. When cancer is being diagnosed and disclosed, despite the depth of involvement of the person with cancer and their relatives and friends, the context for the management of emotion is often dominated by staff in health service organisations, resulting in deferential divisions of emotional labour.

A third key element in the division of emotional labour associated with the disclosure of a diagnosis of cancer is separation brought about by active, day-to-day involvement in the regulation and management of emotions. As report 1 illustrates, although the context was set by the consultant surgeon, it was the patient, relatives, nurses and junior doctor who were doing the ongoing work of managing emotions. Thus, while there has been a rhetoric of hierarchical, male dominated, information-giving disclosure which limits emotional expression, in practice information and feelings are mixed. In this system those who have been perceived as passive, deferential inheritors of 'given' roles (junior staff, patients, unwaged carers) play a key part in fulfilling or challenging the workplace, hierarchical norm. The result is that deferential divisions of emotional labour in the disclosure of cancer are currently subject to negotiation, change and 'de-differentiation'. Although the medical/organisational shaping of diagnosis and disclosure tends to dominate, permeable demarcations and expectations can be, and are, challenged.

In the following section additional interviewee reports and other research data are used to consider who or what is dominant during key aspects of disclosure, and also how the dominance is challenged.

DIVISIONS OF EMOTIONAL LABOUR: METHODS OF CONTROL

The blank numbness of Mrs Jenkins in the report at the beginning of this chapter, the quietness of Bill, the patient; the urgency of the son; the controlled sorrow of the Sister; the embarrassment of the junior doctor at being put on the spot; and the self-congratulation of the surgeon, all attest to the range of sentiments generated by the disclosure of information about cancer. Two further insights that Mrs Jenkins' report highlights are, first, the number and range of people caught up in controlling the emotions and information, and secondly the effects of unwritten rules, status and organisational role in shaping who said what to whom – and how their feelings were expressed. Cumulatively these insights indicate that disclosure of a diagnosis of cancer is a complex process and not a single event, and interventions can be made at various stages in the process.

In the report the interplay of patient/client, family members, doctors and nurses is significant because it illustrates that concentration on any one or two of these groups gives a partial perspective. Further, not only did each family member in report 1 have different ways of handling their painful knowledge, 'don't say anything' (Bill), 'I didn't say anything, naturally' (Mrs Jenkins), 'Mum, don't go thinking the worst' (Robert), but they also all had different roles to play in relation to each other and to the hospital staff. Bill was patient/husband/father, Mrs Jenkins was wife/mother/formal next of kin and Robert was son and a key information route into and out of the formal health system, so that there was potential for a variety of demands and expectations of each person.

Mrs Jenkins' report also indicates how inter- and intra-professional hierarchies of junior and senior doctors and nurses have developed to control the disclosure of life-affecting information, with some resulting demarcation tensions. All those involved were in some way influenced by the view that the senior doctor, the consultant surgeon, was in charge of the diagnosis of cancer. It appeared that until he formally acknowledged the diagnosis of cancer, the emotional labour was carried out in secret or semi-secret. Mrs Jenkins indicated that doctors blocked any contemplation that the diagnosis might be cancer. They had thereby preempted any discussion of associated emotions. Yet the ward Sister appears to have subverted the acknowledged system of consultant disclosure, and ran the risk of incurring the consultant's disapproval. The Sister saved the family a thirty-hour wait for information from the time of the initial post-operative visit until the time when the consultant surgeon was available to see them. In doing so she also gave the family an opportunity to assimilate the information and compose themselves before they saw the surgeon – a factor of which he was probably completely unaware. In this instance, concern that the diagnosis might be cancer was initially unspoken but nevertheless actively managed by health staff, while each family member kept their thoughts to themselves.

The second report is of a mother, Mrs Downie, and her daughter, Mrs Sketty. In addition to the issues mentioned above, this report is an observation of the role of the unwaged carer in recognising the significance of impending diagnosis of cancer and working to support her mother in the period leading up to and during the hospital consultation. It gave rise to the daughter asking a specific question about the consultant's communication skills – a key element in the control of emotions:

> *'Well, I've got an inverted nipple', Mum said. So I said, 'Well in that case we'd better see about it. How long have you had it?' 'Oh about three weeks', she said. And so I took her to the GP who immediately referred her to the hospital and they took her in, and she went to see the surgeon. Well my mum was most annoyed because for a woman of 78 she was very active and very alert. And she went to see the surgeon ... I wasn't allowed in ... My mum said, 'Oh come in with me', and the nurse said, 'Oh you're not allowed ... he likes to examine you on your own'.*
>
> *So ... Mum came out absolutely furious. And I said, 'What's the matter?' And she said – well she didn't actually come out – it was*

> *when we were coming home because I think I would probably have done something about it because, she said, 'I don't know whether he thought I was a complete imbecile', she said, 'but I was sitting on the couch with nothing on, he was sitting the other side of the room with his houseman and said "*That'll *have to come off."' And that was the first indication that my mother had that she ... I mean she knew in her heart of hearts, having gone to the GP who said, oh we're a bit worried about this...*
>
> *'Course when she said to the GP, oh I was ever so annoyed, he said, 'Oh well he's shy, and perhaps he can't ...' But he* should *be able to communicate with his patients, shouldn't he?*
>
> (Mrs Sketty, aged 55, daughter of Mrs Downie. Report 2 – edited interview transcript)

Both the report from Mrs Jenkins and that from Mrs Sketty illustrate the degree to which, as reporters, they were able to reflect on their own role in the process of disclosure. They show how they and their relative were drawn into the bureaucracy of the hospital system where personnel have specific roles to play; and how they were invited into, or excluded from, the private spaces of the hospital. The reports also indicate how invisible their contribution as unwaged carers was to the regulation of emotion, and how they were absorbed into conformity with the hospital organisation while remaining critical of it. For instance Mrs Sketty, herself a radiographer (but acting in the role of daughter and unwaged carer) concurred with the nurse's demand that she let her mother go in to see the consultant by herself because 'he likes to examine you on your own'.

The third report is something of a contrast with the first two, illustrating differential rather than deferential positions. Mr Evans was 79 years old and his account shows that he had less knowledge of cancer than the interviewees in reports 1 and 2. What was significant was his confidence in the control he was able to exert over a number of powerful professionals. He was nursing his wife at home after 57 years of marriage and he was in charge. He asserted his personal knowledge of his wife as a means of controlling the professionals. When his wife was taken into hospital (he had sent the ambulance crew away once) he appeared to relinquish this control without concern, but he left no doubt during the interview that at home, despite considerable unacknowledged help from a niece, he was in charge:

> *Last June she wasn't very well at all. So after a week I told her about going to the hospital. The doctor had been and advised her to have an X-ray. They found a shadow on her lung, so then she had to have the magic eye and took a little piece off her lung and sent it away for examination, and they found out she had a tumour right on the top of*

> *her lung here, which was working towards cancer, probably. She was getting weaker then, but still on her feet ... and going to her meetings most days. In the end she was too weak and had to stay home, and got really ill then.*
>
> *The doctor was calling every week, occasional mornings. I went out with him down the path and I asked him straight. I had a shock. I thought my wife had TB you know. And I asked, 'What is wrong with my wife?' And he said, 'Oh she's got cancer'. And I had a shock with that. Because up until May of that year she had been well, and that was in June...*
>
> *She didn't know what she had, I kept it from her. I wouldn't show her. She always thought she had fluid on the lung, something like that. When she was a young woman she looked after her sister-in-law and she had cancer. She looked after her for a few weeks before she died. And she told me, I hope I never get that.*
>
> *Imagine, I was with her for a month ... and I knew what she had. She didn't know. But she was getting a lot of drugs that was making her feel she couldn't care less. But the doctor told me and my niece, she might live two months. And I was sitting here, and it was exactly like sitting with someone in a condemned cell, waiting to be sent to be hanged. Because it was certain she was going to die.*
>
> *The doctor from Llanbeg came here and I had a good chat to him and I asked him, I asked the family doctor, I asked the head Sister, the nurse, I asked all of them would they please not say a word to my wife, as I had lived with her 57 years and I know her nature ... 'Well, why tell her?', I said. Everybody's of a different nature and some want to know. So the family doctor said, 'If she asks me, I'll tell her'. But she never asked. The last fortnight I think she guessed. I had that feeling. She never had the courage to ask, what have I got, what have I really got, what are they treating me for. She took it marvellous, mind.*
>
> (Mr Evans, aged 79 widower. Report 3 – edited interview transcript)

Mrs. Evans' experience of nursing someone with cancer many years previously had influenced both her own feelings and knowledge about cancer, as well as those of her husband. Unlike Mrs Sketty, Mr Evans was not able to extrapolate the nature of the disease and its progress from the treatment that his wife received. What he did do though was to force the doctor into identifying the doctor's own rule over 'telling'. If Mrs Evans asked, the doctor would tell her. The implication was that he was not prepared to lie or prevaricate if asked a direct question, which contrasts with Mrs Jenkins' experience of evasion illustrated in report 1.

The three reports come from very different types of people: a widow of 69, a daughter of 55 who was a radiographer with her own family, and a widower of 79. Yet the differences in the interviewees' personal perspectives on the process of disclosure help illustrate the divisions of emotional labour. First, the issue of depth of involvement. It is worth noting that the management of emotion takes place day-in, day-out, from the time a diagnosis of cancer is suspected, throughout the actual diagnosis and disclosure. This means that, although the feelings may be denied and the emotional labour unrecognised, both the person with cancer and their unwaged carers may well be involved in the management of emotion before health service staff become dominant participants in the process. Secondly, it is also notable that, in the hospital, doctors are formally dominant in a way that is not necessarily matched when the 'patient' is at home. Thirdly, the reports illustrate that doctors and nurses do not agree about how open to be in discussing cancer, either on an intra-professional basis, or on an inter-professional basis. Nevertheless, their management of emotion affected lay people's willingness to talk about cancer. [...]

Report 1 illustrated the hierarchical organisational rules surrounding disclosure, the precise roles of participants was a matter of each individual's own decision-making process. Report 1 showed that the Sister, the staff nurse and the junior doctor transgressed the unwritten rule of silence. But it is fascinating that, in conversation with the junior doctor, Mrs Jenkins deferentially conformed to his assumption that she did not know the outcome of the operation – thereby protecting the Sister. Further, the son in report 1 sought out information independently from his mother and also tried to assure her that 'Dad's going to be all right'. By pre-empting the surgeon's timing he asserted his right as the patient's son to know what was happening, but then attempted to reintroduce the rule of ignorance to protect his mother from the implications of the diagnosis. Thus it is that each of the participants in the process of disclosure creates their own role and breaks or conforms to the dominant position as they feel is appropriate.

In report 1 the incentives for the Sister to break silence may have been increased by current health service and nursing aspirations toward patient advocacy, delivering 'individual patient care', and considering the 'family as the unit of care'. Such influences run alongside pressures for greater professional accountability and identity (Salvage 1985). Studies by Seale (1991) in Britain and Stein *et al.* (1990) in the United States suggest that there may be some realignment of inter-professional responsibilities. Yet staff and family and patients still act protectively toward their own group and others: misleading, denying and lying where it is thought appropriate, or facilitating 'open-awareness' (Glaser and Strauss 1965) where that is thought preferable.

Like the other elements affecting disclosure, role is organisationally led, but can be subject to individual negotiation, particularly when there are social changes that facilitate this negotiation. Changes in roles that affect the way in which information about cancer is given will also affect the way in which the emotions associated with cancer are managed. Following Heller's speculation (1990) about the re-emergence of an emotional culture, it may be that the consensus will move away from the dominance of senior doctors in setting the context for disclosure. De-differentiation would mean that context setting would no longer be the sole prerogative of senior doctors. Broadening responsibility for it could result in a role realignment affecting the deferential division of emotional labour amongst professionals, and between lay and professional people. [. . .]

NOTE

1 All participants in the interview are given pseudonyms.

REFERENCES

Cancer Relief Macmillan Fund (1988) *Public Attitudes to and Knowledge of Cancer in the UK 1988*, London: Britten Street.

Glaser, B. and Strauss, A. (1965) *Awareness of Dying*, Chicago: Aldine.

Hearn, J. and Parkin, W. (1987) *'Sex' at 'Work': the Power and Paradox of Organisation Sexuality*, Brighton: Wheatsheaf.

Heller, A. (1990) *Can Modernity Survive?*, Cambridge: Polity.

Hochschild, A.R. (1983) *The Managed Heart*, Berkeley: University of California Press.

Hochschild, A.R. (1990) *The Second Shift*, London: Piaktus.

James, N. (1989) 'Emotional labour: skill and work in the social regulation of feeling', *Sociological Review* 37 (1): 15–42.

James, N. (1992) 'Care = organisation + physical labour + emotional labour', *Sociology of Health and Illness* 14 (4): 488–509.

Kfir, N. and Slevin, M. (1991) *Challenging Cancer: from Chaos to Control*, London: Routledge.

Salvage, J. (1985) *The Politics of Nursing*, London: Heinemann.

Seale, C. (1991) 'Communication and awareness about death: a study of a random sample of dying people', *Social Science and Medicine* 32 (8): 943–952.

Sontag, S. (1979) *Illness as Metaphor*, London: Allen Lane.

Stein, L., Watts, D. and Howell, T. (1990) 'The doctor-nurse game revisited', *New England Journal of Medicine* 322 (8): 546–549.

Wouters, C. (1989) 'The sociology of emotions and flight attendants: Hochschild's *Managed Heart*', *Theory, Culture and Society* 6 (1): 95–123.

CHAPTER 28

REDISCOVERING UNPOPULAR PATIENTS: THE CONCEPT OF SOCIAL JUDGEMENT

Martin Johnson and Christine Webb

INTRODUCTION

[...]
The initial purpose of the study was to discover how nurses face the moral problems and conflicts posed by the nature of work in a hospital ward. With this aim in mind I set out in this study to use participant observation to discover something of the moral climate in which nurses work on one medical ward in a Northern Teaching Hospital. [...]

BEING POPULAR: 'HE'S A LOVELY MAN'

I did my best to focus on situations where the nurses were faced with difficult moral choices. It soon became clear, however, that people in the ward were commonly discussed in terms that were other than purely functional or 'professional'. On my second day I made a note in my book as follows:

Some patients are distinctly popular and some unpopular. This does not easily fit them as stereotypes however. Neil (a 23-year-old with

Source: *Journal of Advanced Nursing* (1995) 21: 466–475.

complications of a sexually transmitted disease) has an arguably stigmatising illness, and (being rendered very immobile from arthritis) is very demanding in the sense of knowing what he wants. He seems very popular however.

Other entries in my field diary confirm these impressions. 'He's a good lad' and 'a nice patient' were two other opinions of Neil given to me within hours by different qualified nurses. [...]

Neil, a 23-year-old young man suffering Reiter's syndrome had much to endear him to nursing staff. He was polite, thanked the nurses after they had helped him, and was roughly the same age as the qualified nurses and many of the students. Some clearly felt pity for his situation, describing it as 'very sad'. Somehow it was easy to see Neil fitting the traditional criteria for likability, similarity of age and politeness being examples, despite the possibility of stigma arising from his previous genital infection. Popularity as a patient was not confined to Neil, however.

An 82-year-old man with congestive heart failure, who smoked heavily, smelt very strongly of tobacco and who refused point blank all requests for baths, was nevertheless commonly seen as 'charismatic'. He would entertain nursing staff with stories and photographs of his early life on an ocean liner and was clearly popular.

Many studies suggest that deviant or rule breaking behaviour results in staff perceiving patients as bad. Indeed, Kelly and May (1982) refer to 11 papers which suggest that patients who persistently fail to conform to the clinical regime 'will be regarded unfavourably'. This man smoked very heavily indeed. He smoked roll-ups virtually constantly and spent almost all of every day and night in the day room in which he and others were allowed to smoke. This behaviour was clearly contra-indicated in his condition and the fact that he regularly refused to take a bath or be bathed would, according to many studies, lead him to be negatively evaluated by staff (Kelly and May 1982).

Being seen as a good patient was not at all unique and sometimes good patient labels were applied in a very ambiguous way, one in which differing opinions were expressed at the same time. One example of this was Jimmy MacKindoe, a Glaswegian who had, despite spending most of his adult life in England, never lost his regional Scottish accent. Jimmy had had a stroke and being rather disabled was consequently quite dependent for some weeks. He later began to improve quite remarkably but it was discovered that he also had a malignant tumour of the lung which was inoperable. Jimmy did not know this latter diagnosis (which troubled many of us) and seemed to be trying very hard to develop enough mobility to be accepted in an old people's home. Somehow, the personal evaluations of Jimmy were ambiguous in a way which my conversation with third-year student nurse Olivia crystallised very well:

OLIVIA: . . . I find him quite . . . I'm jumping the gun here . . . I mean he's a great bloke, he is attention-seeking, again who isn't? Losing half your body is a horrible thing to happen to you, and I think he's played a blinder to be quite honest. You should have seen him five weeks ago . . . everybody seems to have quite a negative attitude to him because, I don't know why, usually if someone was like that and they were getting over a stroke, and they [staff] found out the patient had cancer, they'd be absolutely mortified. If it was anyone else they'd be really upset. But I don't know what it is about him that nobody gives a monkey's really.

Olivia seemed to convey the definite ambivalence and, to some extent, the guilt the nurses felt about labelling Jimmy in the way they did. They seemed to be identifying the reasons why they should like him, and then trying to explain the fact that they did not. This complexity is hard to understand in terms of straightforward criteria of likability and unpopularity and is extended by the notion of covert liking which seemed to exist.

COVERT LIKING

Some nurses felt disposed to stress to me both in my informal discussions with them and in the interviews that they somehow liked patients when no one else seemed to:

HELEN: I do find it very strange because we have a very casual report, so these things do come across, and while I don't want the report to be formal, there is too much favouritism. A gentleman on this ward a few weeks ago, everybody hated him, personally I found him very appealing because he reminded me of my father, and that did upset me to hear them talking about him like they did.

This conception of liking was common, but had an 'off the record' quality. By this I mean that it was implied that I could use the idea, but that I must protect anonymity scrupulously in doing so. Among others, a second-year student, Theresa summed up the risks attached to liking people whom others did not:

THERESA: . . . I feel sorry for the people who feel unpopular and no-one likes them and we [nurses] often feel reluctant to come out in the open and say 'I like this or that person'. I just keep my head down really.

This idea, of keeping one's head down, seems to be a common feature of the student nurses' experience despite the apparent 'friendliness' and approachability of the staff. Even staff nurses sometimes felt that they could not challenge the dominant conception of a patient's social worth as expressed, say, in the ward report. Instead they liked people secretly.

I have alluded to some properties of liking such as ambiguity, and covert liking. Indeed, such complexity defies any simplistic notion of 'popularity'. A further dimension of liking was its changeability over time and under differing conditions. Discussing the factors which promoted likability, third-year student Louise pointed this out to me, noting also the need to keep dissident views to oneself:

LOUISE: ... And then I've noticed that the attitude has changed on occasion, not because the patient's behaviour has changed, but because their condition may have worsened, the attitude toward them may change.

MI: Suddenly people feel kindlier toward them ...?

LOUISE: Yeah! I think it's a shame because, like I say, I don't feel on this ward now, that I ... I've spoke up on occasions and don't feel it's been accepted, and it's been very hard to sit there and stand up for what you think has been said that shouldn't have been said. You know you might be put down.

BEING UNPOPULAR

My early fieldwork was confirming that evaluative labels were an important way of managing interpersonal relations. Both my fieldnotes and the interviews were conveying the distinct impression that, although some labels were positive, those about which my informants felt most strongly were of a different sort. Nurses at all levels of experience knew precisely what I meant when I asked about popularity and unpopularity. Their responses at interview were immediate and as if I had, in each case, touched a nerve.

They wanted to tell me about their experiences:

MJ: You seem to be saying that some patients, Jimmy [MacKindoe] in particular, are less popular than others.

OLIVIA: Yeah, I mean he does ask for things if you pass him but he goes out of his way now to say 'If you don't mind, I won't take long' and all this. It's shocking really... how just one person can colour everybody's opinion. It's happened a lot in the case of Jimmy. He's not a bad bloke, and he does really try, unlike a lot of people. He doesn't need a kick up the arse at all.

MJ: So you think that the kind of informal labelling that goes on is quite powerful really?

OLIVIA: Yeah, I think I do it as much as everybody else really.

Olivia brought the issue into the discussion unprompted, and was clearly concerned about its potential effects. Yet she had a lively appreciation of her own role in labelling and was commenting upon the lack of a simple explanation for it. Interviewing my next respondent, it came up quite early in our discussion:

BILL: I've never seen it affect the nursing care as such, maybe on a personal cleanliness level it hasn't, but on a psychological level it does because they [nurses] don't spend as much time with the patient or find time to chat. They just want to get the job over and done with in a way, and then move on...

The data began to yield a large number of examples of labels with which nursing staff communicated their negative social evaluations of the people in their care.

BEING DEMANDING: 'OH, HE'S A RIGHT ONE'!

I began to explore the nature, or the properties of these 'negative' labels, so that I could formulate some notion of their place in managing care on the ward.

BILL: ...I mean, I was surprised myself really coming to the wards, you know, hearing people literally slagged off, and it seemed really strange to me at first, but you get used to it.

Bill's experience was fairly typical. He had anticipated that there would be fewer personal evaluations used in discussing patients, but had begun to accept this norm. I could not help noticing, however, in working with the students, that Bill, a first-ward student, was widely perceived as able to disregard the general opinion of patients and give them as much attention as he felt appropriate. Indeed one of my third-year informants was keen to point this out:

OLIVIA: You know, people in the office [qualified nurses] were saying 'Jimmy Mackindoe's getting far too demanding' and Bill didn't discriminate, he had time for him. And I thought 'that's good, you haven't coloured his opinion'.

Olivia, with three years' experience of differing ward cultures, was aware of the process of negative labelling and its potential to affect the quality and intensity of care. Being 'far too demanding' seems at first like a condition under which a negative attitude might arise. Being demanding did, however, convey a meaning beyond this. Demanding can mean being challenging but not necessarily unpleasant, as in a difficult game or sport. It can also mean asking for that which is due, but in a fairly aggressive manner.

My observations gave me the impression that being demanding was a descriptive label not necessarily related to the holder's propensity to ask for things. It was subtly different. Being demanding was a term used to convey dislike, although it often did apply to those who knew what they wanted and made a point of telling us. It conveyed not merely the fact that an individual was likely to make their expectations of the nurse very clear, it meant that they would do more than this. They were likely to 'overdo it'. An example from my field notes illustrates this:

> *Charles Eastwood is fairly unpopular! He's 60(ish), has severe pneumonia and chronic airways disease. He's very 'demanding' (word used in ward report) and the nurses are easily irritated by him. He leaves sputum-ridden tissues lying all over (which stick to you when you attempt to turn him) and has no humility at all in telling nurses where and how to wipe his bottom (he leaks constantly due to chronic constipation). He is clearly very ill and I'm doing my best to keep an open mind with him…*

This fieldnote reveals my assumptions about how people should ask to have their bottoms wiped! I imply in my hastily written fieldnote that he should have been more humble. On reflection I cannot justify this assumption. Indeed this sort of incident sensitised me to the interplay between my own need to evaluate and label people and their behaviour, and my discovery of this tendency in others.

However, my feelings about it were not unusual, and so the sense in which Charles was 'overdoing it', at least as far as nurses were concerned, is evident. It is interesting that this quite special use of the word 'demanding' stands up to international comparison rather well. Wolf (1988) undertook an ethnography of a medical ward in a large urban hospital in the United States of America using participant observation. She describes nurses routinely complaining about their patients in change of shift reports as follows:

> *Most of these patients were labelled 'demanding'. Jenny Fister, an elderly patient with advanced heart disease, was dying slowly. Known as a demanding or complaining patient, she engendered anger and frustration in the nurses who cared for her. Mrs Fister had been a*

patient on 7H for over a month; her outlook was grim and her nursing care a challenge. She never claimed to feel better. Her nurses felt encouraged that what they did for Mrs. Fister made a difference. Although they cared for Mrs. Fister daily, she never acknowledged their care.

This use of the word 'demanding' reflects very accurately that emerging from my fieldwork. It is a pejorative rather than merely a functional label.

Bill, the first-ward nurse, indicated the way in which some labels are almost permanent and can be based upon previous opinions of an individual:

BILL: ...Some of the patients have been in time and time again, so when you first come they say 'Oh, he's a right one him' and when you see for yourself you think 'he's not that bad really', but you've still got this preconceived idea of what he's like. You can't make your own judgement sometimes.

This suggests that labels are sometimes carried for long periods and can be reintroduced when patients are readmitted. Some labels used a terminology much less genteel than 'he's a right one' or 'he's demanding', but this depended very much upon the nurse using it. Conventional wisdom has it that in their 'professional context' nurses use relatively polite language. I had found personally that in the majority of settings this was the case. Only once in my career, working in an intensive care unit, had I been surprised by colleagues of both sexes using 'strong' or 'barrack room' language to describe their patients. This sort of language was not very common, and certainly was uttered with the aim of being out of earshot of patients in particular and also those nurses perceived to be of more delicate constitution.

One of the staff nurses used this type of language, referring to one patient as 'an old bastard'. The use of such terms carried a high degree of risk both for the user and, it seems to me, for those about whom it was used. It could be seen to break norms of 'professional conduct'. Out of context, for example as evidence in a disciplinary hearing, such language about patients would be hard to justify. The risk to patients that the attitude of other nurses would harden toward them was always present. However, although such labels were sometimes used, in context and with knowledge of the behaviour and commitment of the nurse using them, it was hard to discover any greater degree of malevolence in these labels than others such as 'he's a right one' or 'demanding'.

The discussion of 'unpopular' labels so far has focused upon some types of relatively permanent labels. Others had a more transient nature, seeming to be used to deal with specific events or moods the patient might be perceived to be in. 'He's really grumpy today' was an example of a label used about an elderly patient with an untreatable malignant tumour whom many nurses liked, because he was stoical and needed relatively little attention. On the day in question, however, he had been talked into a colonoscopy and gastroscopy to investigate loss of blood. He was undertaking strong laxative treatment to 'clear his passages' and, being already ill, was not in the best of moods.

This patient, Jack Redford, recovered from these investigations. Later, however, he wanted to go home, seeing little point in further investigations, and made his view known very clearly. This led to him being categorised as 'in a real strop today'.

'IT'S GETTING WORSE'

Labels can change. Catherine was a staff nurse with a quiet and thoughtful temperament. She seemed patient and unlikely to respond inappropriately to provocation. Furthermore, she had considerable ability to articulate her insight into the moral dilemma of labelling. During my fieldwork we had conversations about a number of issues and she seemed very ready to be more formally interviewed with the tape recorder:

MJ: Do you think some of the patients are unpopular?

CATHERINE: Definitely ... It's on the verge of becoming a problem actually, because he [Albert Littlewood] has been in hospital for now, over a week, and it's getting a lot worse and he's getting a lot worse. I don't know if he's feeling a lot of antagonism. I mean I know I've got a lot of antagonism and find him hard to deal with, and I think I'm fairly tolerant. I don't get riled that easily.

Catherine seemed to be saying that a person's popularity can change over time, so I asked her to clarify this for me:

CATHERINE: I think it's easier to be reasonably popular and become unpopular, than to be unpopular and become popular. I think at first Albert Littlewood wasn't unpopular at all.

MJ: No?

CATHERINE: And it's just got worse, and it's getting into quite a bad situation. I can't remember when it was like this. It makes you think, 'well if I'm a professional I'm not reacting in a professional way because I'm letting my feelings affect my behaviour'.

Catherine felt the dilemma acutely, even more because she saw herself as a role model for students and felt that she was letting down both patients and students in betraying her feelings about this patient. She seemed to use the notion of professionalism to mean being in control, not letting her personal feelings affect the care she gave. The consequences of labelling can be deeply felt.

Judgemental social evaluations of inpatients, then, were common. Some were temporary and in some cases labels became relatively permanent. Some labels were subject to change over time.

'YOU'RE ONLY HUMAN'

I will now focus upon the role and influence of nurses in the social construction of patient identity. My staff nurse informant, Neil, was always very keen to keep me in touch with the issues as he perceived them and was very open about some of his feelings. I was impressed by his honesty in admitting quite easily that liking everyone was unrealistic and that we all bring with us prejudices and irritations that are hard to ignore:

NEIL: I think patients can be unpopular for a number of reasons and not just being 'moaners'. I think that, for whatever reason, you just don't like the patient, and then from your point of view that patient is not number one in the popularity stakes.

Third-year student Olivia, also something of a key informant, agreed that whilst it was unrealistic to be able to get on with everyone, it was even less so to keep these opinions private:

OLIVIA: I don't think you can help it because you're only human. If someone's getting on your nerves there's no point in not admitting it, that's even falser.

These nurses clearly espoused a sort of realism, an appreciation that it was inevitable that people will have likes and dislikes and that at least among peers it would be alright to mention them. Other nurses were worried by it, however. Elaine, who felt that it might be necessary to discuss opinions of patients with other qualified nurses, was clearly concerned that as a role model for student nurses she should avoid judging or pre-judging patients in this way:

ELAINE: It's personal really, you can have personal differences, and that can make an unpopular patient. If they've got a personality that you don't 'gel' to. But I don't think you should voice them. Other than like qualified members of staff, I don't think students should ever be there when someone ... but it's difficult when someone gets on your nerves very much.

Clearly Elaine's ideal would be to avoid labelling patients negatively or perhaps positively when students are around. Catherine, among others, echoed similar views, and guilt that on one notable occasion and in the presence of students she had been particularly disparaging about Albert Littlewood (a patient who later died of heart failure). She too seemed to see no alternative to 'segmenting' her behaviour, whenever she had the emotional resources, so that students would not be exposed to what she felt was a negative role model. Melia (1987) utilises the concept of segmentation to explain the different ways in which student nurses behave in order to 'fit in' with two very different areas of their work, the college and the ward.

It seems that some of the qualified nurses also have this sort of conception of the ideal or 'professional' way of working, and the real or ward way. For some of the qualified nurses this segmentation is between two general ways of communicating. One, which is realistic and 'only human', is that in which they betray their perceptions of patients as good and bad. The alternative, of communicating only 'objectively', they see as morally and, therefore, educationally, superior since they are employed at least partly as role models for student nurses. That they cannot achieve this ideal seems to lead to guilt or 'moral dissonance'.

Staff nurses, then, were conscious of their responsibility, in lieu of their formal status, to behave 'professionally', that is in accordance with the ideal. Students were also aware of the power of some individuals to initiate and then promulgate a particular view of someone. Third-year student Anita suggested that certain members of staff had special powers to define the ward view of patients and sometimes other people such as nurses and doctors:

MJ: What do you think it is that gets people labelled as unpopular?

ANITA: It tends to come from a dominant personality among the staff. Expressing a sort of dislike of somebody, and then that tends to get picked up by others, personally I tend to like the ones people don't like.

Anita certainly felt that one or more 'dominant' figures on the staff had special authority to cause labels to stick. She, along with many others, also felt that whilst she might privately disagree, she would normally be unable to challenge this dominant orientation. I had my hunches about which of the nurses had this power, but Anita was reluctant to confirm them herself, and I was reluctant to ask. Anita felt that individuals with dominant personalities and perhaps formal status, could set the values of the group and, further, that dissidence was very difficult to sustain in the role and position of student.

DISCUSSION

Social judgement (or moral evaluation) has been widely discussed in a large number of works (Roth 1972, Kelly and May 1982, English and Morse 1988). However, during my work as a participant observer in this medical ward, the concept assumed an importance I could not ignore. As the data make clear, the expression of evaluations of social worth was widespread on the ward, whether in terms of 'good and bad patients' (Kelly and May 1982) or 'popular and unpopular' ones (Stockwell 1972).

Our argument is that social evaluations are not, in any clear way, tied to traits or variables which patients do or do not possess. Rather, evaluations of people in the ward were socially constructed in relation to a complex web of powerful social influences. Key threads in the web are power, status, the management of uncertainty and negotiation, through which evaluative labels become flexible and changeable, depending upon the social context.

This argument, which is developed more fully elsewhere (Johnson 1993), is effectively a refutation of the dominant view in previous nursing literature, which is that personal biographical variables such as diagnosis or social class are in some way predictors of particular forms of evaluation of social value or worth. [...]

POWER

A more radical explanation of the place of social judgement in the nurse's repertoire for managing social relations in the ward would derive from the perspective of Michel Foucault (1991). He argued that the power of health professionals is expressed through the 'clinical gaze'. By this he means the power to define reality in the professionals' own terms and to examine, diagnose, observe and even restrain all those within our sphere of influence.

At one time this restraint and social control were exercised through severe physical measures such as torture and incarceration in locked institutions. Now the process of control is more subtle. It involves the use of constant observation and humiliation, such as the lack of privacy in toilet activities that Littlewood (1991) documents. These and other measures enable nurses and other professionals to define the social reputation of clients so that they remain vulnerable and compliant to the achievement of nursing and medical goals.

Such a viewpoint, if tenable, shows immediately why we continue to express value judgements in the management of patient care even when we are 'self-aware'. This does not mean necessarily that we are bad people. It simply means that we have been socialised to use these tactics and to play this role in the interests of powerful and dominant groups in society, not least the medical profession. [...]

REFERENCES

English, J. and Morse, J.M. (1988) 'The "difficult" elderly patient: adjustment or maladjustment?' *International Journal of Nursing Studies* 25 (1): 23–39.

Foucault, M. (1991, first published 1975) *Discipline and Punish*, Harmondsworth, Middlesex: Penguin.

Johnson, M. (1993) 'Unpopular patients reconsidered: an interpretive ethnography of the process of social judgement in a hospital ward', Unpublished PhD thesis, Manchester: University of Manchester.

Kelly, M.P. and May, D. (1982) 'Good and bad patients: a review of the literature and a theoretical critique', *Journal of Advanced Nursing* 7: 147–156.

Littlewood, J. (1991) 'Care and ambiguity: towards a concept of nursing', in Holden, P. and Littlewood, J. (eds) *Anthropology and Nursing* London: Routledge, 170–189.

Melia, K.M. (1987) *Learning and Working: The Occupational Socialisation of Student Nurses*, London: Tavistock.

Roth, J.A. (1972) 'Some contingencies of the moral evaluation and control of clientele', *American Journal of Sociology* 77: 839–856.

Stockwell, F. (1972, reprinted 1984) *The Unpopular Patient*, Beckenham, Kent: Croom Helm.

Wolf, Z.R. (1988) *Nurse's Work: The Sacred and the Profane*, Pennsylvania: University Press.

CHAPTER 29

STEVEN

Valerie Sinason

[...] Steven was the second of three children. At the time of his birth, his parents' marriage was already in difficulties owing to the strain caused by the deteriorating physical condition of the oldest daughter, Mary, who was born with a physical handicap. (She has since died.) Depression over the serious illness of the daughter meant that there was little time for Steven and he adapted to this, being seen as a 'perfect quiet' baby. Only a routine clinic visit picked up his cerebral palsy.

When Steven was two, Carole, a healthy daughter, was born. Although there was relief she was normal, the pregnancy had not been consciously planned and the new arrival added to marital strain. Father's unemployment was an extra difficulty. Placed in a daycare nursery so his mother could manage the new baby and the older sibling, Steven displayed aggressive behaviour. By the time his father left home, when he was three, Steven's attacks on himself were so dangerous he was admitted to hospital.

Father had behaved violently to mother prior to their breakup and there was some worry that Steven might have been hurt as well as having witnessed violence. Each time Steven left hospital his attacks on himself recurred. Behaviour therapy helped temporarily but in the end only changed the part of his body he attacked. At six he was admitted to a residential home for severely multiply handicapped children but his violence continued and was so great both to himself through headbanging and to staff through biting that there was fear of what would happen when he was older and stronger. [...]

Steven was finally referred to me when he was ten. [...]

Source: *Mental Handicap and the Human Condition: New Approaches from the Tavistock.* (1992) London: Free Association Books.

FIRST MEETING

In the waiting room, a slumped, twisted, ferocious-looking boy was jammed between his mother and a key worker. I could not see his face. When I introduced myself his legs went into an amazing forceful action as if they had a life of their own. Realising I would not be safe on my own with him I asked his mother and worker to bring him to my room and to stay with us. I tried to sound casual, as if that had been my plan all along, but I felt most fearful. I was not only frightened by the violence of this child whose face I had yet to see, my fear had also eroded my professional confidence. I also felt apologetic to the home staff. When the referral letter had mentioned that his violence meant two staff were needed to be with him at all times I had responded disbelievingly. Now I understood.

Steven grunted and screamed all the way to the room but once inside he moved into a foetal position and then said clearly and distinctly the word 'shy'. His voice was low and guttural and there was a slur from his brain damage but there was no mistaking the word. The social worker looked sad and I felt immensely moved. His mother said he had never said the word 'shy' before, she did not even know he knew it. Steven started ferociously banging his head. The sound really hurt but I restrained his mother from moving to hold his hands.

I started talking, saying how he had said he was 'shy' and that wasn't surprising as I was a stranger to him. He didn't know me. His fist stopped in mid-air. I carried on speaking, saying he was telling all of us that he knew his mum and key worker and all the people at the children's home. He was used to seeing lots of people. But he didn't know me. His hand flopped onto his lap and I was then at peace, knowing that meaning was there and I was at work.

I then explained why he was coming, how people were worrying about him hurting his head and how they felt he was sad. I explained he would come to this room a few times and that there were toys on the table. The moment I mentioned toys he ferociously banged his head. When I said he was worried at being in this new room with toys he stopped banging. Other features of this first session were that he banged his head whenever there was a sound from outside the room. Alternatively, he would curl up and close his eyes like a baby. When I said there were five minutes left he moved the vestigial fingers of his deformed hand and hid them under his head. I wondered aloud whether he was showing me his struggling handicapped hand now it was time to go and maybe there was a struggle with the Steven who had powerful legs and could run and a handicapped Steven. When it was time to stop he kicked the table at me with great force.

SECOND MEETING

At the second meeting, again with his mother and worker present, he screamed and banged all the way to the room but was quiet on sitting down. He did not utter a word, but fell asleep, only to stir to bang his head whenever the wind blew or there were footsteps. At one time when there was a loud noise he fell into a newborn falling reflex. This is the involuntary survival response a tiny baby instinctively demonstrates when startled. I wondered here whether the tiredness was because of all the energy that went into maintaining an unborn state where no other life existed.

THIRD AND FOURTH SESSIONS

It took me until the third session to tell Steven I did not feel ready to see him on my own until I felt I could protect him and me from his violence. I thought we must be connecting more for him to allow me to have that thought and utter it and for him not to bang his head when I said it. Fifteen minutes before the end of the session he fell asleep. I was taken by surprise by my own difficulty in saying aloud that I did not feel safe. I learned a lot from this experience. When I have seen any violent patient since I have always commented on why we are not going to meet on our own. As professionals who pride ourselves on understanding the meaning of violence we can rather stupidly at times consider that means we do not need to fear it. At a meeting in Leeds, with Yorkshire psychologists in mental handicap who work psychodynamically, to look specifically at issues involved in treating violent patients with handicaps, Dr Nigel Beaill, Mrs Pat Frankish and I all agreed that fear in the therapist was a major anti-therapeutic factor and could in fact drive a patient even madder with fear.

During the fourth session a major change happened. For the first time, with his head twisted away from me, Steven held up both his hands to show me not just the difference between his handicapped and non-handicapped hand, but also the secondary handicap he had inflicted by his own banging. He held up that hand in a way that only I could see it. There was a huge swelling on each knuckle with a red bruise at the tip of each. I was aware of the thought that he had made two breasts, that maybe he was attacking his mother in fury at the handicapped body he had been endowed with, but also adding to his body at the same time. I did not feel I could make such a comment in front of his mother and worker. As that was the first private thought I'd had I felt the time must therefore be right for me to see him on his own. What I said was that he was showing me how angry he was about being handicapped and that when he banged his head he also made his knuckles larger. I then said, feeling terrified and daring, that I would see him on his own the next week but his mother and worker would bring and collect him. As usual he fell asleep fifteen minutes before the end of the session.

FIFTH SESSION: ON HIS OWN

The fifth session was the first on his own. It was crucial as it would determine whether therapy was possible. After the usual banging and kicking he was put on the chair by his mother and worker, who then left quickly, looking relieved and apprehensive at the same time. Steven was in his usual foetal position. It was only in this session that I became aware that he always curled up with the normal side of his face showing and his handicapped side hidden. I looked sadly at the dark brown curls of his hair on the 'normal' side of his face. Gritting my teeth, I wondered this aloud. For a moment I sat in terror. To my amazement he suddenly sat up bolt upright and faced me. He looked proud and furious. I felt overwhelmed. A ten-year-old boy with brown curly hair and dark brown eyes gazed intently at me. The effect of the brain damage was, of course, noticeable, but nowhere as noticeable or grotesque as his twisted posture had somehow indicated.

The feelings he evoked in me at that moment made me realise that the twisted postures he took up were a terrible self-made caricature of his original handicap, so he could not be seen as he truly was. I was filled with images from subnormality hospitals and all the twisted movements and guttural speaking which I had previously taken as inevitable consequences of retardation. I found myself wondering about that. I said he was now able to show me how he really was and that he was less handicapped than he made himself look, perhaps as protection. Steven fell asleep at his usual time fifteen minutes before the end of the session and this time I was able to comment to him that he knew the time was coming to an end and he wanted to be asleep.

He would spit quietly and wake up when I spoke. I was also struck again by the unborn state he seemed to remain in where living tired him so enormously. The home staff said he spent long hours sleeping as well as catnapping. Right at the end I asked him if he wanted to continue seeing me. There was no reply. I asked him to raise a finger if he wanted to carry on seeing me. He raised a finger and he continued coming for six years with only two absences for colds, both on the last session before a holiday.

THE NEXT THREE MONTHS

Once long-term therapy for Steven was agreed on I arranged a meeting with the head of his residential home, his key worker and his mother. In this meeting his mother was able to make clear that although she was willing to travel with Steven for his therapy she would in no way manage his living at home with her. In addition to the work she had looking after her two daughters, one of whom required constant attention when she was at home, she was, not surprisingly, frightened of Steven and his violence. 'If he was the only child I had I still couldn't manage him'.

There was a big change in Steven over the next few weeks. In the waiting room he could be seen sitting upright or standing hugging his mother. Several therapists told me their patients were mentioning this boy in the waiting room who used to look terrible but was really nice looking. The home commented he was calm for the rest of the day after coming to see me and for the next day. We agreed that the next important stage would be for me to take him to and from the therapy room. After two months I did this, feeling extremely frightened the first time. However, he managed then and ever after apart from a regression following the death of his sister. The triumph Steven and I felt at our both managing the fear of his violence was visible in the proud way he hugged his mother and worker on his arrival back after going it alone with me. His mother even said, 'Well done, you brave boy'.

The changes that came in the next three months (after which we decided to continue therapy indefinitely) were at one level slow and yet they were immensely exciting and moving. My own affective responses were a mixture of hope and terror. The changes chart gradual movements towards closeness. Here are some examples:

Session 10: He says 'hello' and I can understand despite his speech defect.

Session 11: He asks, 'Time yet'? just before the end of the session. He already has an accurate internal clock. Also, he looks briefly at the toys. (He has not touched them yet.)

Session 12: He says his longest sentence as we walk back to the waiting room together. 'Hello, did you see my mum'?

Session 13: He looks at the toys all the time.

Session 14: His nose runs and he looks desperately at the box of tissues on the table. He cannot bear to reach for it. I offer him one. He says 'No, thank you' slowly.

Session 15: He kicks the toy bag over in order to see the toys. I comment that the table is too far away for him to be able to reach it without walking. I had moved it after our first session as a protection against his violence but now felt ready to manage.

Session 16: I move the table nearer him. He kicks the toy bag accurately so the toys fall over right near him and he can see them carefully without touching them.

GIVING UP SELF-INJURY

The next major change was after one year of once-weekly therapy. I was suddenly aware that when Steven banged his head he was making enormous spitting noises and sound effects but in fact he was miming banging his head. When I said he was not hurting his thoughts so much and he was thinking more about what I said, he lifted his hand to show me the bumps had subsided. I told the home staff about my observation and they then realised it was true in their environment too.

It is important to mention that I had been in a fortunate position with regard to Steven's self-injury. For 50 minutes it was tolerable for me to not restrain his self-attacks unless I felt he could knock himself out. My aim had been to understand the meaning of the different bangs. However, for the residential staff who were with him all day it was another matter. Had he been allowed to continue unhampered there was no doubt that he would have died. I therefore suggest to staff who want to think dynamically about self-injury that they find a five- or ten-minute regular observation point in the week in which they can observe without needing to restrain movement, to make room for thought when otherwise they have to take action.

In the absence of painful circumstances, such as staff leaving for shift changes, Steven's headbanging stopped except for one occasion. I was surprised to see him one week with the old familiar red swelling on his forehead. He looked embarrassed and covered it up. I could not understand the meaning of it. His key worker later embarrassedly explained to me that a staff member had kicked the television when it was not working. Steven had apparently watched this very quietly. The kick knocked the television into correct action and Steven started knocking at the interference in his own brain. I felt like laughing and crying.

I was unable to write up the session until I had written [...] a poem [which] linked together some of the emotions I was experiencing, allowing me then to recall the session.

'OLD MACDONALD': THE SECOND YEAR

After one and a half years Steven stopped falling asleep during sessions and I realised how sleeping must have been a protection for all the exhaustion he felt at being in the world, trying to control all the noises and actions around him. When I gave a comment he did not like he would mime a headbang and then mime sleeping and then open his eyes and say 'shut up', one of the few phrases he ever said to me. He was losing his secondary handicaps, his defences against meaning, and he felt very mixed and exposed about it.

It was at this point that he suddenly burst into a terrible caricature of handicapped singing of 'Old MacDonald had a farm' – or rather, I was only at that moment aware that it must be a caricature. He was singing in the guttural voice I had often felt was intrinsically linked with handicap, just as I had felt previously the twisted postures were. But there was something in the meaning he was conveying that made me say, with trepidation, that maybe he felt there was room here for the animal noises and feelings in him; but maybe too he wanted to see if I was an idiot who thought that was his real singing voice. He looked at me in a startled but proud way. I sat bracing myself, ready for a blow or some catastrophe. He whispered 'Old MacDonald had a farm' in a normal voice that conveyed just a slight slur of brain damage, and then started to cry terribly and deeply.

This pitiful crying was a strong feature for the next six months and it is difficult to put into words. It is not crying that is asking for a word or a hug. It is a weeping to do with a terrible sense of aloneness and the reality of that. Neville Symington has commented (personal communication, 1984) that weeping comes when there is a breakthrough with this kind of patient and represents a real awareness of all the meaning that has been lost in the years up to that moment as well as the aloneness of handicap. His mother and worker were very distressed to see the weeping state Steven was in. They were worried therapy might be too cruel for him. I felt worried at the pain he was in and when he desperately wept 'See Mummy, go now' on one occasion I was in a dilemma. I said that he was able to stand up and leave the room and I could help him but I thought too that he needed to know I could bear his distress. It took the combined strength of myself and Steven's drive for truth to keep him in the room at this stage.

I needed the support of my own personal psychoanalysis and the Workshop to manage emotionally and deal with the ethical [dilemmas involved]. [...]

However, I believe that truth is worth pain. Steven was emotionally able to move through this state and the crying stopped. It was heralded by a session in which, when I said it was time, Steven reached in his pocket and threw a toy watch at me. There was a lot of anger and accuracy in his throw but I was delighted. It was a toy he had brought from his children's home, not one of the therapy toys provided, nor could it exactly be seen as a symbolic use of time. Time was flying! And it was flying at me! But I had borne his weeping and loneliness and so had he and he also trusted that I could survive his anger.

After this, the crying stopped and Steven became more affectionate and responsive. He stopped injuring himself. However, he was still violent to staff and was more dangerous. Previously he just had to be sat in a chair and he would fall asleep; now he would stand up again immediately and attack as he did not mind physical changes so much! He was no longer startled by external noises and slept the ordinary amount for a boy of his age.

This has been a regular pattern in long-term treatment with self-injuring, severely handicapped boys. It requires discussion with the key staff or families concerned because it does not feel like an improvement to them. One father commented, at a similar stage of therapy, 'You've turned my son from a violent sleeping zombie to a violent mobile psychopath'!

After two years of therapy there was a session in which, in the silence, my stomach gurgled loudly. 'Your tummy'? he asked. I said yes, it was my tummy. He giggled. I said he knew the sound was inside my tummy. He nodded. It started raining. 'Rain outside', he commented. There was a startled pause. A telephone rang next door. Steven put a hand to his ear. 'Outside the room', he pronounced. From that moment there was an extra degree of hope and aliveness in the session. Steven had differentiated between inside and outside and had achieved a 'psychological birth' (Mahler *et al.* 1975).

Shortly after this I bought a soft toy, a bear, for the therapy room as Steven always gave me a Christmas card with a bear on it and because he had not touched the other toys. On the first occasion that he saw it, having been told several weeks in advance of its arrival, he held it to him and hugged it with his back to me, not uttering a single word or sound the whole session. He has never managed to touch it since, only to look at it wistfully.

When I commented on his fear of getting close to me, to the bear and the toys, his fear that he will be violent, he said 'stupid'. He knows the meaning of the word 'stupid' because he knows that is not what he really is. After this he started whispering to the blanket, the chair and the bear, so softly I could not hear. It felt as if he had managed to make a move to the bear and have a first embryonic transitional object. From that first tentative link there was a transitional talking space he had made. At the home the staff commented that he spent a lot of time talking to all the objects in his room. He was then able to spend an hour on his own with his mother each week but his violence continued to be a problem with staff needing stitches for bites and treatment for violent kicks.

After he had been in therapy for three years his home sent a report, stating:

> *Since his visits to the Tavistock, staff have noticed progress in his development. He is sometimes able to warn of his aggression and is now guilty for some of the hurt he causes. He has started to say who he will miss and asks questions about staff who leave. He has been able to get closer to his mother and sisters when he goes home for hour-long visits at the weekend. However, although he shows he can develop through understanding, his violence can be so great it is difficult to restrain him. He is 13 now and there is concern for how to manage him when he is older and stronger.*

THE THIRD YEAR: BEREAVEMENT

At this point, when Steven had been in therapy for three years, his oldest sister Mary had an acute deterioration in her condition. She had no use of her legs or arms and it became clear she was dying. There was a temporary return of his headbanging and staff reported he had kicked the television as well as a new worker. Carole also was showing signs of emotional disturbance at school...

I was ... frightened that when faced brutally and clearly and irrevocably with the incurable nature of his primary handicap he would not stand it and would explode. The deterioration of his sister from an incurable physical illness and disability clearly carried his pain at his own condition too.

Although he had cerebral palsy, he did not have too severe a form and was able to walk. I found myself thinking of his strong kicking legs and his sister's dying ineffectual ones for several sessions. It took a while for me to understand my thoughts. We had been so preoccupied with Steven's handicaps, his defences, his fears of speaking that his position as a sibling had been buried. At the next session Steven came in and curled up very quietly. Suddenly his left leg reached out to kick the table. It was not an aggressive act. It was as if he was wanting to show me a problem he had about why his legs could work like that when his sister's legs could not. I faced a difficult technical dilemma. Bringing in outside information could be intrusive and anti-therapeutic. However, with some handicapped patients who cannot think or speak easily I have considered it important to be the voice of these events when I think they are playing a major part in my countertransference feelings.

I said maybe it felt strange being a Steven with legs who had an older sister whose legs did not work. Steven went rigid with attention. I said he was reminding me of what a quiet baby he was when his parents were so busy with Mary and how angry that might have made him. Maybe sometimes he felt he had to sit very quietly so he wouldn't know his legs did work and then he would not be so cross with his parents, Mary and Carole.

He slowly stretched out his legs alternately. I said he was checking each of them to see they were still there and they were working. He could stretch his legs and walk and Mary couldn't, but then again, Mary did not bang her head or have a hard time getting words to come out and Carole did not have either of those problems. He looked at me alively but then banged his head.

I said he could hear my words and think about them for a bit but then they could hurt. He stopped banging and was very still. The week after, Mary died. Mother did not want the word 'death' mentioned to Steven and she did not want him to come to the funeral. She felt she had enough to cope with looking after herself and Carole. This is a regular problem in mental handicap. Sometimes the parent projects his or her own inability to manage into the handicapped member of the family, who is then denied access to something, such as the funeral in this case, so that the rest of the family can manage. I am not here, of course, talking about the mentally handicapped who are also mentally ill and whose particular behaviour would make an undertaking such as the funeral too difficult.

However, mother did not want to speak to anyone about this further tragedy in her life. The residential staff did not know what to do as they were sure Steven understood and would be in a worse state if the knowledge was withheld. Steven eventually solved their problem for them by staring avidly at a soap opera on television in which a baby died. 'Baby dead. Mary dead', he said. After he showed he knew what had happened mother allowed the residential staff to take him to the cemetery.

A terrible period of headbanging followed. And then suddenly he became quiet in the sessions. He would come in, curl up on the armchair and hide his face in his arms or under a blanket. He did not utter a word or sound. For several weeks I interpreted the different shades of silence.

Then there was a change. At a certain moment I lost concentration on Steven. My mind had in fact gone to the shopping I needed to do before I got home later that day. For a moment I wanted to edit out cosmetically that moment of unprofessional deviation. But, of course, thinking about it was crucial. I realised that Steven was being as good as dead precisely so I could think about shopping lists, or indeed anything except him. I wondered aloud whether he was being so silent, as if he were dead, so that he would not be a burden to me. Perhaps he worried I too had a dead Mary daughter and would be angry he was alive instead of her. There was a riveting silence and then he burst into floods of tears. Unlike the lonely devastating weeping of two years ago, this was a mourning for the loss of someone else, not the loss of his own abilities.

When he then cried, 'Mum, now, please', I interpreted it was not just Mum in the waiting room he was calling for but a longed for Mum-in-the-room who might be so upset about a dead Mary and a furious husband leaving home that she just wanted a good quiet dead baby Steven. At the end of the session Steven held his hand for me to hold. He had never done that before. As I reached for it he looked at the untouched toy bear and then said 'Arm hurts' and cried. He kicked the toy mother and father dolls lying on the floor from his earlier throw. It had taken three years to move through the secondary handicap to the trauma of the organic handicap, his hurt arm, and his family life. The hurt arm seemed to be symbolic both of the organic primary handicap that had affected his arm, the couple who had created him and the traumatic violence of his early home life.

FOURTH YEAR: ANNIVERSARY REPETITION

The next year was taken up with his mourning processes for Mary. Unlike his first three years of therapy, where he only had one minor cold, Steven now had severe chest and throat infections. Moving into greater humanness also seemed to make him more vulnerable to infection. The work was all connected with his guilt at being alive.

Having a handicapped sibling is painful for everyone. A child wants to beat his brother or sister in a fair fight and prove he is the favourite, the one who is really the parents' best child. Where a sibling is handicapped there has been a terrible triumph. Where the sibling dies the pain and guilt are even stronger (Judd 1989). I was concerned for Carole and mother too at this point but mother did not wish for any family work.

For the next six months Steven was largely silent and still. In his children's home he was increasingly violent again. Around this time I decided I needed some extra supervision to help me understand why therapy was not progressing. I went to see psychoanalyst Dr Susannah Isaacs-Elmhirst (now vice-chair of the British Psycho-Analytical Society), who had been a consultant of the Child Guidance Training Centre at the Tavistock Centre. She had heard my first assessment meetings with Steven over four years ago. After hearing the description of his pale face and increased violence she wondered when the anniversary of Mary's death was. To my shock, I discovered it was only one week away.

Ready to make amends on the next session, I was extremely worried when Steven did not arrive on time. After 25 minutes I phoned the home to hear the car had arrived for him on time so there must be a traffic jam. Steven arrived with only ten minutes of his session left. I could hear him screaming and banging along the corridor and flinched. When I went to meet them his worker said there had been a terrible traffic jam and Steven was in a terrible mood; I might not be safe on my own with him. I said I would persevere.

Steven looked appalling. He was extremely white and his face had broken out in spots. His forehead was red and swollen again from his renewed headbanging. 'Poor Steven'. I said. 'How awful having such a big traffic jam today'. He shouted 'No'! and started spitting but I felt safe. Inside my room his worker thrust him into a kneeling position on the floor, trying to stop his headbanging. I said they should go.

Steven looked intently at me while banging his head. The sound of flesh hitting bone and flesh hurt particularly today and I wondered if that was because of Mary's painful death. I said he had felt terrible the last few weeks and only now did I realise why. Tomorrow would be the first anniversary of Mary's death. There was a riveting pause. For a moment I feared Steven would throw himself at me to attack me.

However, he carefully lifted himself so he could sit down as usual and continued to stare at me hungrily, his eyes not leaving mine for a moment. I said perhaps he had felt frightened the traffic was bad today; perhaps he was worried I might be cross he was late and then I would say, 'Why is Steven coming when Mary is dead'? Maybe he felt very bad about Mary dying when he would not die from cerebral palsy. He could hurt his head badly when he banged it and he could get bad colds, especially when he was miserable, but he would not die from it.

Steven continued to fix his eyes on mine. I said he was really looking at me today, keeping my face in sight and letting me see his eyes and face as if he especially needed to see me when I was talking about things like this. He made a sound – 'Errr'. Silence. He relaxed again and continued looking at me. I said there was a sound inside him that had wanted to come out into a word but it had not managed to. I wondered what he would want to say if he could speak.

There was a long companiable silence. I found myself recounting our joint history to Steven; how he had been ten when he first came and now he was over 14. How his little sister was 12 and she was two years younger than he, and how Mary had been two years older, and how in just one year he would be the age Mary had been when she died. I said perhaps his colds were his way of seeing if he ought to die to be like Mary and die at 15 as she had done.

A couple of minutes before the end of time two workers urgently knocked on the door and came in before waiting for a reply. They were clearly expecting they would have to rescue me and were surprised to see a thoughtful peaceful Steven sitting down. When his mother came in I told them all about the anniversary of Mary's death and they, like me prior to my supervision, had all obliterated it. Since then, I have been most careful about remembering birthdays and anniversaries.

THE END OF THERAPY

For the next two years Steven faced different external difficulties. There were many staff changes and finally his home was closed, and with only two weeks' warning he was moved to another placement. That was too far away to accommodate weekly therapy, although I remained in telephone contact. After six years in therapy Steven could warn staff when he was feeling violent, could maintain relationships and ask about changes in the staff shifts. With me, right to the last session, he was largely mute. At each new blow the environment offers he returns to banging his head but stops once the situation changes. I feel he will always find life a painful experience but he is now able to gain more from his surroundings.

REFERENCES

Judd, D. (1989) *Give Sorrow Words: Working with a Dying Child*, London: Free Association Books.
Mahler, M., Bergman, A. and Pine, F. (1975) *The Psychological Birth of the Human Infant*, New York: Basic.

PART IV

COMMUNICATION AND RELATIONSHIPS IN ORGANISATIONS

Sheila Barrett

Health and social care organisations form one of the contexts in which care takes place. The chapters in Part IV explore how the organisational context impacts on the relationships and communications that are part of the work of providing care, at the individual, group and wider institutional level.

The first two chapters describe the contexts of care work and discuss the effects of working in these contexts. In Chapter 30 'Some unconscious aspects of organisational life', William Halton, a psychoanalytic psychotherapist and organisational consultant, explores the nature of organisations in health and social care with particular reference to the work of the influential psychoanalytic theorist Melanie Klein. Tom Kitwood, a psychologist who worked in services for older people, has explored one of the potential negative effects of working in care organisations – burnout. In Chapter 31 'The caring organisation' he points to changes in organisational practice that can help prevent and address the negative influences on staff.

The next two chapters focus on working in groups and teams. Most people have experience of living and working in groups, beginning with the family or other group in which they were brought up. There, they learned how to relate to each other as group or family members, and how to relate to individuals and groups outside of that unit. Some perspectives on groups, in particular psychodynamic approaches, would say that these early experiences form the basis of how we relate in work groups. They would also suggest that we often fall back on these patterns, without our knowing, especially when present day experiences remind us of the past. In Chapter 32 'The unconscious at work in groups and teams', Jon Stokes, a clinical psychologist and organisational consultant, explores some group processes from a psychoanalytic perspective. In particular he looks at the work of the psychoanalytic theorist Wilfred

Bion on basic assumptions and how these can operate to the benefit or detriment of the work and the experience of the individual. By contrast, Gareth Morgan, an academic and organisational consultant who works within a social constructionist perspective, describes how metaphor can be helpful in understanding group relations and communications. Chapter 33 'Imaginising teamwork' provides illustrations and offers the reader a chance to explore their own organisation from this perspective. The way in which care services are organised can have a major impact on the type and quality of relationships and communications. The overall values, task and outcomes of an organisation, as well as how they are operationalised through structures, the cultures that develop and what happens when these change, all influence interactions with users of the service, with colleagues and others. Chapter 34 'Going home from hospital – an appreciative inquiry study' by Reed *et al.*, a group of writers concerned in different ways with the care of older people, describes how a social constructionist approach was used in a piece of action research to bring about change in one part of an organisation. It illustrates one approach to understanding and bringing about change.

The last two chapters in Part IV explore the notion of leadership. Talk about leadership and concerns about leadership are currently prevalent in health and social care services and national leadership programmes are committed to developing this quality among practitioners. Despite the widespread attention that it receives, understanding exactly what effective leadership is and how it works remains elusive. Early research sought to identify personal characteristics and behaviours of leaders. What was intrinsic to these people that made them so great? Later there was a focus on environmental or situational factors that influenced leaders. More recently there has been an interest in 'followership' and the relationship between followers and leaders, and with this the question how is power used to enable leadership. Psychologists and academics Beverley Alimo-Metcalfe and Robert Alban-Metcalfe have explored the attributes of leadership from the perspective of those being led. Chapter 35 'Heaven can wait' summarises research which has since been developed into an organisational tool to develop leadership in the National Health Service. Chapter 36 'Why should anyone be led by you'?, written by Robert Goffee, an academic from the London Business School and Gareth Jones, formerly of the BBC, illustrates that even today there is still a focus on the so-called 'Great Man Theory' of leadership.

CHAPTER 30

SOME UNCONSCIOUS ASPECTS OF ORGANISATIONAL LIFE: CONTRIBUTIONS FROM PSYCHOANALYSIS

William Halton

'None of your jokes today', said an eight-year-old coming into the consulting room. Interpretations about the process of the unconscious may often seem like bad jokes to the recipient, if not frankly offensive. Although some elements of psychoanalysis have become part of everyday life, psychoanalysis as a treatment for individual emotional problems remains a minority experience. As a system of ideas it has adherents, sceptics and a multitude of indifferent passers-by.

Despite the fact that there is no exact parallel between individuals and institutions, psychoanalysis has contributed one way to approach thinking about what goes on in institutions. This approach does not claim to provide a comprehensive explanation or even a complete description. But looking at an institution through the spectrum of psychoanalytical concepts is a potentially creative activity which may help in understanding and dealing with certain issues. The psychoanalytical approach to consultation is not easy to describe. It involves understanding ideas developed in the context of individual therapy, as well as looking at institutions in terms of unconscious emotional processes. This may seem like a combination of the implausible with the even more implausible or it may become an illuminating juxtaposition.

Source: Obholzer, A. and Zagier Roberts, V. (eds) (1994) *The Unconscious At Work. Individual and Organizational Stress in the Human Services*, London: Routledge.

THE UNCONSCIOUS

As Freud and others discovered, there are hidden aspects of human mental life which, while remaining hidden, nevertheless influence conscious processes. In treating individuals, Freud found that there was often resistance to accepting the existence of the unconscious. However, he believed he could demonstrate its existence by drawing attention to dreams, slips of tongue, mistakes and so forth as evidence of meaningful mental life of which we are not aware. What was then required was interpretation of these symbolic expressions from the unconscious.

Ideas which have a valid meaning at the conscious level may at the same time carry an unconscious hidden meaning. For example, a staff group talking about their problems with the breakdown of the switchboard may at the same time be making an unconscious reference to a breakdown in interdepartmental communication. Or complaints about the distribution of car-park spaces may also be a symbolic communication about managers who have no room for staff concerns. The psychoanalytically oriented consultant takes up a listening position on the boundary between conscious and unconscious meanings, and works simultaneously with problems at both levels. It may be some time before the consultant can pick up and make sense of these hidden references to issues of which the group itself is not aware.

THE AVOIDANCE OF PAIN

Like individuals, institutions develop defences against difficult emotions which are too threatening or too painful to acknowledge. These emotions may be a response to external threats such as government policy or social change. They may arise from internal conflicts between management and employees or between groups and departments in competition for resources. They may also arise from the nature of the work and the particular client group. Some institutional defences are healthy, in the sense that they enable the staff to cope with stress and develop through their work in the organisation. But some institutional defences, like some individual defences, can obstruct contact with reality and in this way damage the staff and hinder the organisation in fulfilling its task and in adapting to changing circumstances. Central among these defences is *denial*, which involves pushing certain thoughts, feelings and experiences out of conscious awareness because they have become too anxiety-provoking.

Institutions call in consultants when they can no longer solve problems. The consultant who undertakes to explore the nature of the underlying difficulty is likely to be seen as an object of both hope and fear. The conscious hope is that the problem will be brought to the surface, but at the same time, unconsciously, this is the very thing which institutions fear. As a result, the consultant's interpretations of the underlying unconscious processes may well meet with *resistance*, that is, an emotionally charged refusal to accept or even to hear what he or she says. The consultant may only gradually be able to evaluate the nature of the defences, reserving interpretation until the group is ready to face what it has been avoiding and to make use of the interpretation.

A symbolic communication may occur just at a point where the consultant's understanding of the hidden meaning coincides with the group's readiness to receive it. The following example illustrates a symbolic communication occurring in a group unable to accept the reality of a threat from an external source:

> *The Manfred Eating Disorders Unit at Storsey Hospital was conducting a last-ditch campaign against closure, and had engaged the help of a consultant. The campaign had been running for several months, with the staff working late and over weekends organising a local petition and lobbying professional colleagues, local councillors and MPs. Public opinion was on the side of keeping the unit open; closure seemed unthinkable. New patients were still being admitted and no preparation had been made for transferring existing patients. Only the consultant did not share the excited mood and felt depressed after each meeting.*
>
> *At one meeting the discussion strayed to the apparently irrelevant topic of the merits of euthanasia. The consultant heard this as an indirect expression of the anticipated relief which the completion of closure would bring, and said this to the group. Their first reaction was one of shock. However, over time the interpretation led to a more realistic attitude to the possibility of closure, which made it possible for the staff to begin to think and plan for the patients.*

In this example, the staff had been responding to the threat of closure with angry and excited activity aimed at saving the unit. By relating only to the possibility of winning their fight for survival, they resisted and denied the possibility of closure, ignoring the reality of financial cuts which had already closed other local units. The motivation behind this resistance was not only the wish to save the unit for the benefit of patients; closure would also hurt their pride, cast doubts on the value of their work, and cause other emotional pain. But insofar as they had lost touch with reality, they had also failed in their responsibility to prepare patients for the possibility of closure. As an outsider, the consultant felt the depression which was so strikingly absent in the group; this was an important clue to what was being avoided. The euthanasia discussion indicated that previously denied feelings were moving towards the surface as a symbolic communication, and that the group was ready to acknowledge them.

THE CONTRIBUTION OF MELANIE KLEIN

In play, children represent their different feelings through characters and animals either invented or derived from children's stories: the good fairy, the wicked witch, the jealous sister, the sly fox and so on. This process of dividing feelings into differentiated elements is called *splitting*. By splitting emotions, children gain relief from internal conflicts. The painful conflict between love and hate for the mother, for instance, can be relieved by splitting the mother-image into a good fairy and a bad witch. *Projection* often accompanies splitting, and involves locating feelings in others rather than in oneself. Thus the child attributes slyness to the fox or jealousy to the bad sister. Through play, these contradictory feelings and figures can be explored and resolved.

Through her psychoanalytic work with children in the early 1920s, Melanie Klein developed a conceptualisation of an unconscious inner world, present in everyone, peopled by different characters personifying differentiated parts of self or aspects of the external world. Early in childhood, splitting and projection are the predominant defences for avoiding pain; Klein referred to this as the *paranoid-schizoid position* ('paranoid' referring to badness being experienced as coming from outside oneself, and 'schizoid' referring to splitting). This is a normal stage of development; it occurs in early childhood and as a state of mind it can recur throughout life. Through play, normal maturation or psychoanalytic treatment, previously separated feelings such as love and hate, hope and despair, sadness and joy, acceptance and rejection can eventually be brought together into a more integrated whole. This stage of integration Klein called the *depressive position*, because giving up the comforting simplicity of self-idealisation, and facing the complexity of internal and external reality, inevitably stirs up painful feelings of guilt, concern and sadness. These feelings give rise to a desire to make reparation for injuries caused through previous hatred and aggression. This desire stimulates work and creativity, and is often one of the factors which leads to becoming a 'helping' professional.

THE PARANOID-SCHIZOID POSITION

The discovery from child analysis that the different and possibly conflicting emotional aspects of an experience may be represented by different people or different 'characters' is used in institutional consultancy as a guide for understanding group processes. In play, the child is the originator of the projections and the play-figures are the recipients. In an institution, the client group can be regarded as the originator of projections with the staff group as the recipients. The staff members may come to represent different, and possibly conflicting, emotional aspects of the psychological state of the client group. For example, in an adolescent unit the different and possibly conflicting needs of the adolescent may be projected into different staff members. One member may come to represent the adolescent's need for independence while another may represent the need for limits. In an abortion clinic, one nurse may be in touch only with a mother's mourning for her lost baby, while another may be in touch only with the mother's relief. These projective processes serve the same purpose for the client as play does for the child: relief from the anxieties which can arise from trying to contain conflicting needs and conflicting emotions. It is hard to contain mourning and relief simultaneously, or to experience the wish for independence and the need for limits at the same time. The splitting and projection of these conflicting emotions into different members of the staff group is an inevitable part of institutional process.

Schizoid splitting is normally associated with the splitting off and projecting outwards of parts of the self perceived as bad, thereby creating external figures who are both hated and feared. In the helping professions, there is a tendency to deny feelings of hatred or rejection towards clients. These feelings may be more easily dealt with by projecting them onto other groups or outside agencies, who can then be criticised. The projection of feelings of badness outside the self helps to produce a state of illusory goodness and self-idealisation. This black-and-white mentality simplifies complex issues and may produce a rigid culture in which growth is inhibited.

> *A student occupation protesting against the effects of government cuts was condemned by the college authorities as a ludicrous and irrational waste of resources. They were quoted in the press as saying: 'The question remains as to who was leading this disruption. We have had complaints from students suggesting that outsiders and non-students took active parts in proceedings in meetings and occupation action ... there was no apparent agenda other than disruption.*

The implication was that inside the college there were good students and good managers. Outside there were bad people who contaminated and disrupted the institution, manipulating its members for destructive purposes. Splitting and projection exploits the natural boundary between insiders and outsiders which every institution has. In this example it led to a state of fragmentation because contact was lost between parts of the institution which belonged together inside its boundary. There was no dialogue possible between the conflicting points of view within the college, and so change and development were frustrated.

Sometimes the splitting process occurs between groups within the institution. Structural divisions into sections, departments, professions, disciplines and so forth are necessary for organisations to function effectively. However, these divisions become fertile ground for the splitting and projection of negative images. The gaps between departments or professions are available to be filled with many different emotions – denigration, competition, hatred, prejudice, paranoia. Each group feels that it represents something good and that other groups represent something inferior. Doctors are authoritarian, social workers talk too much, psychotherapists are precious, managers only think about money. Individual members of these groups are stereotyped like the characters playing these roles in children's games and stories. The less contact there is with other sections, the greater the scope for projection of this kind. Contact and meetings may be avoided in order unconsciously to preserve self-idealisation based on these projections. This results in the institution becoming stuck in a paranoid-schizoid projective system. Emotional disorder interferes with the functioning of an organization, particularly in relation to tasks which require co-operation or collective change.

ENVY

On occasion, difficulties in collaboration arise not so much from the desire to be an ideal carer or a more potent worker, but from a sense of being an inevitable loser in a competitive struggle. In the current climate of market values and shrinking budgets, the success of one part of the organization can be felt to be at the expense of another. The survival-anxiety of the less successful section stimulates an envious desire to spoil the other's success. This spoiling envy operates like a hidden spanner-in-the-works, either by withholding necessary co-operation or by active sabotage.

A group of lecturers at Branston Polytechnic were organizing a money-raising short course out of term-time. They found it impossible to gain the co-operation of the catering department, who refused to provide tea and coffee for course participants. Then, on the first day of the course, despite the lecturers' having requested a delay, mainte-

nance work was started on the toilet facilities, putting them out of action. Both the catering and maintenance departments were about to be closed down, their services to be taken over by private organisations following tendering. Their unco-operativeness led to considerable inconvenience for the participants, who blamed the course organisers and left the course very critical of the polytechnic as a whole.

Catering and maintenance staff felt devalued by the decision to 'sell off' their services, and envious of the academic staff's protected status. This kind of spoiling envy often gives rise to hostile splits between parts of an organisation such that the enterprise as a whole is damaged.

PROJECTIVE IDENTIFICATION AND COUNTERTRANSFERENCE

Although psychoanalysis is based on the idea that the behaviour of an individual is influenced by unconscious factors, the psychoanalytic view of institutional functioning regards an individual's personal unconscious as playing only a subsidiary role. Within organisations, it is often easier to ascribe a staff member's behaviour to personal problems than it is to discover the link with institutional dynamics. This link can be made using the psychoanalytic concept of *projective identification*. This term refers to an unconscious inter-personal interaction in which the recipients of a projection react to it in such a way that their own feelings are affected: they unconsciously identify with the projected feelings. For example, when the staff of the Manfred Eating Disorders Unit projected their depression about closure into the consultant, he felt this depression as if it were his own. The state of mind in which other people's feelings are experienced as one's own is called the *countertransference*.

Projective identification frequently leads to the recipient's acting out the countertransference deriving from the projected feelings. For example, the staff of an adolescent unit may begin to relate to each other as if they were adolescents themselves, or may act in adolescent ways such as breaking the rules and otherwise challenging authority figures. Such behaviour indicates that projective identification is at work, but the true source of their feelings and behaviour is likely to remain obscure until staff achieve a conscious realisation that they have become trapped in a countertransference response to a projective process.

It is also through the mechanism of projective identification that one group on behalf of another group, or one member of a group on behalf of the other members, can come to serve as a kind of 'sponge' for all the anger or all the depression or all the guilt in the staff group. The angry member may then be launched at management by the group, or a depressed member may be unconsciously manoeuvred into breaking down and leaving. This individual not only expresses or carries something for the group, but may be used to export something which the rest of the group then need not feel in themselves. Similarly, a group may carry something for another group or for the institution as a whole. If there is something which a group cannot bear at all, like the depression about the closure of the Manfred Unit, it may call in a consultant to carry that feeling on its behalf.

THE DEPRESSIVE POSITION

When we recognise that our painful feelings come from projections, it is a natural response to 'return' these feelings to their source: 'These are *your* feelings, not mine'. This readily gives rise to blaming, and contributes to the ricocheting of projections back and forth across groups and organisations. However, if we can tolerate the feelings long enough to reflect on them, and *contain* the anxieties they stir up, it may be possible to bring about change. At times when we cannot do this, another person may temporarily contain our feelings for us. This concept of a person as a 'container' comes from the psychoanalytic work of Bion (1967). He likened it to the function of the mother whose ability to receive and understand the emotional states of her baby makes them more bearable.

Certainly, both psychoanalysts and psychoanalytical consultants aim to identify the projective processes at work and trace the projections to their source, but this in itself is not enough. What was previously unbearable – and therefore projected – needs to be made bearable. It is painful for the individual or group or institution to have to take back less acceptable aspects of the self which had previously been experienced as belonging to others: for example, that legitimate criticisms may arise from within a college, and not simply as intrusions by malicious outsiders; or that no psychiatric unit is so ideal that it cannot be closed; or that in adolescents the need for independence and the need for limits are equally valid concerns and should be held in a complementary tension; or that abortion gives rise to both mourning and relief; or that good managers and good caretakers are both necessary to make a healthy organisation; or that authorities who implement cuts and students who protest may both care about the education system.

The consultant's willingness and ability to contain or hold on to the projected feelings stirred up by these ambiguities until the group is ready to use an interpretation are crucial. Otherwise the interpretation will be experienced as yet another attack. However, when the timing is right, some of the projections can be 're-owned', splitting decreases, and there is a reduction in the polarisation and antagonism among staff members themselves. This promotes integration and co-operation within and between groups or, in psychoanalytic terms, a shift from the paranoid-schizoid to the depressive position.

In a group functioning in the depressive position, every point of view will be valued and a full range of emotional responses will be available to it through its members. The group will be more able to encompass the emotional complexity of the work in which they all share, and no one member will be left to carry his or her fragment in isolation. Furthermore, in order to contain the tendency towards splitting in the client group, the staff group must be able to hold together the conflicting elements projected into them, discussing and thinking them through instead of being drawn into acting them out. This requires being aware of the particular stresses involved in their work, as well as recognising its limitations. The lessening of conflict may then open the way to better working practices and greater job satisfaction, as staff process and integrate their collective work experience. However, the depressive position is never attained once and for all. Whenever survival or self-esteem are threatened, there is a tendency to return to a more paranoid-schizoid way of functioning.

CONCLUSION

Psychoanalytical concepts make a particular contribution to thinking about institutional processes, though contributions from other conceptual frameworks are also necessary to understand institutional functioning. Psychoanalysis is concerned with understanding the inner world with its dynamic processes of fragmentation and integration; key concepts include denial of internal and external reality, splitting, projection and idealisation.

Psychoanalytically oriented consultants extend these concepts to understanding unconscious institutional anxieties and the defences against them. Besides concepts, they bring from psychoanalysis a certain stance or frame of mind: to search for understanding without being judgemental either of their clients or of themselves. This enables them to make themselves available to receive and process projections from the institution. The feelings experienced by the consultant or, indeed, by any member of an institution, while interacting with it, constitute the basic countertransference response on which the understanding of unconscious institutional processes is based.

At its best, such understanding can create a space in the organisation in which staff members can stand back and think about the emotional processes in which they are involved in ways that reduce stress and conflict, and can inform change and development. The ideas discussed in this and subsequent chapters can be used to develop a capacity for self-consultation: for observing and reflecting on the impact unconscious group and organisational processes have on us all, and our own contribution to these processes as we take up our various roles.

REFERENCES

Bion, W. (1967) 'Attacks on linking', in *Second Thoughts: Selected Papers on Psychoanalysis*, London: Heinemann Medical (reprinted London: Maresfield Reprints, 1984).

Klein, M. (1959) 'Our adult world and its roots in infancy', in Colman, A.D. and Geiler, M.H. (eds) *Group Relations Reader 2*, A.K. Rice Institute Series [Washington, DC], 1985.

CHAPTER 31

THE CARING ORGANISATION

Tom Kitwood

Whenever people join together to perform a complex task, a number of questions inevitably arise. How is the task to be divided up? Is there any way of ensuring that people do their jobs correctly? Who is accountable, to whom, and for what? How much scope is to be given for individual creativity and initiative in each role? Who holds authority, and over what domains? Questions such as these apply to all types of context (production, communication, human services, etc.) and to all types of organisation, from the small and informal (such as a family) to the large and bureaucratic (such as an international bank or the entire civil service). Many of the older theorists of management held the view that there was one best way for all organisations to function. Now, however, it is generally accepted that there is a valid place for many organisational forms, and that it is necessary to find the form that is best fitted to the task.

Dementia care brings its own special organisational issues, although these generally have not been addressed with the depth and thoroughness that they deserve. The crux of the matter is this. Caring, at its best, springs from the spontaneous actions of people who are very resourceful and aware, able to trust each other and work easily as a team. However, employees vary greatly in their experience and skill, and in their motives for being involved in this kind of work. Thus the organisation has to find a way to set each person free to do his or her best work, while also safeguarding against slovenliness and inconsistency; there are standards to be maintained. An optimum solution has to be found, and in a general economic context of limited resources.

Source: *Dementia Reconsidered: The Person Comes First* (1999) Maidenhead, Open University Press/McGraw-Hill.

In any organisation that delivers a human service, there will be a close parallel between the way employees are treated by their seniors, and the way the clients themselves are treated. If employees are abandoned and abused, probably the clients will be too. If employees are supported and encouraged, they will take their own sense of well-being into their day-to-day work. Thus if an organisation is genuinely committed to providing excellent care for its clients – if it is committed to their personhood – it must necessarily be committed to the personhood of all staff, and at all levels. [...]

STRESS, STRAIN AND BURN-OUT

The condition we have come to know as burn-out was first described as a loss of energy, enjoyment, vision and commitment, and as a general sense that it is impossible to do a job as it should be done (e.g. Freudenberger 1974; Maslach 1982). Burn-out is clearly different from simple exhaustion, which is remedied by rest and recreation. In some instances the onset of burn-out is dramatic; a person may feel, quite suddenly, that they cannot face going to work. It is more common, however, for the process to be gradual, happening over a period of months or even years. Factors of a personal kind are, of course, involved in burn-out. A considerable body of research on this topic, however, comes strongly to the conclusion that the main causes lie in the way organisations function, particularly inadequacies in the design of jobs, the lack of support structures, and in the workload itself.

Burn-out is particularly likely in occupations that have a strong vocational quality, and a close study has been made of it in the caring professions (e.g. Chernis 1980). It has not been subjected to close research, however, in the field of dementia care, although there is good reason for believing that it is a serious problem here. Burn-out is more likely when there is a very needy client group (Maslach 1978).

Three main stages have been identified in the development of burn-out, the first of which is stress, as shown in Figure 31.1. Here there is a serious attempt to do the job, giving close attention to all its aspects. An employee has vision, energy and determination, and for a short time it seems to be possible to do the job well. The output of good work is high. The demands, however, are too great for this effort to be maintained. A state develops in which the body is in a more or less permanent state of over-arousal. Health may begin to be affected, with a lowered resistance to viral infections, or such symptoms as headaches or lower back pain. There may be an experience of recurrent anxiety; patterns of sleep may be disturbed. Stress arising from the workplace tends also to have secondary effects; for example a deterioration in close relationships, or a loss of interest in leisure pursuits. A sensitive person may be inclined to internalise the

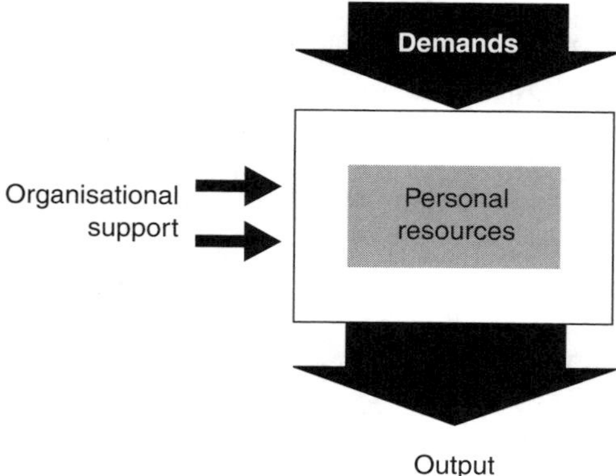

Figure 31.1 Stress: The first of the three main stages of burn-out.

problem, and frame the state of stress as a consequence of personal inadequacy. This, unfortunately, is a view with which some organisations very readily collude.

The second stage is often described as one of strain, as shown in Figure 31.2. Now the output of good work declines, as the recognition grows that the job as originally envisaged is impossible. As with stress, strain has its counterpart in changed body chemistry, particularly in enduring adverse changes in hormone balance. It is as if the body has been constantly on the alert, but never identified what it has to fight against or run away from. Prolonged strain seems to be associated with a greater susceptibility to serious illness such as cancer, ulceration of the gut and heart disease (e.g. Cooper 1984). The chronic fatigue syndromes, which are still only very poorly understood, may also have some connection with continued strain.

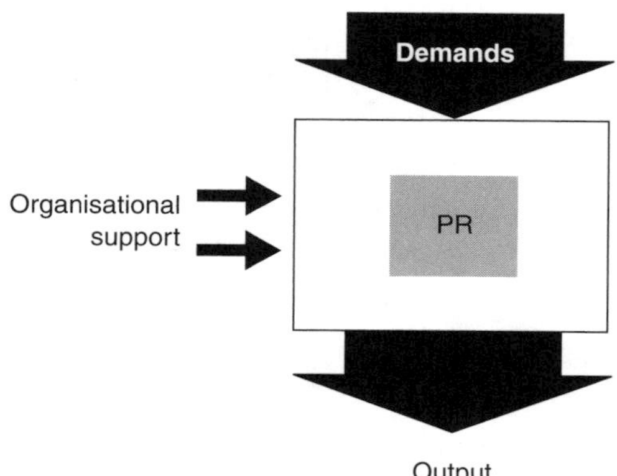

Figure 31.2 Strain: The second of the three main stages of burn-out.

The third stage is one of more steady low-level functioning, as shown in Figure 31.3. Now there is no longer an attempt to do all that the job really requires. A new equilibrium is established between personal resources and organisational demands. Many tasks are performed in a minimal way, and in care work there is a tendency to withdraw once the basic tasks are done. The idea of attempting to meet the full range of clients' needs is abandoned, and there is a kind of psychological disengagement.

Burn-out is expressed in different ways. The obvious initial signs are lateness, absenteeism, carelessness, disowning of responsibility, and high rates of sickness. Often there is a cynical or resentful attitude, with criticism directed at anyone who does more than the accepted basic minimum. Much of this resembles the state of 'learned helplessness' (Mukulineer 1995); a person has discovered that efforts at bringing change are futile, and that the outcomes are out of his or her control. The third stage, then, is a kind of stalemate, which has evolved as a form of self-protection by employees. Perhaps it is the only way they have of coping while the organisation sets up their work in such an unrealistic way.

This account of burn-out in the caring professions may shed light on what has been happening in dementia care. In the tradition of practice that we have inherited, where staff were given very little support or help in their work, it is possible that the majority of those who survived had moved into a chronic state of low-level burn-out. The situation was all too easily accepted, and transformed into the idea that a basic minimum of physical care was all that people with dementia needed. It is essential, then, as we seek to improve dementia care, that organisations take on the full range of psychological and moral responsibilities, and create conditions where their employees can flourish.

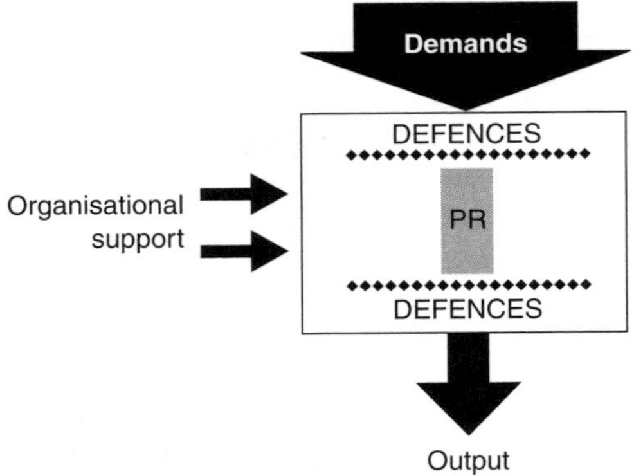

Figure 31.3 Steady low-level-functioning: The third of the three main stages of burn-out.

TAKING CARE OF STAFF

Thus far the improvements that have been made in dementia care have been far more concerned with the quality of life of the clients than with that of staff. The well-being of care assistants, especially, has been sadly neglected. Sooner or later, however, it becomes clear that there is a close connection between the personhood of clients and that of the staff; it is only a short-term expedient to ignore the latter issue. There are many ways in which an organisation can take care of staff, and we will look briefly at eight of these. What follows is based on a document written by Robert Woods and myself for a charity wanting to improve its dementia care; it draws in part on our own experience, and in part on consultation with several very experienced practitioners (Kitwood and Woods 1996).

Pay and conditions of service

The central point is simple and obvious. Staff should be properly rewarded for their work. A good organisation makes provision for sickness and holidays, and gives the opportunity for those who wish it to contribute to a pension scheme. Where these arrangements are not made, the organisation is expressing to staff that they are little more than casual labour; it is not surprising if they, on their part, show casual attitudes and low commitment. A sound framework of pay and conditions, on the other hand, creates security and conveys to staff that they are valued.

Induction

Experience in the first few weeks after starting work deserves very careful attention. It is easy to underestimate the apprehension and lack of confidence that many new employees feel. A well-designed induction process might take place over, say, two months, giving time for the newcomer to assimilate all necessary information and learn all the basic tasks. One possibility is to have two induction packs. The first contains details of conditions of service, pay and pensions, health and safety, fire precautions, disciplinary procedures, etc. The other is more related to the job itself, with a clear statement of what is expected in a particular role, and information on care planning, supervision and quality standards. It might also have some material on the nature of dementia and dementia care. During the induction period an employee will need a higher level of supervision, and should have ready informal access to an experienced person who can give guidance and support.

Creation of a team

Care is much more than a matter of individuals attending to individuals. Ideally it is the work of a team of people whose values are aligned, and whose talents are liberated in achieving a shared objective. It is unlikely that this will happen just by chance; if teambuilding is neglected it is probable that staff will form their own small cliques, and begin to collude in avoiding the less obvious parts of care. Some developmental group work may be necessary, in order to facilitate self-disclosure and to lower interpersonal barriers. The formation of a close-knit senior care team is especially important, with a consensus about the nature of good practice, and a common framework for their supervisory work. As new employees arrive, they should be properly integrated into the team.

Supervision

In an area so fraught with uncertainty as dementia care it is vital that staff should be given regular feedback about their work, and have the opportunity to discuss issues from it with someone who has greater experience. In the best care settings all employees, including the manager, receive regular supervision. A good arrangement is for there to be an hour of supervision per month, and for new members of staff to have an hour per fortnight during their first few weeks in employment. Effective supervision involves forming a kind of 'learning alliance', with a clear understanding of the purpose and the format (Hawkins and Shohet 1989). A rough boundary should be drawn between issues that are genuinely work-related, and those of a more personal kind (which might need to be dealt with through counselling outside the workplace). However, it is appropriate for supervision to provide some kind of 'containment' for painful feelings arising directly from work. Supervision might lead to agreements about what action is to be taken, for example if it has become clear that a particular skill is missing. In some settings supervisees are given the opportunity to give feedback to their supervisors; it is almost a supervision in reverse. There is also a place for some small group supervision, perhaps in order to learn from a critical incident of a positive or negative kind.

In-service training

In care work at all levels, the proper aim is to promote the formation of a 'reflective practitioner' (Schön 1983) – one whose work is flexible, assured and full of understanding. A mechanised approach, which merely deals with acquiring 'competences', does not go nearly far enough. The training of staff, if well designed, will set up a process of experiential learning, involving a cycle of action, reflection, and consolidation of better practice (Kolb 1992).

Much of the in-service training can be carried out by the manager and senior care team if the organisation has enabled them to learn how to do this work. Training is better done with teams than individuals, because members develop shared goals, and can support each other in the improvement of their practice. Single 'shots' of training are relatively ineffective, because the learning cycle is unlikely to be completed. A structured programme of, say, six two-hour sessions over six months, is far more likely to bring about creative change. The content of training should never be merely theoretical as has often happened with dementia. It should stimulate staff to subject their practice to continuing reflection.

Individual staff development

Over and above the more obvious training issues, there is the question of how to enable each member of staff to flourish in his or her own unique way. In any care team there is likely be a rich array of abilities and interests, which could be drawn into the work. When staff are simply made use of, or when care is defined in too narrow a way, these remain largely hidden. A caring organisation will make it possible for staff to take courses, offer more flexible hours so that a special interest can be pursued, encourage innovations in the activities arranged for clients, and allow jobs to be redesigned so as to take new interests into account.

Accreditation and promotion

An organisation that is concerned for its staff will make it possible for those who are highly committed to gain some form of accreditation, and will have a route for promotion out of the care assistant grade. Several programmes are available for enabling people to gain nationally recognised accreditation in dementia care, through to university level qualifications. If individual accreditation is to become an established practice, it will probably involve one or two members of the senior care team themselves becoming qualified as assessors, tutors or mentors, in addition to their ordinary role in supervision. Indirectly, the heightened level of activity will improve the quality of care. Also, as more opportunities are provided for staff members to gain qualifications specifically related to dementia care, the general status of this work is likely to rise.

Effective quality assurance

Generally quality assurance is viewed as a way of protecting the needs and interests of clients, and of satisfying inspectors and senior managers that basic standards of care are being met. The whole process also has another function; it is a way of giving systematic feedback to staff, and hence, if handled rightly, of giving them assurance in their work. In all assessment of care practice, then, great attention should be paid to the 'developmental loop'; that is, data collected should be made available to staff as a basis for discussion, in order that a plan can be drawn up for the improvement of care. Ideally each quality assurance round will generate such a plan, and the next round will provide information on whether the plan has actually been effectively implemented. There is an insincere way of going about quality assurance, which consists essentially of 'being seen to be doing the right thing'. It is more challenging by far to confront the realities, and in particular to assess what is actually occurring to the clients in the process of care. When this is done it will be necessary to face up to some issues that had been avoided, but there is the possibility of setting a virtuous circle into motion, with huge increases in job satisfaction. [...]

REFERENCES

Chernis, C. (1980) *Staff Burnout: Job Stress in the Human Services*, Beverly Hills: Sage.

Cooper, C.L. (ed.) (1984) *Psychosocial Stress and Cancer*, Chichester: Wiley.

Freudenberger, H.J. (1974) 'Staff burn-out', *Journal of Social Issues* 30 (1): 159–165.

Hawkins, P. and Shohet, R. (1989) *Supervision in the Helping Professions*, Buckingham: Open University Press.

Kitwood, T. and Woods, R.T. (1996) *A Training and Development Strategy for Dementia Care in Residential Settings*, Bradford: Bradford Dementia Group.

Kolb, D.A. (1992) *Experiential Learning: Experience as a Source of Learning and Development*, London: Prentice Hall.

Maslach, C. (1978) 'The client role in staff burn-out', *Journal of Social Issues* 34 (4): 111–123.

Maslach, C. (1982) 'Understanding burn-out: definitional issues in analysing a complex phenomenon', in Paine, W.S. (ed.) *Job Stress and Burnout: Research Theory and Intervention Respectives*, Beverly Hills, CA: Sage.

Mukulineer, M. (1995) *Human Learned Helplessness*, New York: Plenum.

Schön, D. (1983) *The Reflective Practitioner*, London: Temple Smith.

CHAPTER 32

THE UNCONSCIOUS AT WORK IN GROUPS AND TEAMS: CONTRIBUTIONS FROM THE WORK OF WILFRED BION

Jon Stokes

Our experiences of being and working in groups are often powerful and overwhelming. We experience the tension between the wish to join together and the wish to be separate; between the need for togetherness and belonging and the need for an independent identity. Many of the puzzling phenomena of group life stem from this, and it is often difficult to recognise the more frequent reality of mutual interdependence. No man is an island, and yet we wish to believe we are independent of forces of which we may not be conscious, either from outside ourselves or from within. At times we are aware of these pulls within ourselves; at other times they overwhelm us and become the source of irrational group behaviour. While most obvious in crowds and large meetings, these same forces also influence smaller groups, such as teams and committees. This chapter will focus on groups at work, and how they are affected by unconscious processes.

The psychoanalytic study of unconscious processes in groups begins with Freud's *Group Psychology and the Analysis of the Ego* (1921). Essentially, Freud argued that the members of a group, particularly large groups such as crowds at political rallies, follow their leader because he or she personifies certain ideals of their own. The leader shows the group how to clarify and act on its goals. At the same time, the group members may

Source: Obholzer, A. and Zagier Roberts, V. (eds) (1994) *The Unconscious At Work. Individual and Organisational Stress in the Human Services*, London: Routledge.

project their own capacities for thinking, decision-making and taking authority on to the person of the leader and thereby become disabled. Rather than using their personal authority in the role of follower, the members of a group can become pathologically dependent, easily swayed one way or another by their idealisation of the leader. Criticism and challenge of the leader, which are an essential part of healthy group life, become impossible.

WILFRED BION AND BASIC ASSUMPTIONS IN GROUPS

A major contributor to our understanding of unconscious processes in groups was the psychoanalyst Wilfred Bion, who made a detailed study of the processes in small groups in the army during World War II, and later at the Tavistock Clinic. On the basis of these, he developed a framework for analysing some of the more irrational features of unconscious group life. His later work on psychosis, thinking and mental development (Bion 1967, 1977) has also contributed much to our understanding of groups and organisational processes. Bion himself wrote little further on groups as such, preferring to concentrate on the internal world of the individual. In fact, as he himself argues, the group and the psychoanalytic pair of psychoanalyst and analysand actually provide two different 'vertices' on human mental life and behaviour. Each is distinct but not mutually incompatible, just as, for example, physics and chemistry provide distinct levels of understanding of the material world. Indeed, the whole matter of the relationship between the individual and the group is a central theme throughout both Bion's work and his life (Armstrong 1992 and Menzies Lyth 1983 – for a further understanding of Bion's work see Anderson 1992; Meltzer 1978; and Symington 1986). This chapter concentrates solely on some of the implications for understanding groups and teams based on the ideas contained in Bion's *Experiences in Groups* (1961).

Bion distinguished two main tendencies in the life of a group: the tendency towards work on the primary task or *work-group mentality*, and a second, often unconscious, tendency to avoid work on the primary task, which he termed *basic assumption mentality*. These opposing tendencies can be thought of as the wish to face and work *with* reality, and the wish to evade it when it is painful or causes psychological conflict within or between group members.

The staff of a day centre spent a great deal of time arguing about whether or not the clients should have access to an electric kettle to make drinks with. Some were strongly of the opinion that this was too dangerous, while others were equally adamant that the centre should provide as normal an environment as possible. While there was a real policy issue, the argument was also an expression of the difficulty the staff were having with their angry and violent feelings towards their clients, who were behaving in ways that frustrated the staff's wish that they 'get better'. The fear of the clients' scalding themselves also contained a less conscious and unspoken wish to punish them. However, it was too painful for the staff to face these feelings. Instead, each time the ostensible problem was near to solution, some new objection would be raised, with the result that the group was in danger of spending the whole of its weekly team meeting on the matter of the kettle. An interpretation of this problem by the consultant enabled a deeper discussion of the ambivalent feelings, and a return to the group's work task: the exploration of working relations and practices in the centre.

In work-group mentality, members are intent on carrying out a specifiable task and want to assess their effectiveness in doing it. By contrast, in basic assumption mentality, the group's behaviour is directed at attempting to meet the unconscious needs of its members by reducing anxiety and internal conflicts.

THE THREE BASIC ASSUMPTIONS

How groups do this varies. According to Bion, much of the irrational and apparently chaotic behaviour we see in groups can be viewed as springing from *basic assumptions* common to all their members. He distinguished three basic assumptions, each giving rise to a particular complex of feelings, thoughts and behaviour: *basic assumption dependency*, *basic assumption fight-flight* and *basic assumption pairing*.

BASIC ASSUMPTION DEPENDENCY (baD)

A group dominated by baD behaves as if its primary task is solely to provide for the satisfaction of the needs and wishes of its members. The leader is expected to look after, protect and sustain the members of the group, to make them feel good, and not to face them with the demands of the group's real purpose. The leader serves as a focus for a pathological form of dependency which inhibits growth and development. For example, instead of addressing the difficult items on the agenda, a committee may endlessly postpone them to the next meeting. Any attempts to change the organisation are resisted, since this induces a fear of being uncared for. The leader may be absent or even dead, provided the illusion that he or she contains the solution can be sustained. Debates within the organisation may then be not so much about how to tackle present difficulties as about what the absent leader would have said or thought.

BASIC ASSUMPTION FIGHT-FLIGHT (baF)

The assumption here is that there is a danger or 'enemy', which should either be attacked or fled from. However, as Bion puts it, the group is prepared to do either indifferently. Members look to the leader to devise some appropriate action; their task is merely to follow. For instance, instead of considering how best to organise its work, a team may spend most of the time in meetings worrying about rumours of organisational change. This provides a spurious sense of togetherness, while also serving to avoid facing the difficulties of the work itself. Alternatively, such a group may spend its time protesting angrily, without actually planning any specific action to deal with the perceived threat to its service.

BASIC ASSUMPTION PAIRING (baP)

BaP is based on the collective and unconscious belief that, whatever the actual problems and needs of the group, a future event will solve them. The group behaves as if pairing or coupling between two members within the group, or perhaps between the leader of the group and some external person, will bring about salvation. The group is focused entirely on the future, but as a defence against the difficulties of the present. As Bion puts it, there is a conviction that the coming season will be more agreeable. In the case of a work team, this may take the form of an idea that improved premises would provide an answer to the group's problems, or that all will be well after the next annual study day. The group is in fact not interested in working practically towards this future, but only in sustaining a vague sense of hope as a way out of its current difficulties. Typically, decisions are either not taken or left extremely vague. After the meeting, members are inevitably left with a sense of disappointment and failure, which is quickly superseded by a hope that the next meeting will be better.

RECOGNISING BASIC ASSUMPTION ACTIVITY

The meetings of a group of psychologists to which I consulted would often start with a discussion of their frustration at decisions not having been implemented. At one meeting, the main topic for a considerable time was the previous meeting, whether it had been a good meeting or a bad meeting – it being entirely unclear what this meant. When I pointed this out, there followed a lengthy debate about the relative merits of various chairs, seating arrangements, and, finally, rooms in which to hold the meeting. Various improved ways of organising the meeting were proposed, but no decision was reached. I suggested there was a fear of discussing matters of real concern to the members present, perhaps a fear of conflict. At this point it emerged that there was indeed considerable controversy about a proposed appointment, some favouring one method, others another. Eventually a decision was almost reached, only to be resisted on the grounds that one significant member of the team was absent.

When under the sway of a basic assumption, a group appears to be meeting as if for some hard-to-specify purpose upon which the members seem intently set. Group members lose their critical faculties and individual abilities, and the group as a whole has the appearance of having some ill-defined but passionately involving mission. Apparently trivial matters are discussed as if they were matters of life or death, which is how they may well feel to the members of the group, since the underlying anxieties are about psychological survival.

In this state of mind, the group seems to lose awareness of the passing of time, and is apparently willing to continue endlessly with trivial matters. On the other hand, there is little capacity to bear frustration, and quick solutions are favoured. In both cases, members have lost their capacity to stay in touch with reality and its demands. Other external realities are also ignored or denied. For example, instead of seeking information, the group closes itself off from the outside world and retreats into paranoia. A questioning attitude is impossible; any who dare to do so are regarded as either foolish, mad or heretical. A new idea or formulation which might offer a way forward is likely to be too terrifying to consider because it involves questioning cherished assumptions, and loss of the familiar and predictable which is felt to be potentially catastrophic. At the prospect of any change, the group is gripped anew by panic, and the struggle for understanding is avoided. All this prevents both adaptive processes and development (Turquet 1974). Effective work, which involves tolerating frustration, facing reality, recognising differences among group members and learning from experience, will be seriously impeded.

LEADERSHIP AND FOLLOWERSHIP IN BASIC ASSUMPTION GROUPS

True leadership requires the identification of some problem requiring attention and action, and the promotion of activities to produce a solution. In basic assumption mentality, however, there is a collusive interdependence between the leader and the led, whereby the leader will be followed only as long as he or she fulfils the basic assumption task of the group. The leader in baD is restricted to providing for members' needs to be cared for. The baF leader must identify an enemy either within or outside the group, and lead the attack or flight. In baP, the leader must foster hope that the future will be better, while preventing actual change taking place. The leader who fails to behave in these ways will be ignored, and eventually the group will turn to an alternative leader. Thus the basic assumption leader is essentially a creation or puppet of the group, who is manipulated to fulfil its wishes and to evade difficult realities.

A leader or manager who is being pulled into basic assumption leadership is likely to experience feelings related to the particular nature of the group's unconscious demands. In baD there is a feeling of heaviness and resistance to change, and a preoccupation with status and hierarchy as the basis for decisions. In baF, the experience is of aggression and suspicion, and a preoccupation with the fine details of rules and procedures. In baP, the preoccupation is with alternative futures; the group may ask the leader to meet with some external authority to find a solution, full of insubstantial hopes for the outcome.

Members of such groups are both happy and unhappy. They are happy in that their roles are simple, and they are relieved of anxiety and responsibility. At the same time, they are unhappy insofar as their skills, individuality and capacity for rational thought are sacrificed, as are the satisfactions that come from working effectively. As a result, the members of such groups tend to feel continually in conflict about staying or leaving, somehow never able to make up their minds which they wish to do for any length of time. Since the group now contains split-off and projected capacities of its members, leaving would be experienced as losing these disowned parts. In work-group mentality, on the other hand, members are able to mobilise their capacity for co-operation and to value the different contributions each can make. They choose to follow a leader in order to achieve the group's task, rather than doing so in an automatic way determined by their personal needs.

THE MULTIDISCIPLINARY TEAM

I wish now to look at the effects of the interplay between work-group mentality and basic assumption mentality functioning in a particular situation – the multidisciplinary team. Such teams are to be found in both public and private sector settings. For example, a health centre may be staffed by several doctors, a team of nurses, social workers, counsellors, a team of midwives and a number of administrative staff. In industry, management teams will consist of individuals from production, marketing, sales, audit, personnel and so on. In universities and schools, teams consist of staff teaching a range of subjects, the heads of different departments, together with administrators and others.

Teams such as these often have difficulty developing a coherent and shared common purpose, since their members come from different trainings with different values, priorities and preoccupations. Often, too, team members are accountable to different superiors, who may not be part of the team. This is an important and yet often ignored reality which leads to the illusion that the team is in a position to make certain policy decisions which, in fact, it is not. Considerable time can be wasted on discussions which cannot result in decisions, instead of exploring ways the actual decision-makers can be influenced in the desired direction.

The meetings of such teams typically have a rather vague title such as 'staff meeting' or 'planning meeting'. Their main purpose may well be simply for those present to 'meet' in order to give a sense of artificial togetherness and cohesion as a refuge from the pressures of work. The use of the word 'team' here is somewhat misleading: there may be little actual day-to-day work in common. Indeed, because of a lack of clarity about the primary task, confusion, frustration and bad feeling may actually be engendered by such meetings, interfering with work. The real decisions about work practices are often made elsewhere – over coffee, in corridors, in private groups, between meetings but not in them. Furthermore, such decisions as are taken may well not be implemented, because it is rare for anyone in the group to have the authority to ensure they are carried out.

Task-oriented teams have a defined common purpose and a membership determined by the requirements of the task. Thus, in a multidisciplinary team, each member would have a specific contribution to make. Often, the reality is more like a collection of individuals agreeing to be a group when it suits them, while threatening to disband whenever there is serious internal conflict. It is as if participation were a voluntary choice, rather than that there is a task which they must co-operate in order to achieve. The spurious sense of togetherness is used to obscure these problems and as a defence against possible conflicts. Even the conflicts themselves may be used to avoid more fundamental anxieties about the work by preventing commitment to decisions and change.

BASIC ASSUMPTIONS IN DIFFERENT PROFESSIONS

So far I have referred to basic assumptions as defensive or regressive manifestations of group life. However, Bion (1961) also refers to what he termed the *sophisticated use of basic assumption mentality*, an important but lesser-known part of his theory. Here, Bion suggests that a group may utilise the basic assumption mentalities in a sophisticated way, by mobilising the emotions of one basic assumption in the constructive pursuit of the primary task.

An example of such sophisticated and specialised use of baD can be found in a well-run hospital ward. An atmosphere of efficiency and calm is used to mobilise baD, encouraging patients to give themselves over to the nurses or doctors in a trusting, dependent way. BaF is utilised by an army to keep on the alert, and, when required, to go into battle without disabling consideration for personal safety. In social work, baF supports the task of fighting or fleeing from family, social and environmental conditions or injustices which are harmful to the client. BaP finds a sophisticated use in the therapeutic situation, where the pairing between a staff member and a patient can provide a background sense of hope in order to sustain the setbacks inevitable in any treatment.

In trying to understand some of the difficulties of multidisciplinary work, it is helpful to understand the different sophisticated uses of basic assumption mentality adopted by the various professions or disciplines that make up a team. Fights for supremacy in a multidisciplinary team can then be viewed as the inevitable psychological clash between the sophisticated use of the three basic assumptions. Each carries with it a different set of values and a different set of views about the nature of the problem, its cure, what constitutes progress, and whether this is best achieved by a relationship between professional and client involving dependency, fight-flight or pairing. Furthermore, individuals are drawn to one profession or another partly because of their unconscious predisposition or *valency* for one basic assumption rather than another. As a result, they are particularly likely to contribute to the interdisciplinary group processes without questioning them.

Put another way, one of the difficulties in making a team out of different professions is that each profession operates through the deliberate harnessing of different sophisticated forms of the basic assumptions in order to further the task. There is consequently conflict when they meet, since the emotional motivations involved in each profession differ. However, conflict need not preclude collaboration on a task, provided there is a process of clarifying shared goals and the means of achieving these. However, difficulties in carrying out the task for which the team is in existence can lead to a breakdown in the sophisticated use of the various basic assumptions, and instead *aberrant* forms of each emerge. Examining these can illuminate some of the frequently encountered workplace tensions in teamwork.

For instance, medical training involves an institutionalised, prolonged dependency of junior doctors on their seniors over many years, from which the medical consultant eventually emerges and then defends his new independence. This can degenerate into an insistence on freedom for its own sake. The doctor may then operate from a counterdependent state of mind, denying the mutual interdependency of teamwork and the actual dependency on the institutional setting of hospital or clinic. This can extend to other professionals, each arguing for their own area of independence, with rivalry and embittered conflict impeding thought and work on establishing shared overall objectives for the team.

By contrast, the training of therapists – whether of psychological, occupational, speech or other varieties – tends to idealise the pairing between therapist and client as the pre-eminent medium for change. Aberrant baP can lead to collusion in supporting this activity, while refusing to examine whether or not it is in fact helping, or how it relates to the team's primary task. Indeed, therapist and client may remain endlessly 'glued' together as if the generation of hope about the future were by itself a cure.

In social work, the sophisticated use of baF in the productive fight against social or family injustices can degenerate into a particular kind of litigious demand that justice be done, and on 'getting our rights'. Responsibility for improvement is felt to rest not at all with the individual, but solely with the community. Projecting responsibility in this way then disables the client and social worker from devising together any effective course of action: it is only others that must change.

These are examples where the capacity for the sophisticated use of basic assumption activity has degenerated, and the professional's action and thought becomes dominated by its aberrant forms. Each then produces a particular group culture. Aberrant baD gives rise to a *culture of subordination* where authority derives entirely from position in the hierarchy, requiring unquestioning obedience. Aberrant baP produces a *culture of collusion*, supporting pairs of members in avoiding truth rather than seeking it. There is attention to the group's mission, but not to the means of achieving it. Aberrant baF results in a *culture of paranoia and aggressive competitiveness*, where the group is preoccupied not only by an external enemy but also by 'the enemy within'. Rules and regulations proliferate to control both the internal and the external 'bad objects'. Here it is the means which are explicit and the ends which are vague.

CONCLUSION

In a group taken over by basic assumption mentality, the formation and continuance of the group becomes an end in itself. Leaders and members of groups dominated by basic assumption activity are likely to lose their ability to think and act effectively: continuance of the group becomes an end in itself, as members become more absorbed with their relationship to the group than with their work task. In this chapter, we have seen how the functioning of teams can be promoted by the sophisticated use of a basic assumption in the service of work, or impeded and distracted by their inappropriate or aberrant use. [. . .]

REFERENCES

Anderson, R. (ed.) (1992) *Clinical Lectures on Klein and Bion*, London/New York: Tavistock/Routledge.

Armstrong, D. (1991) 'Thoughts bounded and thoughts free', paper to Department of Psychotherapy, Cambridge.

Bion, W. (1961) *Experiences in Groups*, New York: Basic Books (see 'Selections from: Experiences in Groups', in A.D. Colman and W.H. Bexton (eds) *Group Relations Reader 1*, A.K. Rice Institute Series [Washington, DC], 1975).

Bion, W. (1967) 'Attacks on linking', in *Second Thoughts: Selected Papers on Psychoanalysis*, London: Heinemann Medical (reprinted London: Maresfield Reprints, 1984).

Bion, W. (1977) *Seven Servants*, New York: Jason Aronson.

Meltzer, D. (1978) *The Kleinian Development*, Perthshire: Clunie Press.

Menzies Lyth, I.E.P. (1983) 'Bion's contribution to thinking about groups', in Grotstein, J.S. (ed.) *Do I Dare Disturb the Universe?*, London: Maresfield Library.

Symington, N. (1986) *The Analytic Experience: Lectures from the Tavistock*, London: Free Association Books.

Turquet, P. (1974) 'Leadership: the individual and the group', in Colman, A.D. and Geller, M.H. (eds) *Group Relations Reader 2*, A.K. Rice Institute Series [Washington, DC], 1985.

CHAPTER 33

IMAGINISING TEAMWORK

Gareth Morgan

In this chapter, my aim is to throw light on some taken-for-granted images that shape how we think about teamwork and to offer some fresh ideas for developing teamwork in practice.

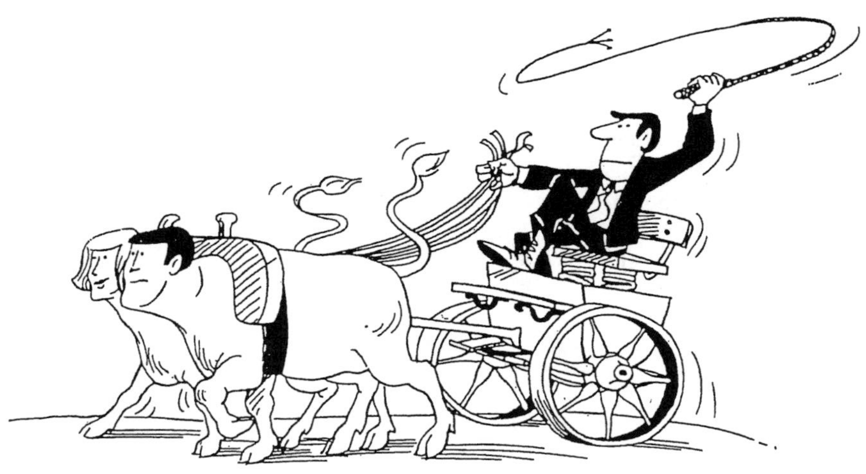

Source: *Imaginization: The Art of Creative Management* (1993) London: Sage, 195–213.

TEAM METAPHORS

'Come on, Jack. You're not being a team player'. It's one of the ultimate corporate insults.

The accusation has great normative power, because teamwork has become a sacred aspect of management. It conveys the idea that Jack, like every reasonable person, *should* be 'pulling his weight' or devoting himself to the cause.

Yet what does teamwork mean? In what ways is Jack out of line?

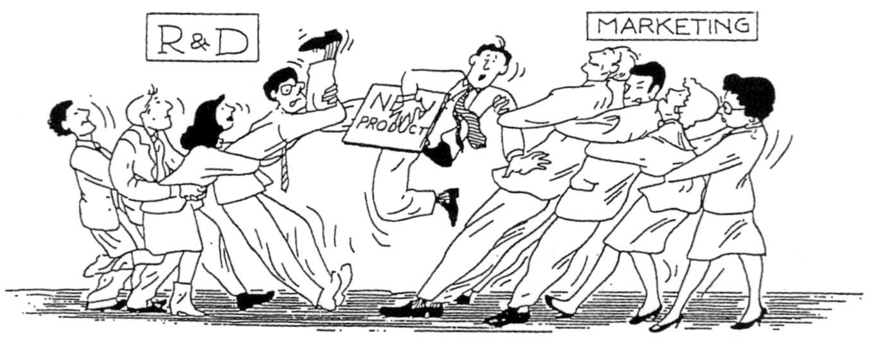

The word *team* was originally used to describe a 'family or brood' or a set of draft animals like oxen, horses, or dogs harnessed to pull and work together.

Is that what we have in mind? Are we asking Jack to act like one of the family? To pull like an ox or draft horse? Or, as is more common nowadays under the influence of sports culture, are we asking him to play some kind of game?

If so, what's the game?

- American football?
- Soccer?
- Basketball?
- Baseball?
- Hockey?
- Rowing?
- Volleyball?
- Rock climbing?
- Tug-of-war?

As Robert Keidel shows us in his book *Corporate Players*, each image carries very different implications for the role of team members, for the role of 'coach' or manager, and for how the detailed 'game' unfolds. [...]

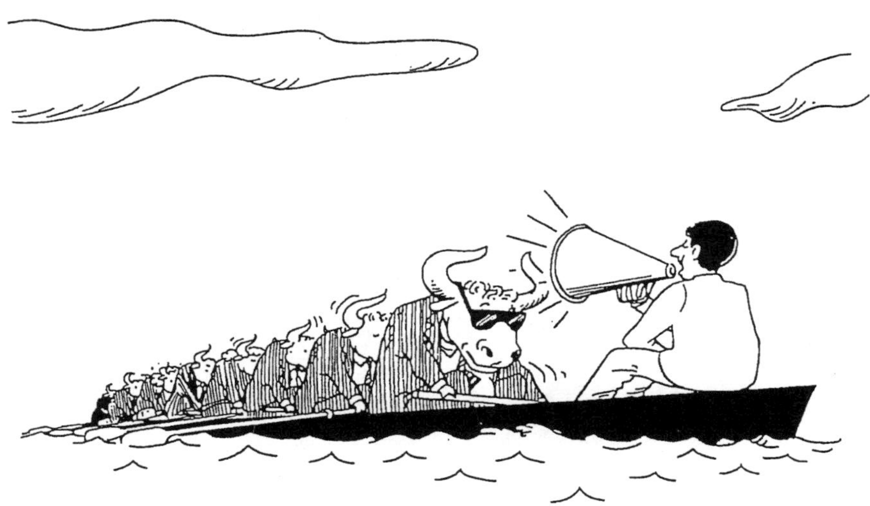

In any organisation of any complexity, there may be a need for different kinds of teamwork. Some areas may need to have the direction and synchronicity of a rowing crew; others may need to be guided by the strong hand of a football coach. Others, as in baseball, may need to cultivate cooperation between a group of solid players who rely for their ultimate success on the unpredictable efforts of a few true stars. Others may need the self-organising qualities of volleyball, soccer, or basketball. Others may need to develop the organisational equivalent of rock climbing, creating a sense of interdependence and mutual trust that will allow people to take great personal risks. And so on!

Each of these images of teamwork implies a very different strategy for creating effective teamwork in practice. So, as suggested in Figure 33.1, it's often a good idea to think quite systematically about the kind of teamwork that's required and about the team metaphors through which it is best shaped.

That's one of the central messages of this chapter, and it helps to explain why so many attempts at creating teamwork have run into trouble. The harsh reality in many organisations is that, while teamwork is a high priority and has often been the focus of massive expenditures, results are mediocre. Indeed, in many organisations, the concept of *teamwork* has become discredited; it exists as an empty buzzword.

Yet, to find the reasons, one only has to look at the incongruities that are usually reflected in the results of an exercise like that in Figure 33.1 and identify where the ruling team metaphor breaks down.

I don't think we need to say any more about the oxen. For who, after all, wants to be driven in this way?

Here's a simple exercise for thinking about teamwork:

What team-building metaphors are appropriate in *your* organisation and *where*?

	Appropriate metaphors
Organisational unit	
Type and quality of existing teamwork	
The teamwork we should be aiming for	

Figure 33.1 Teamwork can take many forms.

But, when it comes to the failure of sports metaphors, the situation is a little more interesting. One important factor, as I've mentioned above and illustrated through some of the cartoons, is that people are not always playing the right game or even the same game. Another rests in the fact that managers can easily get carried away with the kind of experience that

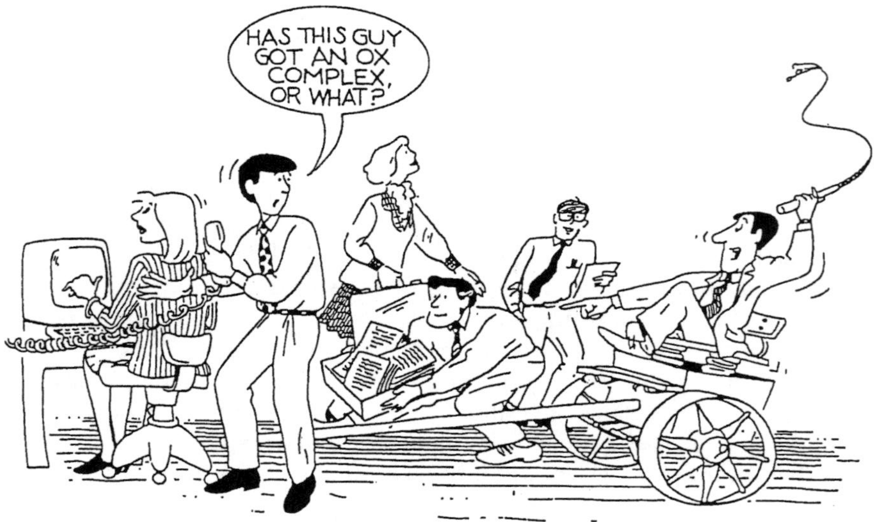

they've had of teamwork in sports settings. It's great to be on a team that's playing well. And knowledge of great games, great teams, and great coaches can provide wonderful role models and points of reference for shaping activities in one's organisation.

Hi ! I'm the New Manager.
WHAT THE HELL IS GOING ON?

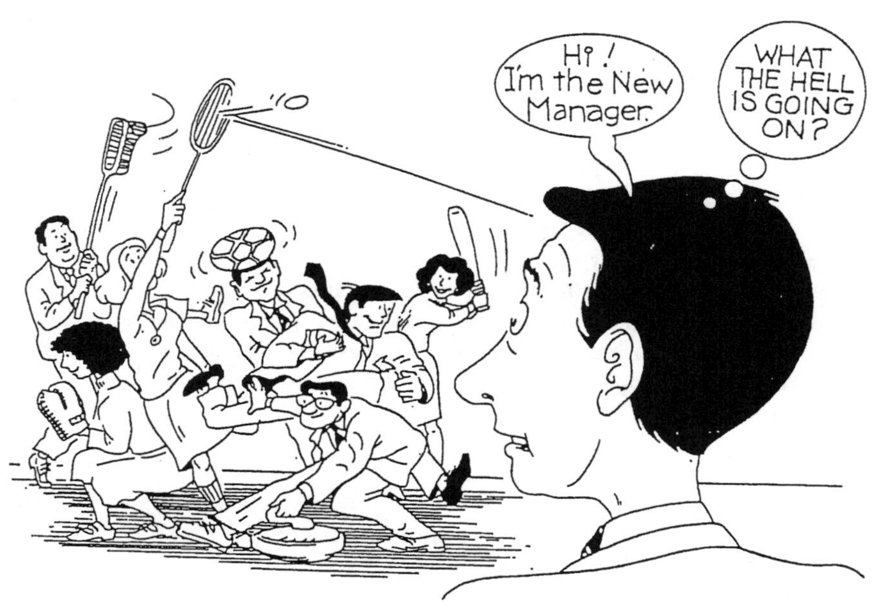

But it's easy to forget that there's an enormous distance between 'the big game' on the television, or on the sports field, and the humdrum existence in the factory or office in which the team metaphor is to be applied.

The situation here can be completely different:

- No big game atmosphere;
- Sometimes, no obvious competition in sight;
- Diffuse, ambiguous goals;
- Political conflicts;
- Divergent interests.

[. . .]

BUILDING TEAMWORK IN DIFFICULT SITUATIONS

The reality facing many managers is that simple calls for teamwork are likely to fall on deaf ears...

Most employees are far too sophisticated to take such calls seriously, especially if they are working in difficult, fragmented, and politicised contexts or where diversity and creative dissent are essential to the work being done. Simple sports metaphors or packaged approaches to teamwork don't resonate. They tend to be too superficial. And they tend to stress and encourage more uniformity and coherence than the nature or demands of many situations allow.

In these circumstances, it is often much more productive to turn our capacities for imaginisation in a new direction. Instead of just calling for teamwork, or extolling the virtues of great causes, great games, or great players, it may be much more effective to initiate processes that create new patterns of shared understanding that address the barriers and blocks to teamwork in practice and find realistic ways of mobilising and coordinating efforts.

To illustrate, I will draw on the work of Michael Walton, a British management consultant who uses a highly visual method of imaginisation to explore organisational problems and to find ways of building team cultures in difficult settings. One of his approaches involves creating a context where individuals and groups can develop independent and shared images of their situation and explore common and divergent understandings in novel ways. [...]

The following illustration of the method in practice involves the Personnel Department of a large energy company.

FOOTBALL, SKIERS, ROCKETS, AND RACING CARS

[...]

The Personnel Department, which was responsible for the whole spectrum of human resource management functions, had been charged with helping the company adjust to major new changes in management practice. Its task was to develop a corporate culture that encouraged managers to help, encourage, support, motivate, and coach their staff rather than just to engage in 'top-down' evaluations focusing on 'bottom line performance'.

But Personnel was in a state of major disarray itself. The department was internally fragmented and overloaded with work. There had been an influx of new staff, and there was a wide variety of skill levels. Internal cohesion was at an all-time low.

To remedy the situation, Michael was invited to help. Fourteen senior managers attended a two-and-a-half-day meeting to set the stage for a formal review of the department's role and responsibilities and to explore links with the rest of the organisation. [...]

After a brief introduction from Michael, two groups of seven managers were set to work imaging current and future realities.

One of the groups represented the current reality within Personnel as the dismembered football player illustrated in Figure 33.2. As can be seen,

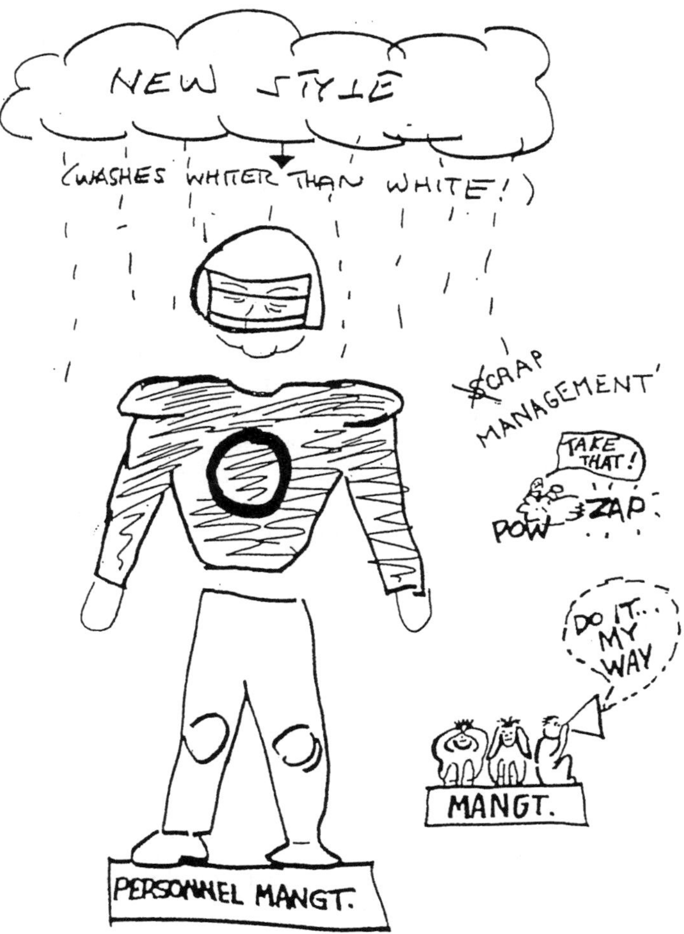

Figure 33.2 The dismembered football player.

NOTE: The illustrations presented in this and the next three figures were originally drawn on large sheets of flip chart paper with coloured pens. They have been reproduced to scale.

each part of the body is solid and well proportioned but disjointed. The strong, capable image stands on a firm base of professional personnel management, but, as the group reported, it couldn't get its act together because the legs are not connected with the trunk, and the trunk is not connected with the head, the directing force. There was a real sense of surprise and shock when the image was disclosed. It immediately seemed to make sense, but there was embarrassment about being so split into separate parts. At the same time, there was deep recognition of the inherent strength of the image and an immediate sense of just how able, powerful, and influential the department *could* be if it could find a way of working together.

The group went on to describe the effect of the current organisational changes in terms of the motifs surrounding the football player. The new management style was presented as a dark rain cloud accompanied by the cryptic comment: 'Washes whiter than white'. The slogan played on the laundry detergent commercials that promise perfect results. Cynicism was rife. The group felt that management were making great promises but, in a way, whitewashing the reality. It took more than words on paper, or a directive from above, to create a new culture. They felt that top management would have to show their continuing commitment to the desired change, through deeds as well as words. There would have to be new recognition of the importance of collaboration and rewards for working in a different way.

Further aspects of this cynicism are captured in the side comments around the football player: about 'scrap management' and 'crap management' and the accompanying fighting motifs of 'Pow', 'Zap', and 'Take That'. These slogans were used to convey the macho bottom line culture that dominated the current organisation with its win-lose undertone. A clash with the more collaborative culture that management was now calling for seemed inevitable. The organisation was very macho, a point captured in the very idea of representing the department as a football player. It was unlikely that the strengths of the current style of organisation would be thrown away lightly, so the Personnel group felt quite intimidated by its task.

Further concerns and cynicism were symbolised through the famous image of the three monkeys – one closing its eyes to what was happening, the other refusing to hear what was happening, and the third shouting, 'Do it my way'!

The image of current reality produced by the second group featured the chaotic ski school illustrated in Figure 33.3. Skiers on all three runs, coloured green, blue, and black to characterise three levels of increasing difficulty, are in various states of disarray. Those on the beginner's green run are confused and calling for help. Those on the blue run are crashing and buried in snow. Those on the experienced black run are having a better time, negotiating their obstacle course, enjoying the risk, and moving toward the finish. Meanwhile, the instructors are shown removed

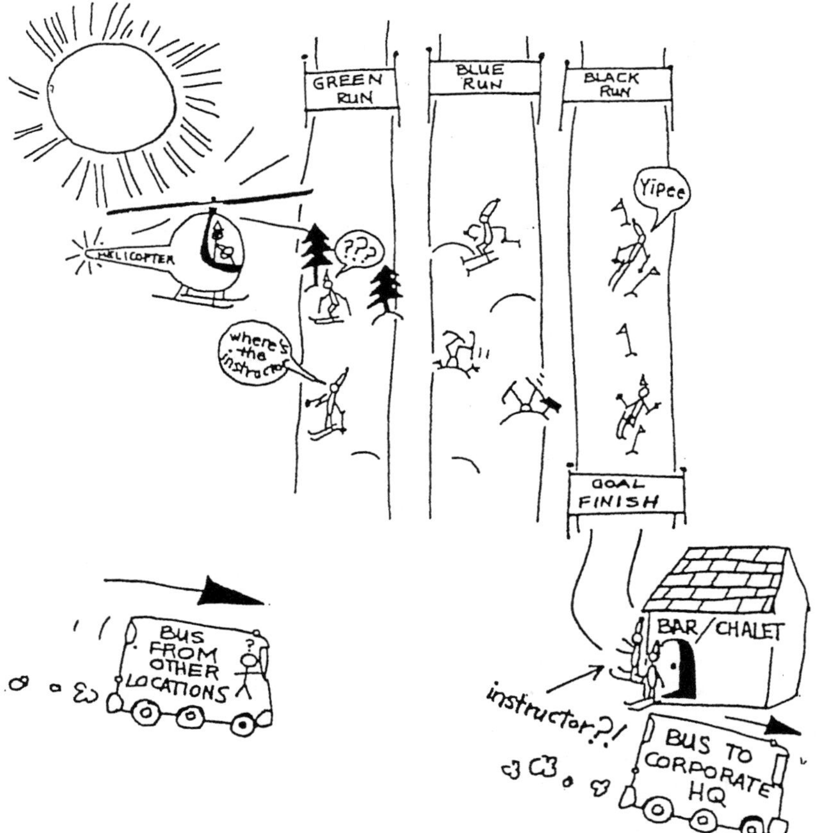

Figure 33.3 The chaotic ski school.

from the immediate problems and concerns, enjoying the bar and chalet. The recent movement of staff in and out of the department was represented by two buses, one bringing people in from other locations in the company, the other taking them to company headquarters. Meanwhile, the sun shines in the top left-hand corner, and a helicopter is hovering overhead, ready to remove casualties when necessary.

Michael Walton reports that the overall mood of this group's presentation was one of anger and great annoyance with senior management. There was a feeling that those at the top perceived them as novices and that inadequate support was being given to them in undertaking what was an extremely difficult task. This is reflected throughout their image of the ski slopes and in the separation of interests between the instructors in the bar and the people on the ski hills. The mood was one of great worry, concern, and conflict. Even though top managers regarded Personnel Department staff as novices or, at best, as intermediates, they *still* expected them to deliver the new culture in a 'hard-bitten' and 'hostile' environment.

Here was the contradiction between the macho and supportive cultures highlighted by the first group, but in a new form. It was believed that top management, critical and judgemental in the manner encouraged by the old culture, could not be counted on for support in developing the new. They were 'boozing it up in the bar', waiting for people to either crash or make it down the hills by themselves. Given these circumstances, the group felt that it was vital for the Personnel Department to become as professional and mutually supportive as it could in approaching the current challenge.

The images created by both groups thus had a great deal of consistency, speaking to the stress, division, contradiction, and frustration inherent in the current state of affairs as well as to the challenges that lay ahead. There was an emotional atmosphere, with the main messages ringing clear and true. With appropriate integration and development of their fragmented skills and abilities, and support from top management, staff believed that they *could* make a major contribution. But the route was uncertain and paved with problems. The imagery helped to express many of the hidden feelings and insecurities that were lurking in the group.

With these feelings fully vented, and the issues placed clearly on the table, attention was then directed to the future. Following individual reflection and group desired discussion, the two groups produced the imagery presented in Figures 33.4 and 33.5.

The dismembered-footballer group developed the theme 'Personnel Strikes Back' (Figure 33.4). Their image, rich in bright, fluorescent colour, created an overall shining effect, with a rocket ship being launched toward the organisational problems, represented by a planet in space, but supported by mission control (top management) back on the ground. Flowers bloom in red and yellow. The person riding the rocket ship (symbolising the staff of the department) and the senior manager, in mission control, are smiling and positive, approaching the organisational problems directly, together, and with confidence. But the image also recognises some of the difficulties. Parts of head office are still lost in space, symbolised by the person riding the set of golf clubs. The mood of the group was, however, optimistic and communicated its hope for an integrated and well-focused department.

The image of the desired future situation produced by the second group (Figure 33.5) was also very positive. It showed the company winning the 'Energy Grand Prix' as a powerful, smart, effective, well-tuned racing car about to take the checkered flag. Personnel is depicted as the racing support team in the pits, providing the 'Superlube' and the 'Can Do' attitude required to make the car run well. The staff are smiling. The spectators are supportive, enjoying the achievements of the number-one car as

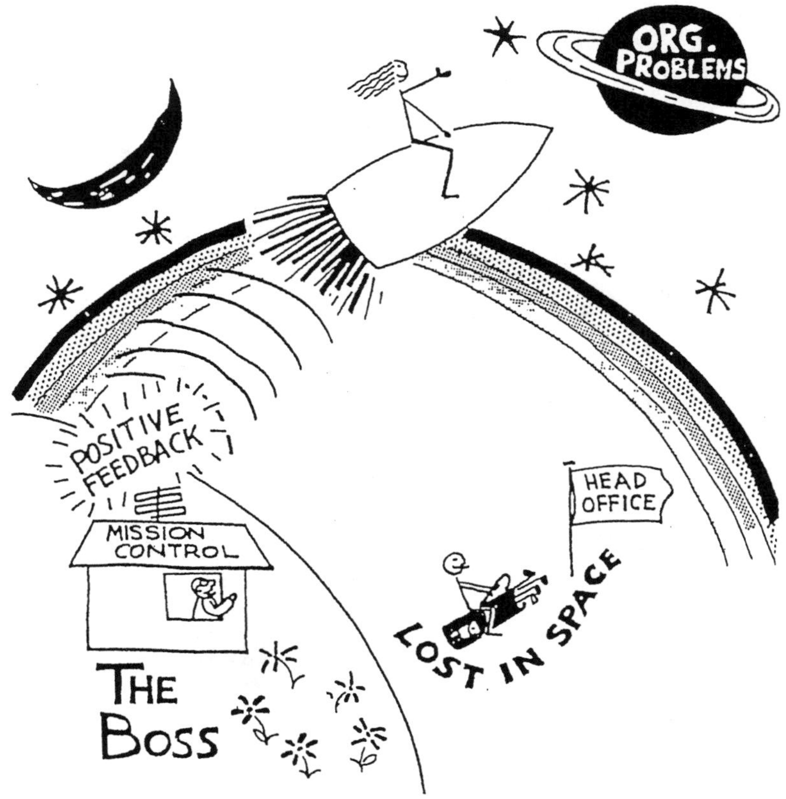

Figure 33.4 'Personnel strikes back'.

it speeds ahead of its rivals, the firm's main competitors. The competitors' cars are smaller, less glamorous, and less colourful, and one is skidding off the track.

In this way, both images emphasised a sense of integration, momentum, direction, and collaboration – qualities that were conspicuously absent in both groups' descriptions of their current reality. The images were still very macho and closely linked with the current culture but were much more colourful, positive, and optimistic in basic orientation.

The team-building session had a major catalytic effect on those present. It surfaced key problems and provided vivid illustrations of what people

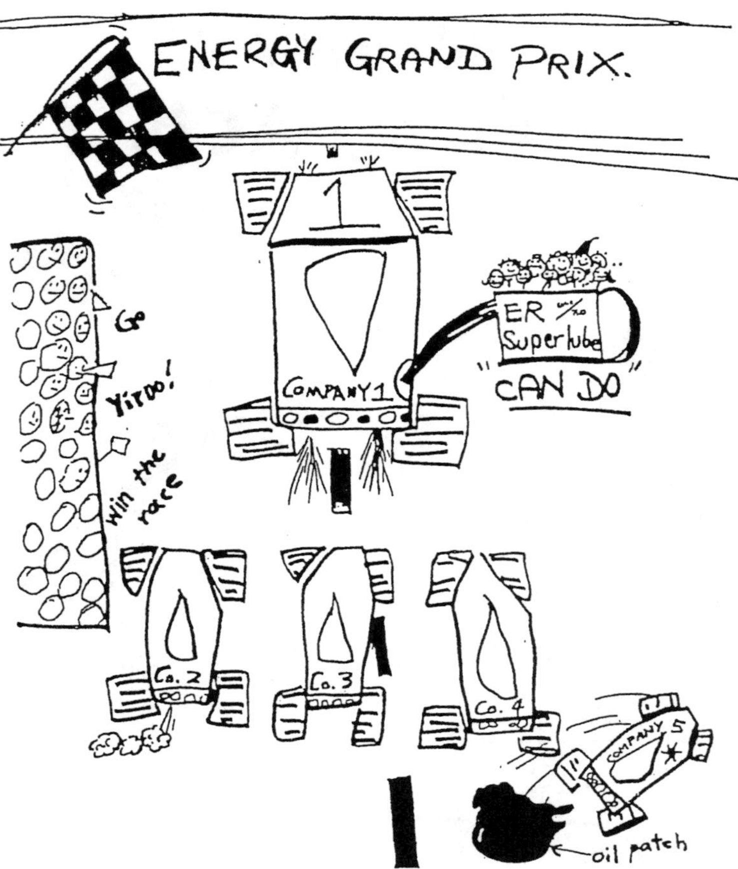

Figure 33.5 'Energy grand prix'.

wanted to achieve. In just a few hours, Michael was able to take a group that was cynical and divided and help them talk frankly and freely about the difficulties in their situation. As Michael puts it:

> *It was as if a curtain had been drawn back as they confronted what they were dealing with. They were fragmented, drifting, and faced with an extremely difficult task. The imaging process allowed them to develop a deeper shared understanding of what lay ahead ... The humor lightened the atmosphere, and helped to release a positive energy that began to create a feeling that 'we're a team; we can work together to overcome our difficulties'! It was as if a magnet had been introduced into the situation, and all the iron filings that were lying in different directions came together.*

The process helped to draw the head of the department closer to his staff and allowed them to work on the challenges being faced. They now had common reference points that they didn't have before and began to become much more collaborative and cohesive. The positive energy also spread beyond those involved in the exercise. As new staff picked up on the energy, a new team culture began to emerge. The whole experience became a major staging point in the development of the department. [...]

In many organisations, teamwork has become trapped by formal team building, because, in more ways than one, it has become just a game! In such circumstances, it is much more powerful to develop processes of imaginisation that will help people build from their own feelings and experiences, so that they can create a truly shared understanding of problems and challenges rather than operating within frameworks imposed by others.

REFERENCES

Keidel, R. (1988) *Corporate Players*, New York: John Wiley.

Taylor, F.W. (1911) *Principles of Scientific Management*, New York: Harper & Row.

CHAPTER 34

GOING HOME FROM HOSPITAL – AN APPRECIATIVE INQUIRY STUDY

Jan Reed, Pauline Pearson, Barbara Douglas, Stella Swinburne and Helen Wilding

INTRODUCTION

This chapter reports on a project (carried out in Newcastle) that involved a number of agencies and groups, including older people, working together to examine and develop practice in an area of shared concern – going home from hospital. The project was stimulated by a 'whole-system event', and was based on appreciative inquiry (AI) methodology, which has roots in both action research and organisational development. In AI, the research is directed towards appreciating what it is about the social world that is positive, and exploring this. The study was planned around three workshops to streamline data collection and analysis. Group members were also required to carry out some activities between workshops. Invitations were sent out to groups and individuals previously identified as involved or interested in the discharge process across one health district ($n = 71$). Workshop one discussed the planned research schedule, and introduced the basic concepts of AI. This workshop also took participants through the interview process. Each participant was asked to undertake two interviews. Thirty-five individual interviews and one focus group were completed. At workshop two, interview data were analysed by the group using the nominal group technique. Subsequent group discussion produced 'provocative propositions'. At the third workshop, provocative propositions were developed into

Source: *Health and Social Care in the Community* (2002) 10 (1): 36–45, Oxford: Blackwell.

action plans. This paper gives an overview of the study, and explores some of the issues involved when working with service users and providers as co-researchers. [...]

METHODOLOGY – APPRECIATIVE INQUIRY

Appreciative Inquiry (AI) has roots in both action research and organisational development (Bushe 1995). Cooperrider and Srivastva (1987) have argued that action research is restricted by its implicit positivist assumptions about a world 'out there' that can be described objectively and engineered effectively. AI, on the other hand, represents a move towards a social constructionist position in which the social world is created and constructed by the debates that we have about it (Steier 1991) and the method of enquiry used to explore a social world is part of this debate. In AI, as the term indicates, the research is directed towards appreciating what it is about the social world that is positive and exploring this.

Bushe (1995) cautions against offering a 'recipe' for how to do AI, given that it is an approach in its early stages of development. However, he does offer a summary: 'Appreciative Inquiry, as a method of changing social systems, is an attempt to generate a collective image of a new and better future by exploring the best of what is and has been' (Busche 1995: 14).

He goes on to refer to Cooperrider and Srivastva's (1987) description of four basic principles: that research should begin with appreciation, should be applicable, should be provocative (i.e. stimulate fresh thinking) and should be collaborative. Translating these principles into a process of enquiry, Bushe has described how a project would proceed, going through the following stages:

> *A grounded observation of the 'best of what is', then through exercises in vision and logic collaboratively articulate 'what might be', developing consensus and obtaining the consent of those in the system to 'what should be' and collectively experimenting with 'what can be'.*
>
> (Bushe 1995: 15)

As an aid to this process, AI projects use specific exercises. For example, a 'miracle question' is used to generate ideas of 'what might be': after identifying the best of what is, participants are asked what the world would look like if a miracle occurred overnight and they woke up to find a world in which everything was in place to support the best happening all of the time. In another exercise, participants are asked to generate 'provocative propositions', statements of aspirations that challenge (rather than conform with) the way that things currently happen in the system (Hammond 1996). As an approach to organisational and community development, AI has been used with a variety of different groups, from religious and legal organisations to one project that tried to create new ways of improving life across Chicago (Ludema 1993).

Therefore, AI offered a framework that had been successfully used in large and complex systems, and that reflected the aims of the group – to explore the innovations and developments that were taking place across the system – in a way that would not become problem-focused and prevent the ability to move beyond this. However, agreeing on this basic framework still involved the research team in a complex process of planning in order to make the group project effective and systematic.

THE DESIGN OF THE STUDY

Invitations to participate were sent out to a range of different agencies and individuals who had been involved in the 'going home from hospital' event, or had expressed interest in these activities. Seventy-one individuals responded to say that they would be interested in taking part in a study to explore ways of improving the experience of going home from hospital. [...]

In order to streamline data collection and analysis, the study was planned around three workshops, to which all participants in the original group were invited to participate. The workshops would also require group members to carry out some activities between workshops. However, the design of the study could not be determined precisely before the study began, as the nature of collaboration (across agencies and groups) meant that flexibility and responsiveness had to be an important theme of the study – attempts to rigidly specify study design would alienate participants and reduce the ability of the study to respond to emerging ideas. Therefore, the core group developed an overall plan, but realised that the study would develop organically as participants developed ideas about the way in which it should be carried out. Thus, the workshops were as detailed in Table 34.1.

WORKSHOP ONE

This workshop was attended by people from 37 different organisations, including older people's groups, hospital and community trusts, the local authority, voluntary agencies and the private care sector. The purpose of

Table 34.1 Workshop sequence

Workshop	*Activity*	*Data generated*	*Stage of AI*
One	Introducing the project and developing AI interview skills	Workshop interviews and subsequent interviews that group members carried out in the workplace or peer groups	Appreciating the best of 'what is'
Two	Group members analysed interview data to develop a series of 'provocative propositions' about goals and aims expressed in the interviews	List of 'provocative propositions'	Envisioning 'what might be' and 'what should be'
Three	Group members looked at provocative propositions to develop a series of action plans.	Action plans	Planning 'what could be'

the workshop was to present and discuss the planned research schedule and to introduce the basic concepts of AI. The workshop was also a training session, which took participants through the process of carrying out AI interviews, so that they could then carry these out in the workplace or with their peer group. Because of the large number of people involved as data collectors, there was potential for interviews, and therefore data, to vary considerably. Group members practiced their interview techniques, but also requested guidelines to take with them; these were subsequently developed and distributed.

The interviews were semi-structured using a common schedule that began with interviewers asking people to tell them about a time when they felt that a hospital discharge had gone well, and then included some probing questions to explore what people had valued about their contribution to it and what they felt had helped them to contribute. They were then asked the 'miracle question' (Hammond 1996) – they were asked to imagine that a miracle had occurred overnight that had helped discharge to go well every time. They were then asked to tell the interviewer what would be different about the world after the miracle, what would be in place, what would be happening and what the results would be. The responses to the interview questions were recorded in interviewers notes (as tape recording equipment was not available for all the interviewers), and these were passed back to the interviewee for confirmation. Where there were differences in interpretation between interviewer and interviewee, researchers were asked to record the interviewees' views.

In the workshop, participants found the interview process comfortable and effective, and felt confident about carrying out further interviews. Those who were working for a helping agency were asked to interview a colleague and/or a client. Some people felt that this might be difficult, either because their colleague was senior to them or because clients might feel inhibited; in these cases, the older people in the group were asked to carry out these interviews. The older people in the group also interviewed friends and members of organisations, such as church groups, to which they had access. Participants were asked to send their interview notes to the co-ordinating group so they could be copied and distributed to members before the next workshop. As tape-recording interviews was not possible because of resource constraints, there was discussion in the workshops about the importance of making clear and accurate notes, and confirming these with interviewees.

WORKSHOP TWO

At this workshop, the data from the interviews were analysed by the group. Thirty-five interviews had been conducted by the group, and notes were brought to the workshop. The processes of analysis with such a large number of researchers was likely to prove very complex, and so a structured approach was needed to ensure consistency. The use of multiple researchers to analyse data is not as well explored in methodological literature as is analysis by single researchers – Miles and Huberman's (1994) text on qualitative data analysis, for example, does not mention analysis by multiple researchers at all. While data collection and analysis by single researchers is an individual activity that requires an analytical or theoretical framework in order to ensure validity (Miles and Huberman 1994), applying these frameworks to analysis by a group presents particular problems. The group had different views and experiences, and in this study did not have any research training; this meant that they approached the data from many different perspectives. Therefore, it was necessary to identify a strategy for analysis that would encompass the diversity of views and ideas, and to build from these to come to a consensus about the implications of the data for change. The workshop therefore began by using nominal group technique (Delbecq 1975) to identify what the group thought were the key themes in the data. In nominal group technique, the aim is to explore the range of views within a group and arrive at a consensus that reflects this range and also identifies priorities that the group share. Participants were therefore divided into three groups, each with a facilitator, and were asked initially to simply write down three key themes or ideas that they had identified in the data. These were all recorded on a flip chart, and a process of refinement and clarification was carried out through group discussion, with some points being 'collapsed' as they were very similar or closely related, and others being expanded in order to be more specific.

Following nominal group technique procedures, the results of the small group discussions were displayed to the whole group, and a process of grouping took place, in which individual themes were linked together by participants. The areas agreed upon are reproduced in Table 34.2, along with some illustrative quotes, and these were used as the basis for the next exercise, where groups then tried to develop 'provocative propositions' from them. Provocative propositions (Hammond 1996) are challenging statements of goals developed in the AI process; participants are encouraged to think creatively and radically and to move beyond the restrictions of current practice and constraints in order to articulate ideal states. This involved taking the area, revisiting the responses to the miracle questions in the interviews, drawing on members' own personal experiences and translating these into statements about what the ideal would be. For example, if the area was 'working across agencies', the group might develop a provocative proposition that 'everyone in the system should understand everyone else's role'. A list of the provocative propositions that resulted is given in Table 34.3.

WORKSHOP THREE

In the third workshop, the provocative propositions were pinned on the walls, and participants were asked to choose one that they felt most

Table 34.2 Key themes identified from the interviews by the research group

Theme	*Illustration*
Understanding	In many of the positive instances cited by people in the initial AI interviews, a factor that they identified was the knowledge that they had of the system outside their own particular group or organisation. Knowing what roles and functions other organisations and workers had was valued as an aid to planning and organising discharges. 'If I were running the Health Services I would train everybody in the importance of talking to each other – I mean the hospitals and the people outside'.
Co-ordination	Making sure that the right things happened at the right time was important, and also the avoidance of gaps in support or overlaps. 'Good practice doesn't depend on money or resources, but on systems being organised and working well'.
Empowerment	Some participants remarked that a feature of the good discharge they remembered was that the patients and carers felt 'in charge'. Other participants also remarked that they themselves had felt empowered, had been allowed to organise the discharge in the way that the older person had wished. 'We were considered, our opinion counted for something'.
Evaluation/ feedback	One of the features of a good discharge mentioned by participants was that they had been able to check up on how it had gone, and were able to evaluate their care in the light of this. Older people felt reassured when services had checked up on them. 'I recommend that professionals review cases and offer contact numbers, so even if a patient/carer initially refuses help, the situation will be reviewed'.

Table 34.3 Provocative propositions and key themes

	Provocative proposition	*Key theme*
1	Every worker/patient/carer knows exactly what other workers do	Understanding
2	Every worker has the opportunity within their job to develop and use networks across the system	Understanding, co-ordination
3	Every worker takes responsibility to act on information that they hold or receive about the person and their circumstances	Empowerment, co-ordination
4	There is a process for checking up to ensure that the person going home is managing and has received all the services they were expecting	Feedback/evaluation
5	There is co-ordination of the process of going home to avoid duplication and/or gaps in the services and support provided	Co-ordination
6	Resources and funding are co-ordinated to avoid disputes or time-consuming negotiations	Co-ordination
7	All patients are given individually tailored information and support to ensure choice and ownership of their own health/social care	Empowerment
8	There are joint care plans (held by the patient and shared documentation/information	Co-ordination, empowerment
9	Care is flexible and responsive and there is a fall back strategy	Understanding, co-ordination, feedback/evaluation

interested in, and join the group that was considering that proposition. The task of these groups was to develop an action plan, either in their own organisation or across the system. The provocative propositions and action plans are presented in Table 34.4.

At the end of this workshop, participants were asked to complete feedback forms, giving their comments on being involved in the appreciative inquiry project. These were collected by the core group and analysed to identify key themes and issues.

FINDINGS

The AI process generated many ideas and debates that could be treated as findings, but for the purposes of this paper the discussion of findings will focus on the key themes that were identified in descriptions of discharges that went well, with other issues arising from the action plans being discussed under the section of methodological issues. Table 34.2 summarises the themes identified by the group from the AI interviews, and provides some illustrative quotes. The four themes in Table 34.2 can be discussed further here, in particular the links between the themes.

The theme of understanding was a central one, reflecting the import-

Table 34.4 Action plans and provocative propositions

Action plan	*Provocative propositions*
The development of an information pack, to be accessible to all patients, carers and agencies, about support services and resources for people going home from hospital. This material would be used flexibly, as patients' circumstances changed, and would include different media. Work is currently underway on collecting material for this.	1, 2, 7
Holding an event for people involved in training and staff development. This event would include discussions of pre-qualification training, induction courses and 'on-the-job' training. The latter might include 'shadowing' schemes, job rotation, interagency training and networking opportunities.	2, 5
Each agency should identify key people to oversee the process, including follow-up. People being discharged should identify an important person to be notified of their discharge, and be given a contact number of a key person who would know about them, to ring if things don't go to plan.	3, 4, 5, 7
A person-centred care plan should be developed that was easy to understand and that included the views of users and carers. The group knew of some developments in this area, and agreed to explore them further.	5, 8

ance that participants placed on developing knowledge of the whole system. While professionals could feel that they understood their own service very well, they were often mystified by the services that they linked with. For older people, whose contact was often fragmented and transitory, their understanding could be broader, in that they had experience of a wider range of services, but did not develop detailed knowledge about them.

For professionals, understanding of the whole system allowed them to co-ordinate their activities with those of others. The temporal or sequential element of discharge planning could be extremely complex, with agencies unable to do their part until others had done theirs. This meant that multiple schedules had to be met and followed, as well as those of other agencies and the participant's own agency. Understanding these timescales was important in making sure that things progressed as quickly as possible – understanding what happened to an equipment request, for example, allowed staff to judge how long the process would take, so that they could plan their work to fit in with this. For older people, co-ordination meant that there were less points in the discharge process where things were stalled, or things were rushed. Things did not get missed out, and there was no duplication of effort. However, co-ordination was referred to less explicitly by older people than by professionals, perhaps reflecting that when things go well, there is often little to notice, unless one understands the complexity of what is happening and what can go wrong.

The theme of empowerment was important to professionals and older people, and again was connected to understanding the system. A hallmark of a good discharge for many of the interviewees was that the older person and their carer felt in control, and this was linked to their participation in decision making. In order to do this, people had to know about the choices that were available to them and the consequences of those choices. Empowerment for professionals took a slightly different form, in that they felt able to take action that supported the choices of older people and carers, rather than take actions that they – in their professional judgement – felt would be best. Sometimes professionals disagreed with the choices of service users, but still described a discharge as good if they had been able to support them in putting their choice into action.

The fourth theme identified in Table 34.2 is that of Evaluation and feedback. This was mentioned more by professionals than by older people, and was related to the extent to which they had been able to find out how things had gone for the older person going home from hospital. This feedback loop not only had heuristic value, in that professionals could learn from their experiences, but it also gave a sense of completion to the discharge – staff did not feel that people simply disappeared from their service to an unknown fate; they knew the end of the story, or at least this particular chapter. [...]

REFERENCES

Bushe, G.R. (1995) 'Advances in appreciative inquiry as an organization development intervention', *Organization Development Journal* 13 (3): 14–22.

Cooperrider, D.L. and Srivastva, S. (1987) 'Appreciative inquiry in organizational life', *Research in Organizational Change and Development* 1: 129–169.

Delbecq, A. (1975) *Group Techniques for Programme Planning*, Glenview: Scott F Foreman.

Hammond, S. (1996) *The Thin Book of Appreciative Inquiry*, Plano, TX: Thin Book Publishing.

Ludema, J. (1993) *Vision Chicago: a Framework for Appreciative Evaluation*, Cleveland, OH: Case Western Reserve University Department of Organizational Behavior.

Miles, M.B. and Huberman, A.M. (1994) *Qualitative Data Analysis*, California: Sage.

Steier, F. (1991) 'Reflexivity and methodology: an ecological constructionism', in Steier, F. (ed.) *Research and Reflexivity*, London: Sage, 163–185.

CHAPTER 35

HEAVEN CAN WAIT

Beverly Alimo-Metcalfe and Robert Alban-Metcalfe

The requirement for a leader to be a charismatic superman was one of the mythologies debunked in a major survey on qualities needed at the top.

We are seeing major initiatives on developing leadership in the NHS including those related to clinical governance leadership, primary care group leadership and, of course, the chief executives' programme.

The NHS Executive's paper *Leadership for Health: the health authority role* (1999) extols the virtues, and common sense, of adopting a transformational leadership approach to achieving a new NHS. We need to know the behaviours, skills, qualities, and attitudes that reflect this form of leadership.

In 1997 we were commissioned by the Local Government Management Board to undertake a two-year exploratory investigation into the nature of leadership in local government. The Nuffield Institute for Health at Leeds University was keen to co-sponsor the project and, in parallel, to conduct an investigation of its own on the NHS. The end-point of the project was to be the creation of a new 360-degree feedback instrument for measuring the dimensions of leadership identified in the research.

Unlike previous studies of leadership, mostly from the US, we designed a project which would start with no pre-determined notion of what the word meant.

It was evident that as this was an exploratory study, a qualitative methodology was essential for the first stage. The technique we selected

Source: *Health Service Journal* (2000) 12: 26–29, Oxford: Blackwell.

was the repertory grid interviewing process. We decided to interview staff in a dozen organisations in both the NHS and local government. In each case, at least six of the organisations were selected randomly from a national list, and four were organisations which had a reputation for being cutting edge in their respective sector.

We spent a day in each of these organisations conducting one-hour interviews with the chief executive, a director, an assistant director, and a middle-level manager. We asked that both sexes be represented, and that the group would include at least one person from a minority ethnic group. A final sample of 92 individuals was interviewed. The table below shows the breakdown of managers by sector, level, and gender.

First it was necessary to discover what interviewees actually meant by leadership. They were each asked to identify (using initials) on a piece of paper two individuals in the NHS with whom they currently worked, or had worked, who they believed had outstanding leadership qualities. They were also asked to identify two individuals who were average, and a further two who were deemed to have poor leadership skills. These individuals are referred to as the 'elements'. Finally, a seventh element, 'self', is added to the group. The pieces of paper were shuffled, and three were randomly selected. The interviewee was asked to think about the three individuals identified on the pieces of paper, and consider in what way two of them were similar to each other, but different from the third, with respect to their leadership qualities, or lack of leadership. What the interviewee said was recorded as their 'construct', or perception, of leadership.

For example, the individual might say, 'Two of these people are outstanding at developing the confidence of their staff, whereas the third person is totally self-interested'. The perception 'develops staff' versus its opposite pole, 'self-interested', provides us with a construct this particular person has of one aspect of leadership.

The interview continued, using different combinations of elements. Typically, we elicited around 15–20 major constructs from each person interviewed.

To ensure that we had obtained the constructs that doctors held of

Table 35.1 Breakdown of repertory grid interviews by sector, level, and gender

	Local government		*NHS*		*Total*	
Level:	*Female*	*Male*	*Female*	*Male*	*Female*	*Male*
Chief executive	6	5	1	3	7	8
Director	2	8	11	8	13	16
Assistant director	5	6	8	9	13	15
Middle manager	9	2	6	3	15	5
Sub-total	22	21	26	23	48	44
Total	**43**		**49**		**92**	

leadership, we also gathered data from six focus groups of doctors, in which a total of 51 male and female doctors participated.

Content analysis of the 2,000+ constructs, conducted independently by the two authors, led to the emergence of 48 'themes', which formed the basis of items for a pilot leadership instrument.

This list was augmented by a small number of items based on a review of the leadership literature. No significant differences were detected between the range of constructs from NHS and local government managers, nor between men and women, nor between managers at different levels in the organisation.

The range of constructs held of leadership was complex. But fascinating as this data appeared to be, it would have been impossible to generalise from the views of around 150 individuals, of whom around 100 were staff in the NHS, to the wider NHS and local government.

So a 171-item questionnaire was distributed, initially to a sample of 100 managers, who were asked to comment on the clarity and relevance of the questions, and then to two samples of managers, one in the NHS, the other in local government. Participants were asked to rate their current manager, or a previous manager with whom they had worked, on a six-point scale from 'Strongly agree' to 'Strongly disagree': two additional responses were available: 'Don't know' and 'Not relevant'.

In the NHS, around 300 organisations were selected at random and a letter explaining the research was sent to the chief executive, with a request that they return a slip offering their support. Packs of 45 to 60 questionnaires, depending on size, were distributed to trusts. An explanatory letter, and stamped-addressed envelope, were included with each questionnaire. The request was again that the manager receiving the questionnaire anonymously rated their current boss, or a previous boss with whom they had worked in the NHS.

By mid-1999, after a second wave of requests to both organisations, a total of 1,464 usable responses were received from local government, and 2,013 from the NHS. The results were analysed separately for the two public sector organisations.

Among the NHS managers, six factors emerged in the research model, and a further eight factors emerged in a second additional analysis of the data. These were turned into 14 robust leadership scales, with high internal reliability co-efficients, each of which measures a different aspect of leadership. These dimensions will form the basis of a 360-degree feedback instrument, 'The transformational leadership questionnaire © (NHS version)'.

The most obvious implication of these findings is the staggering complexity of the role of leadership in the NHS. Another lesson is that the transactional competencies of management, while crucial, are simply not sufficient on their own.

What is clear is that existing US models of leadership do not encapsulate this complexity. Typically, they place an overwhelming emphasis on charisma and vision: on leaders acting primarily as the role model for their followers. Is this the product of adopting research methodologies which focus solely on the views of top managers, or are the researchers developing models from their own observations?

In contrast, the results which emerge from asking the recipients and ultimate arbiters of leadership effectiveness – namely, the staff who work in the NHS – how they perceive leadership, presents a very different model.

They are clearly stating that the most important prerequisite role for the leader is what they can do for their staff. This is far more reminiscent of the model of leader as servant. But they are not simply stating that leadership is about meeting staff's needs; it is much more than that. The 2,000 staff who participated in this research project are also saying that leadership is fundamentally about engaging others as partners in developing and achieving the shared vision and enabling us to lead. It is also about creating a fertile, supportive environment for creative thinking, for challenging assumptions about how healthcare should be delivered. And it is about much closer sensitivity to the needs of a range of stakeholders inside and outside health care. It is about 'connectedness' – joined-up thinking, even.

Another very positive feature of the findings is that the model significantly reflects aspects of the modernisation agenda, including partnership working, valuing staff, aiming for best practice, removing the traditional barriers between agencies working together within the community.

It would appear that there is a high degree of similarity between what those who work in the NHS believe to be leadership and the espoused leadership tenets of the centre. This can only be very good news.

What needs to be heeded, however, is the nature, and degree of support from the centre to enable this to happen locally.

To make most effective use of the findings, to make a significant impact, it will require NHS organisations to develop a transformational culture which reflects the dimensions of leadership emerging from this research. US scholar Ed Schein believes that probably the most important responsibility of leadership is to create the most appropriate culture for the organisation. We also know from substantial research evidence that there is a highly significant relationship between the leadership style adopted by the top manager and the culture of the organisation.

Here we face, perhaps, the greatest challenge for leadership reform in the NHS, since it is highly likely that the current top and senior managers were not selected for these posts on the basis of possessing a transformational style of leadership. What, then, will happen if the model is not adopted by the top NHS managers?

Clearly the answer is that there will be no cultural infrastructure supporting and nurturing its growth. The noble attempts of managers further down the organisation to practise a transformational approach will be blocked, or even 'punished', by the influence, and perhaps game-playing, of more senior managers.

Will managers who adopt a predominantly controlling, or laissez-faire, style see the need to change? It is likely that these very managers will lack the insight or willingness and commitment to develop transformational leadership. Who holds the responsibility to deal with these powerful blocks to progress? This is a key consideration for the NHS centre, since the government's modernisation agenda will not be achieved unless the NHS recognises that cultures of blame, authoritarianism, narrow-mindedness and reckless disregard for staff are not to be tolerated. Can those managers who wish to strengthen their transformational leadership change? This oft-asked question is still a matter of some debate among organisational psychologists. However, the findings from recent research are heartening.

There is evidence that the use of 360-degree feedback, plus tailored individual support, can lead to sustained positive changes in leadership style.[1] But, like quitting smoking, the all-important prerequisite is the managers' willingness and openness to change.

Another vitally important aspect of the findings is that the model of transformational leadership which emerged does not simply apply to managers, it applies equally to other NHS professionals, including clinicians. Leadership, like communication skills, must be incorporated into doctors' appraisals (both developmental and summative), and those of other staff, including the posts of primary care trust chief executives, and chairs.

NHS organisations can no longer rely on the transactional competencies of management to run the NHS. They must adopt, and be truly committed to incorporating, these dimensions in their recruitment, selection, promotion, performance management and development processes, for all staff whatever the area or level of work.

The human resources professionals will have to think creatively about how these qualities can be measured and developed alongside the transactional competencies of management. It will also require organisations to consider who they use as judges/assessors in such situations. Why should this be important?

The reason is that the chances are very high that those who will occupy the gate-keeping role of assessors have been promoted to those positions on the basis of a track record on the transactional competencies. Given the difficulty HR professionals often say they have in influencing these decisions, it will be beholden on the centre to advise NHS organisations of the importance of ensuring that best practice is exercised here.

As the findings show the local government and NHS models of leadership are virtually identical, it is time to consider seriously joint development and perhaps recruitment since inter-agency working can be strengthened considerably by this approach.

Finally, this study has served to debunk and demythologise the 'heroic' image of leadership which has been so prevalent.

The model which emerges here is one of down-to-earth decency, humanity, humility, sensitivity and respect for others, but this is no soft option.

It is fired with a passionate commitment to living the values, to engaging all in sculpting the vision, to creating an environment where challenging, questioning, and turning mistakes into catalysts for learning are regarded as the norm.

The notion of connection and partnership is a backbone theme of this UK model, and appears to be driving a very new image of leadership for the new millennium.

ASKING THE IMPOSSIBLE? QUALITIES OF LEADERSHIP STAFF WANT

At the very top of the list of dimensions for leadership came genuine concern for others. This includes showing a genuine interest in staff as individuals, seeing the world through their eyes, valuing their contributions, developing their strengths: coaching, mentoring and having positive expectations of what staff can achieve. The others, in order of importance, were as follows:

- **Inspirational communicator, networker and achiever:** This is essentially about communicating the vision of the organisation with passion and commitment. Unlike US models of visionary and charismatic leadership, it stresses the need for partnership in engaging an extensive range of internal and external interested parties in the process by actively networking with them, gaining their confidence and support through sensitivity to their varying needs. It is also about celebrating the accomplishments of the team, department or organisation.
- **Empowering others to lead:** A manager who displays this dimension, trusts staff to take decisions/initiatives on important matters; delegates effectively and encourages staff to develop their leadership by providing opportunities for them to take on increased responsibilities.
- **Transparency:** This relates to the aspect of integrity which is about honesty and consistency in behaviour, but also reflects the attitude of placing the good of the organisation before personal gain. It also involves humanity and humility and willingness to modify one's views after listening to others.

- **Accessibility, approachability and flexibility:** This reflects a style which is not status-conscious, which places great importance on face-to-face, as opposed to distant leadership, and which attempts to ensure that staff at all levels feel comfortable and able to access the individual.
- **Decisiveness, determination, readiness to take risks:** Ability to clarify shared values and a sense of direction. This reflects a strong element of engaging with colleagues. This is another example of how the model differs from major US ones.
- **Ability to draw people together with a shared vision:** This relates to having a clear vision and strategic direction in which the 'leader' actively engages various internal and external stakeholders in developing: drawing others together in achieving the vision. It encapsulates some of the core values and attitudes exhorted by the government's modernisation agenda.
- **Charisma:** This is concerned with exceptional communication skills, ability to keep in close contact with others, encouraging others to join in.
- **Encouraging challenges to the status quo:** This includes clarifying long term corporate direction while encouraging others to challenge the status quo, with respect to traditions and assumptions about what is done, how problems are dealt with, and the quality of the service provided.
- **Supporting a development culture:** This includes empowering individuals to challenge tradition, take risks and express dissatisfaction. In so doing the person presents a powerful role model for leadership.
- **Ability to analyse and think creatively:** This is seen as an essential dimension of a public sector leader. It involves the capacity to deal with a wide range of complex issues and the ability to utilise creativity in problem-solving.
- **Managing change sensitively and skilfully:** This includes being sensitive to the impact which changes in the external environment can have on the organisation; being aware of how these changes will differentially impact on parts of the organisation, being aware of the impact of one's decisions, and having the wisdom to balance the need to change with some degree of stability.

NOTE

1 Alimo-Metcalfe, B. '360-degree feedback and leadership development', *The International Journal of Selection and Assessment* 6 (1): 35–44.

CHAPTER 36

WHY SHOULD ANYONE BE LED BY YOU?

Robert Goffee and Gareth Jones

If you want to silence a room of executives, try this small trick. Ask them, 'Why would anyone want to be led by you'? We've asked just that question for the past ten years while consulting for dozens of companies in Europe and the United States. Without fail, the response is a sudden, stunned hush. All you can hear are knees knocking.

Executives have good reason to be scared. You can't do anything in business without followers, and followers in these 'empowered' times are hard to find. So executives had better know what it takes to lead effectively – they must find ways to engage people and rouse their commitment to company goals. But most don't know how, and who can blame them? There's simply too much advice out there. Last year alone, more than 2,000 books on leadership were published, some of them even repackaging Moses and Shakespeare as leadership gurus.

We've yet to hear advice that tells the whole truth about leadership. Yes, everyone agrees that leaders need vision, energy, authority, and strategic direction. That goes without saying. But we've discovered that inspirational leaders also share four unexpected qualities:

- They selectively show their weaknesses. By exposing some vulnerability, they reveal their approachability and humanity.
- They rely heavily on intuition to gauge the appropriate timing and course of their actions. Their ability to collect and interpret soft data helps them know just when and how to act.

Source: *Harvard Business Review* (2000) September–October: 63–70.

- They manage employees with something we call tough empathy. Inspirational leaders empathise passionately – and realistically – with people, and they care intensely about the work employees do.
- They reveal their differences. They capitalise on what's unique about themselves.

You may find yourself in a top position without these qualities, but few people will want to be led by you.

Our theory about the four essential qualities of leadership, it should be noted, is not about results per se. While many of the leaders we have studied and use as examples do in fact post superior financial returns, the focus of our research has been on leaders who excel at inspiring people – in capturing hearts, minds, and souls. This ability is not everything in business, but any experienced leader will tell you it is worth quite a lot. Indeed, great results may be impossible without it.

Our research into leadership began some 25 years ago and has followed three streams since then. First, as academics, we ransacked the prominent leadership theories of the past century to develop our own working model of effective leadership. (For more on the history of leadership thinking, see the sidebar 'Leadership: A Small History of a Big Topic'.) Second, as consultants, we have tested our theory with thousands of executives in workshops worldwide and through observations with dozens of clients. And third, as executives ourselves, we have vetted our theories in our own organisations.

Some surprising results have emerged from our research. We learned that leaders need all four qualities to be truly inspirational; one or two qualities are rarely sufficient. Leaders who shamelessly promote their differences but who conceal their weaknesses, for instance, are usually ineffective – nobody wants a perfect leader. We also learned that the interplay between the four qualities is critical. Inspirational leaders tend to mix and match the qualities in order to find the right style for the right moment. Consider humour, which can be very effective as a difference. Used properly, humour can communicate a leader's charisma. But when a leader's sensing skills are not working, timing can be off and inappropriate humor can make someone seem like a joker or, worse, a fool. Clearly, in this case, being an effective leader means knowing what difference to use and when. And that's no mean feat, especially when the end result must be authenticity.

REVEAL YOUR WEAKNESSES

When leaders reveal their weaknesses, they show us who they are – warts and all. This may mean admitting that they're irritable on Monday mornings, that they are somewhat disorganised, or even rather shy. Such admissions work because people need to see leaders own up to some flaw before they participate willingly in an endeavour. Exposing a weakness establishes trust and thus helps get folks on board. Indeed, if executives try to communicate that they're perfect at everything, there will be no need for anyone to help them with anything. They won't need followers. They'll signal that they can do it all themselves.

Beyond creating trust and a collaborative atmosphere, communicating a weakness also builds solidarity between followers and leaders. Consider a senior executive we know at a global management consultancy. He agreed to give a major presentation despite being badly afflicted by physical shaking caused by a medical condition. The otherwise highly critical audience greeted this courageous display of weakness with a standing ovation. By giving the talk, he had dared to say, 'I am just like you – imperfect'. Sharing an imperfection is so effective because it underscores a human being's authenticity. [...]

Knowing which weakness to disclose is a highly honed art. The golden rule is never to expose a weakness that will be seen as a fatal flaw – by which we mean a flaw that jeopardises central aspects of your professional role. Consider the new finance director of a major corporation. He can't suddenly confess that he's never understood discounted cash flow. [...]

BECOME A SENSOR

Inspirational leaders rely heavily on their instincts to know when to reveal a weakness or a difference. We call them good situation sensors, and by that we mean that they can collect and interpret soft data. [...]

While leaders must be great sensors, sensing can create problems. That's because in making fine judgements about how far they can go, leaders risk losing their followers. The political situation in Northern Ireland is a powerful example. Over the past two years, several leaders – David Trimble, Gerry Adams, and Tony Blair, together with George Mitchell – have taken unprecedented initiatives toward peace. At every step of the way, these leaders had to sense how far they could go without losing their electorates. In business, think of mergers and acquisitions. Unless organisational leaders and negotiators can convince their followers in a timely way that the move is positive, value and goodwill quickly erode...

There is another danger associated with sensing skills. By definition, sensing a situation involves projection – that state of mind whereby you attribute your own ideas to other people and things. When a person 'projects' his thoughts may interfere with the truth. Imagine a radio that picks up any number of signals, many of which are weak and distorted. Situation sensing is like that; you can't always be sure what you're hearing because of all the static. The employee who sees her boss distracted and leaps to the conclusion that she is going to be fired is a classic example. Most skills become heightened under threat, but particularly during situation sensing. Such oversensitivity in a leader can be a recipe for disaster. For this reason, sensing capability must always be framed by reality testing. Even the most gifted sensor may need to validate his perceptions with a trusted adviser or a member of his inner team.

PRACTICE TOUGH EMPATHY

Unfortunately, there's altogether too much hype nowadays about the idea that leaders *must* show concern for their teams. There's nothing worse than seeing a manager return from the latest interpersonal-skills training program with 'concern' for others. Real leaders don't need a training programme to convince their employees that they care. Real leaders empathise fiercely with the people they lead. They also care intensely about the work their employees do. [. . .]

At its best, tough empathy balances respect for the individual and for the task at hand. Attending to both, however, isn't easy, especially when the business is in survival mode. At such times, caring leaders have to give selflessly to the people around them and know when to pull back. [. . .] It's tough to be tough.

Tough empathy also has the benefit of impelling leaders to take risks. When Greg Dyke took over at the BBC, his commercial competitors were able to spend substantially more on programmes than the BBC could. Dyke quickly realised that in order to thrive in a digital world, the BBC needed to increase its expenditures. He explained this openly and directly to the staff. Once he had secured their buy-in, he began thoroughly restructuring the organisation. Although many employees were let go, he was able to maintain people's commitment. Dyke attributed his success to his tough empathy with employees: 'Once you have the people with you, you can make the difficult decisions that need to be made'.

One final point about tough empathy: those more apt to use it are people who really care about something. And when people care deeply about something – anything – they're more likely to show their true selves. They will not only communicate authenticity, which is the precondition for leadership, but they will show that they are doing more than just playing a role. People do not commit to executives who merely live up to the obligations of their jobs. They want more. They want someone who cares passionately about the people and the work – just as they do.

DARE TO BE DIFFERENT

Another quality of inspirational leaders is that they capitalise on what's unique about themselves. In fact, using these differences to great advantage is the most important quality of the four we've mentioned. The most effective leaders deliberately use differences to keep a social distance. Even as they are drawing their followers close to them, inspirational leaders signal their separateness.

Often, a leader will show his differences by having a distinctly different dress style or physical appearance, but typically he will move on to distinguish himself through qualities like imagination, loyalty, expertise, or even a handshake. Anything can be a difference, but it is important to communicate it. Most people, however, are hesitant to communicate what's unique about themselves, and it can take years for them to be fully aware of what sets them apart. This is a serious disadvantage in a world where networking is so critical and where teams need to be formed overnight. [...]

Inspirational leaders use separateness to motivate others to perform better. It is not that they are being Machiavellian but that they recognise instinctively that followers will push themselves if their leader is just a little aloof. Leadership, after all, is not a popularity contest.

One danger, of course, is that executives can over-differentiate themselves in their determination to express their separateness. Indeed, some leaders lose contact with their followers, and doing so is fatal. Once they create too much distance, they stop being good sensors, and they lose the ability to identify and care. That's what appeared to happen during Robert Horton's tenure as chairman and CEO of BP during the early 1990s. Horton's conspicuous display of his considerable – indeed, daunting – intelligence sometimes led others to see him as arrogant and self-aggrandising. That resulted in overdifferentiation, and it eventually contributed to Horton's dismissal just three years after he was appointed to the position.

LEADERSHIP IN ACTION

All four of the qualities described here are necessary for inspirational leadership, but they cannot be used mechanically. They must become or must already be part of an executive's personality. That's why the 'recipe' business books – those that prescribe to the Lee Iaccoca or Bill Gates way – often fail. No one can just ape another leader. So the challenge facing prospective leaders is for them to be themselves, but with more skill. That can be done by making yourself increasingly aware of the four leadership qualities we describe and by manipulating these qualities to come up with a personal style that works for you. [...]

UNRAVELLING THE MYSTERY

As long as business is around, we will continue to pick apart the underlying ingredients of true leadership. And there will always be as many theories as there are questions. But of all the facets of leadership that one might investigate, there are few so difficult as understanding what it takes to develop leaders. The four leadership qualities are a necessary first step. Taken together, they tell executives to be authentic. As we counsel the executives we coach: 'Be yourselves-more-with skill'. There can be no advice more difficult to follow than that.

INDEX